Killing Yourself

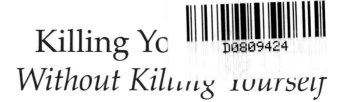

Without Killing Yourself

Using Natural Cures That Work!

Eric,
Peace on the journey!

(first edition)

BEA 2006

An educational guidebook by

Allen S. Chips, DCH, PhD

Allen Chips

Transpersonal Publishing
PO Box 7220, Kill Devil Hills, NC 27948
www.TranspersonalPublishing.com

Orders:
Wholesale—www.TranspersonalPublishing.com
Retail—www.Holistictree.com

Photo Illustrations of Harry Hoxsey and Mildred Nelson, and of the outside of the clinic—used with permission of the Biomedical Center
Photo Illustrations of Edgar Cayce and the 80/20 diet—used with permission of the Association for Research and Enlightenment
All other Photo Illustrations taken by and © Allen S. Chips
Cover Design by Allen S. Chips

First printing, first edition: May, 2006

ISBN 1-929661-24-X (soft cover edition)

Unattributed quotations are by Allen S. Chips

All Transpersonal Publishing titles, imprints, and distributed lines are available at special quantity discounts for bulk purchases for sales promotions, premiums, fundraising, and educational or institutional use. Special book excerpts or customized printings can also be created to fit specific needs. For details, contact the publisher at www.TranspersonalPublishing.com or 800-296-MIND.

Authors seeking a publisher must query this publisher at their web site, only by e-mail, and only through the submission guidelines; all unsolicited query letters and manuscripts are unread and discarded.

Printed in the United States of America
10 9 8 7 6 5 4 3 2 1

Contents

Dedication

To Jane Chips, my mother

Acknowledgments

A special thank you goes to my mother. Years ago, when she was diagnosed with the same type of cancer as I was, she chose radiation therapy and damaged her heart, bones, and immune system. She spent more than 40 years as a career medical professional and was always supportive of my decision to use Hoxsey therapy. Thank you to my traditional medicine oncologist, alias Dr. Ben Fineman, for his friendship, clinical and spiritual support, and for using state-of-the-art testing procedures in documenting my recovery.

Thanks also go to Aida, office manager at the Biomedical Center in Tijuana, Mexico, who helped me locate several current and past Hoxsey patients, and to the dozens of those patients and their families who shared their stories with me. I am also grateful to the doctors at the Biomedical Center, particularly Dr. Gutierrez, who helped ensure the accuracy of the information in this book. Thanks also are due to my editors, Bob and Paula Minaert; my proofreader and indexer, Jana Sheldon (my wife's sister who's in the literary business); and to my long-standing fact checker, final proofreader, and wife, Dee Chips, who was also—most importantly—a wonderful supporter in the quest to save my life.

Disclaimer

It's unfortunate that those who don't want to take responsibility for their own decisions and actions have created the necessity for a disclaimer, and that the legal system in this country has gotten powerful enough to stunt our freedom of speech. However, be that as it may, here is what we Americans must state to other Americans in the process of trying to get information to the public that will help save lives.

The information in this book is for educational purposes. The author and individuals mentioned herein are in no way advising any reader or cancer patient to take any specific medical approach. If you have an illness, you should see a health care professional. However, it is your constitutional and God-given right to choose for yourself treatment programs, medicines, and remedies that are available to you on this planet, whether they are natural/God-made or man-made. Whatever your choices, you automatically assume risks, and they may be considerably greater if you treat yourself from the information in this book without the approval or supervision of a health care professional. The publisher, the author, and the treatment centers written about in this book assume no responsibility for personal recovery choices.

Neither the author nor any of the other patients whose testimonials appear herein has received funding or sponsorship from the Biomedical Center, or any other person or entity, to write or promote this book. Every person interviewed and written about herein has paid for every aspect of his or her treatment program himself or herself and is contributing his or her story out of gratitude for having their lives saved through this approach.

To protect privacy, some of the names of my health care providers and most of the names of the Hoxsey patients I have interviewed for this book have been changed, except whereby permission was granted, or their story was in the public domain.

Preface

I have written this book to document my quest to find a safe and reliable, all-natural cure for cancer that won't make you sick, damage your organs, or give you more cancers in the future. This quest is buoyed by my faith that God put a cure for this disease on planet earth for us to find.

During the first few chapters, you will be taken on a journey with me to meet my alternative health practitioners, my traditional medicine physicians, and my alternative medicine oncologists, in order to experience the crucial decision-making process I used to save my life. Together we will explore information at the National Institutes of Health, the Edgar Cayce Foundation/Association for Research and Enlightenment, and the Biomedical Center in Tijuana, Mexico. At the center, naturopathic cancer research has been extensive and treatment programs typically offer a higher success rate than those achieved through traditional medicine. I will discuss herbal medicines that since the late 1800s have been historically documented and proven to be effective against cancer—that are still used to cure cancer today. We will also explore a Chinese medicine that some researchers and physicians recently have labeled a "miracle cure," yet it is one that not many know about, due to medical politics. We will discuss nutritional supplements and foods that helped my immune system to recognize and destroy the cancer cells in my body, and you will see my medical reports—biopsies, CT and PET scans—that document my illness and its cure.

Thereafter, you will learn about the conditions in the mind and body that contribute to both the contracting and curing of cancer, including body fluid alkalinity, oxygenation, immune system volatility, environmental conditions, and nutritional factors. We will consider the best diet and supplements for both preventing and curing cancer, and we will discuss numerous cases of patients who used the Hoxsey system who are recovering or have recovered, all of whom I met personally. One person had pancreatic cancer and another liver cancer, both conditions for which traditional medicine has no treatment.

Their stories are meant to inspire you and inform you that the war on cancer may have already been won, although the general population involved in cancer recovery is largely unaware of this. We will hypothesize as to why such a highly successful approach was not approved by the FDA, nor accepted by mainstream medicine in the United States. Most of our focus, however, will be on patient education and saving or extending our lives. After reading about dozens of cases where the Hoxsey system of recovery was used successfully, you may find value in the comprehensible basic truths about the human body that I present and the effectiveness of this powerful, all-natural treatment modality. The Hoxsey system has documented hundreds of thousands of cancer cures worldwide for more than 80 years, with an average success rate of 80 percent.

For those with cancer...

Cancer. Just the word brings about fear. It blew *me* away. It changed my life. Contracting it brings up new choices and new directions, and it makes us think about the precious lives we live and the inevitability of the next world. We each need to be ready to fight this thing, keeping our own personal reasons for winning close to our hearts, to live on to fulfill our hopes and dreams, should we get a second chance. In order to do this, we need to become a sponge for information now, a self-educated student of healing in the short time that we have to effectively make the crucial decisions that lie before us.

My hope for this book is that all the research that I conducted during my studies for a doctorate in natural health, which used dozens of traditional and naturopathic books, articles, and interviews, will help others who wish to try the Hoxsey system for themselves, either as a complementary therapy with traditional medicine, or as a stand-alone therapy. I regularly receive many e-mails and phone calls, and people at seminars and conferences come up to me asking how I did it, how I cured myself of a cancer called lymphoma. They want information and understanding, sometimes for themselves and sometimes for people they know—people who are facing the same uncertainties that may have led you to pick up this book.

Whether it's you, a loved one, a family member or a friend, you probably know someone who is staring into the uncertainties of a cancer diagnosis and facing many critical decisions. If you have been diagnosed with cancer, you know that these decisions need to be made quickly. Survival is time-dependent. You can't afford to waste time on approaches that don't work; you need to play your percentages with either the traditional medical or a proven alternative/complementary medical approach, or maybe both.

This book explains how to cure cancer the natural way, with nature's secrets passed down through the ages; it tells us how we can do it without killing ourselves in the process or shortening our lives. The good news is that there is a natural method with a proven track record of success that won't make you more sick, disfigure, or kill you. Yet nothing is 100 percent effective, so if you stand a good chance for survival with a good traditional medical approach, then this book may simply provide information, possibly outlining a backup plan. On the other hand, if your prognosis is not good, or you can't afford to take a year or two of sick leave to do chemotherapy, if I were you I would contact the Biomedical Center in Tijuana, Mexico, book a flight for San Diego, go from there to Tijuana, and read this book on the way.

Instead, you may want to experiment, as I did; then, if you get some positive results, invest in the whole program. Yet I must warn you that I am not a medical doctor and cannot recommend any medical treatment programs. I can only share what I discovered along my own healing journey. Some of this research I conducted during my studies toward a naturopathic doctoral degree.

Keep in mind that your doctors may be against this approach. They may caution you that they don't know anything about it, or they may give you their blessing to try it. Ultimately, the choice is yours. Naturopaths, medical doctors, researchers, or writers like me are all simply sources of information for you to better traverse the jungles on your own unique healing journey.

How can we maximize our chances for success using an alternative/complementary approach? This book will help you answer this question and others. My hope is that it will become a good reference for both cancer patients and the health care professionals who treat them—easy to read as a patient guidebook, but scientific enough for both traditional and naturopathic health care practitioners to consider it clinically viable.

I discovered that patients and their families, when facing this challenge, often feel as if they are swimming up a stream of medical terms and concepts as they try to comprehend the approaches that are best for them. So I have also put together a list of patient education resources at the end of this book that will help patients understand the benefits of both traditional and alternative approaches.

This book was designed to be a story-based reference book, easy enough to read in one day and something that will prove invaluable to cancer patients when *time is of the essence*. Some may want to read this book to patients whose physical or mental condition deters them from doing so themselves. At the very least, this book could bring *hope*, so that if the approach selected is not working, another option may be available that carries a high success rate. But please, don't take my word for it, or anybody else's, for that matter. Instead, examine the wealth of information herein, and listen to yourself and God.

It is important to note that traditional and alternative medical doctors all simply offer what they know. It was my own trusted traditional oncologist who said, "I don't know anything about alternative medicine," when I asked him about alternative approaches to cancer treatment. Not that this was a bad thing. I loved my allopathic (traditional medical) oncologist. He was a godsend, offering sound clinical and spiritual support during my journey. However, he was trained only in traditional medicine, which is still the first line of defense in America. He said, "I am known as a chemo man," but I needed more. I needed answers, quick ones, and I believed there was another way, one that no clinic in America offers at this time.

We are all students of self-curing, because even if we choose to simply have the oncologist turn on the juice (chemo), or blast us (radiation), it's our decision. We make the choices, the doctors don't; they simply offer what they know. We sign off on the procedure because we've done our homework and are playing our percentages...or perhaps, like many people mentioned in this book, we don't use the traditional approach at all. Perhaps we gave up on it, or never started it, for various reasons. Maybe we decide to do both allopathic and naturopathic medicine. Or maybe we choose to rely solely on naturopathics (diet and herbs), or even spiritual healing (God). In the end, the final decision belongs to each of us.

Throughout this book, many questions will be answered. What if alternative approaches, using herbs, supplements, and diet, have been curing cancer effectively for over a hundred years? Would we know about it? What if natural cures for this ancient disease have been effectively documented on the North American continent since the late 1800s, before naturopathic remedies became synthetically manufactured by pharmaceutical companies? Did you know that some very powerful chemo drugs are derived from plants that are available today? Are these plants and herbs still effective by themselves? Did they really need to be synthetically reproduced so they could be patented, sold, and regulated? What if some Native American herbal medicines were just as successful in curing many cancers several hundred years ago as traditional medicine is today, would we know about them?

Why are all the alternative cancer centers located in Tijuana, Mexico, anyway? Are they all effective, or are they just quackery houses getting rich off people's misfortunes? If some of these clinics, which collectively see tens of thousands of cancer patients each year, are really helping people, why are they there and not in the United States? If they work, shouldn't we make this treatment more available to Americans, and people in other countries? Shouldn't our physicians, particularly the ones in medical school, such as some of my family members, be taught these natural cures and be allowed to prescribe them in all of our country's beautiful states? I truly hope this will happen some day in the future.

What condition does a human body need to be in to contract such an illness anyway? Why does one person's immune system recognize cancer cells and destroy them while another person's does not? Does it have to do with stress, genetics, our way of thinking, our attitude, outlook on life, our diet, pollution in our environment, or is it just our time to get sick, our destiny?

Doesn't it make you wonder? Wonder no longer as you keep turning the pages. Begin the journey today into the history of naturopathic oncology and learn about the ability we have to heal ourselves by reading my story and sharing in my discoveries as they unfolded. Put yourself in my shoes for a little while, and dare to think like a survivor.

Introduction

This book is divided into two parts. Part one is a story about the decisions I made that led to my overcoming a life-threatening illness—cancer—and part two describes the natural cures that encompass the most well documented, underground, natural cancer cure of our time, called Hoxsey therapy. It was my editors who suggested two parts, because even though the process of educating myself in how to cure my own cancer was an integral part of my recovery, throwing it all together as one long story, citing my research in the middle of my recovery, would put the reader in the position of a new pilot trying to concentrate on correctly flying a plane in a storm, while at the same time attempting to read the pilot's instruction manual.

Essentially, I was told I actually had written two books, or one long book with two parts. Part one is for the average cancer patient seeking a reliable natural cure, and part two is for research-minded individuals and medical professionals. At the same time, I was told by the Biomedical Center in Tijuana, Mexico that they appreciated how I made Hoxsey therapy so easy to understand so cancer patients could better use it. As a result, as I rewrote, I attempted to keep part two comprehensible for most cancer patients and their families, so they could make educated decisions for themselves about how to use those cancer cures that God intentionally left in nature for us to discover.

In addition, I was also told that the audience for this book would want to know more about who I was before I tell them about my health challenges, so they could better understand how my exposure to alternative medicines and holistic health led me to make the decisions I did for my own recovery.

As the reader proceeds, he or she should keep in mind that the research behind each of the nutritional and herbal medicines mentioned in part one is linked to more documented research in part two. In the process, I've refrained from using footnotes (referencing resource books in the text), so that readers would better comprehend how easy it is to research natural cures for their own health challenges. The scientific basis for these approaches is explained so that the research-oriented patient and the patient's family members, as well as the various medical professionals involved, may comprehend the efficacious aspects of Hoxsey therapy.

Who Am I?

In order for readers to better comprehend what allowed me to walk away from traditional medicine and use my body as a laboratory experiment for testing my theories, I will highlight five major events that led me to shift my personal and professional values and convictions.

First Event

We must go back to the early 1980s, when I was fresh out of college and working at my first job as a medical sales representative in the Midwest.

I promoted germicidal hand cleansers to surgical nurses and pharmaceutical manufacturing operations, a skin care line for decubitus ulcers (bed sores), and more. I appreciated the nurses for whom I'd done presentations, many of whom were genuine humanitarians. But the pharmaceutical manufacturing personnel were strictly business-oriented.

I remember being invited, along with my supervisor, into one of the manufacturing facilities of a major player in the pharmaceutical industry. In the front offices, we discussed our cleanser with a purchasing agent. This particular cleanser would sanitize the skin without water and without chapping when used consistently, which was revolutionary at that time—though products like this can now be found in a cheaper, consumer-based version at many YMCAs.

On the way down to the sterile rooms, where capsules were being manufactured, my supervisor told me, "I'll bet these pills down here cost them about 5 cents each." When we got inside the plant, we peered into a vacuum-controlled, sterile manufacturing room. The production manager, who was well acquainted with his stock options, confirmed that the pills cost about 5 cents each and sold for about a dollar apiece. That's a 2000 percent markup! I was amazed at how the American public was simply being *ripped off!*

At that time, I had a meager health insurance policy with a high deductible, a wife, and a new baby, and I could barely afford our medical expenses, as insurance companies were becoming increasingly parsimonious with their coverage. (The trends of higher medical profits and lower insurance coverage have continued to create the financial health care crisis we are experiencing today). Needless to say, my early belief that American medicine was a humanitarian pursuit was forever changed long ago, as I foresaw a societal disease progressing to epidemic proportions.

Second Event

In 1985, while I was still living in the Midwest, I went to a chiropractor who was very effective with both chiropractic and nutritional remedies. He was a miracle worker, who helped me with a neck problem I'd received from a bicycle accident at age 10. He was very intelligent as well as spiritual, which I believe contributed to his extraordinary gifts. While under his care, I joined a natural health group that met in his office in the evenings. One night, a man introduced himself as one who had worked as a biochemical engineer in the research and development department of a well-known pharmaceutical company. His company was working on a sweetener that I hadn't heard of before when he quit his job.

People asked him more questions, and he told a story about a chemical called aspartame, which was proven in laboratory testing to have serious side effects. He was unable to stop his company from filing for approval with the FDA. When the chemical was approved, his conscience was troubling him, so he resigned from the company and was unemployed at the time I met him. His anguish and concern, his sincerity, and the level of education I perceived in his speech led to me to believe that what he was saying was true.

This event provided yet more proof to me that our capitalist economy, coupled with a government supported by corporate and private interest groups, was largely ignorant of patient-centered health care (unlike systems in some countries with socialized medicine). I was also convinced that the U.S. government's mandate to protect the public was secondary to the American pharmaceutical industry's attempts to line its pockets with the money of those who were sick and desperate. (Needless to say, it didn't take the televised reports of headaches, hyperactivity, loss of concentration, and symptoms of multiple sclerosis and other diseases to convince my family and friends to avoid consuming aspartame.)

Third Event

A merger a few years later led to the elimination of my medical sales position, and I obtained another position with a new company as a pharmaceutical sales representative covering accounts in Pennsylvania, West Virginia, and Ohio. I began giving presentations to prestigious groups of physicians (primarily endocrinologists) in hospitals like the Cleveland Clinic. It was there that I became acquainted with studies that documented the placebo effect: the phenomenon that people who believe they are receiving medicine often begin to heal, even if they are instead given a harmless substance. This is when I began to recognize the power of the mind's ability to affect the body.

I was amazed by scientific documentation showing that the placebo group, which took sugar pills, had relatively the same benefits as the group that took the actual medicine—until the placebo group discovered that the medicine they were taking was nothing more than a sugar pill. At that point, the results dropped off dramatically. I was amazed by the scientific proof of the mind-body connection right in front of our faces, even though the medical establishment focused more on the results of the medicine and dismissed the placebo effect. The results of the placebo group were insignificant to the scientific wisdom of that time.

Shortly thereafter, a medical doctor by the name of Deepak Chopra began to release information to the public that documented the placebo effect and demonstrated that the mind-body connection is a credible, noteworthy aspect of health and wellness. In his early writings, he spoke of the molecular difference between happy tears and sad tears. Dr. Chopra also cited a study in which elderly people in a nursing home were used to prove the mind-body connection. Their environment was decorated with artifacts and music from the 1920s and 30s. They were given physicals before and after the environmental changes, and it was documented that systems in their bodies rejuvenated themselves to reflect an average age regression of 10 years! Dr. Chopra's research began to gain public attention, and the concept of "placebo" began to take on new meaning. Psychosomatics began to become an integral aspect of medical practice for many physicians, particularly those in family practice.

This steady accumulation of proof of the reality of the mind-body connection greatly affected my thinking.

Fourth Event

As I began to ponder the power of the mind-body connection, I was flown up to the International Diabetes Center in Minneapolis, Minnesota, on behalf of the medical company where I was employed, to participate in a series of diabetes patient education classes. Up to this point, our training involved understanding the difference between type one and type two diabetes, the diabetic diet, reactions to medication, glucose tests, jet injection verses bolus (syringe) absorption, and more. However, on this particular trip, we were to learn about the psychological aspects of the disease.

In one session, I was placed with a group of medical professionals. We were lined up on a set of benches, similar to gymnasium bleachers, where we sat and studied people who had recently contracted diabetes. These people were talking to a psychologist about the circumstances of their disease, while we were able to observe them through a one-way mirror. One case in particular struck me.

A woman with thin, short blond hair entered the small cubicle. The psychologist questioned her about the psychosomatic aspects of her illness by asking her to talk about the time she contracted diabetes. She told of how she and her husband were constantly engaged in conflict, until one day he left her without warning. That was the day she contracted insulin dependent diabetes mellitus (IDDM), type one. My mouth dropped open. There I was, observing a direct mind-body connection in action, the power behind the placebo effect fully demonstrated. This woman, unknowingly, changed my life.

Fifth Event

In the mid-1980s, I was moving up fast in the corporate world; I was the number-one sales representative in my company, with a healthy salary to boot. Upper management invited me to a private meeting to pick my brain for tips on how to succeed, because the company was in trouble with its bottom line. They didn't get out of me what they'd hoped for, though, and their verdict, which afterward circulated within the company, was that I was simply a humanitarian, a nice guy, and that was why people liked to buy medical products through me. After that, I knew I was a duck out of water in the corporate world, which focused more on profits and less on patient care. I knew there was something I was supposed to be doing that would help people, but I didn't know what. In the meantime, the company reorganized, eliminated the outside sales force, and I was put on severance pay. This provided an opportunity for me to explore a career change.

I did have some interviews with other pharmaceutical companies, but many of them claimed I made too much money and wouldn't be satisfied with their typical sales rep salaries. But I also knew my interviews were falling flat because of my lack of interest in the corporate game. Then one day I was looking in the newspaper classifieds and I noticed an advertisement that offered certification as a hypnotherapist. This seemed to be was what I was looking for. I drove 5 hours each way to attend the program. This was the beginning of a new career for me, and was the last of the five events that profoundly affected my life.

How I Became Acquainted with Natural Health and Naturopathy

I loved hypnotherapy, because it taps the power of the mind, it is never monotonous—since each individual mind is different—and it was a way to help people. I knew that I wanted to teach and write about this stuff some day, so after becoming a certified hypnotherapist, I decided to enter a clinical doctoral program with an emphasis in hypnotherapy. By 1990, I had two private practices; one was part of a hypnotherapy clinic I owned and the other with a psychiatric counseling group practice. In these clinics, among other things, I treated smoking, weight problems, chronic pain, post-traumatic stress disorder, anxiety, panic attacks, memory and comprehension problems, self-esteem issues, fears and phobias, cancer recovery, and more. In 1991, I received my doctorate.

During this time, my wife started practicing (and later teaching) reiki therapy, an energy therapy that originated in Japan just before World War II. The process involves the practitioner calling on the healing power of the Holy Spirit to help restore the sick person's health. The practitioner uses a hands-over/hands-on technique and often feels the reiki healing energies, called *universal life force*, flow through his or her hands into the parts of the sick person's body that need the most healing. Often the practitioner is a medical intuit (which my wife is) who can hear the voices of guidance and can tell the client what is happening in his or her body.

The reiki approach fit in well with the hypnotherapy sessions I was conducting, so my wife joined my private practice and later began teaching reiki certification programs through the National Association of Transpersonal Hypnotherapists (NATH). We founded this organization in 1994 to promote body-mind-spirit oriented clinical hypnotherapy education and certification. It turned out to be a nice complement to the field of clinical hypnotherapy. NATH quickly grew to offer a variety of mind-body therapies taught by a variety of speakers and authors.

Shortly thereafter, we began offering clinical and personal growth workshop through the Association for Research and Enlightenment (ARE), the home of the Edgar Cayce Foundation. Edgar Cayce was the most well-documented mystic of our time, who did most of his work under a state of self-hypnosis, so this provided a great opportunity for me to satisfy my thirst for more information about the power of the mind. I was also intrigued by other natural health systems housed in the ARE library, the largest holistic health library in North America. Located above ARE's conference center, it contains 14,000-plus Edgar Cayce readings on health remedies, metaphysics, and prophecies about the future.

From 2000 to 2003, with a group of faculty, I spearheaded the implementation of a hypnotherapy degree program for the American Holistic University. As a result, I was well accustomed to researching alternative and holistic health systems. Later, after my experience of curing myself of cancer, I decided to use much of the research I had conducted to direct and co-create a naturopathy / natural health degree path within the university. And, because I had already started the research to earn another doctorate in natural health, I was introduced to a vast number of alternative cancer cures. All in all, several years of natural health research lie within the pages of this book, which highlight those proven to be the most effective alternative cancer cures available today. I not only believe this in theory, but also because of the wisdom I'd gained by documenting the natural remedies that cured the cancer within my own body!

Now, readers can turn the page and walk with me as I grasp for answers, then desperately seek a cure for something growing uncontrollably within my own body.

Part One

My Story

"Seek and ye shall find. Knock and the door shall be opened." Jesus of Nazareth

Chapter 1

In the Beginning

April 2003: Easter's Black Friday

It was Easter weekend. While visiting my parents, my mother asked, "What's that?" and pointed to a swollen protrusion on the left-hand side of my neck.

I responded, "I don't know, what does it look like?"

"That's strange," she said as she felt it with her finger tips. "It feels like swollen lymph nodes. That's the same place where my lymph nodes swelled up on my neck when I got Hodgkin's disease. How old are you now?"

"Forty-one."

"That's the same age I was. You should really have it looked at. I hope it's not what I had, but you're better safe than sorry by having your doctor look at it. How does it feel when I touch them?"

She grasped the two nodes between my neck and collarbone and started to move them around, squinting at the little mass as a seasoned nurse would. In fact, she had worked as a nurse in Cook County Hospital in Chicago earlier in her career, teaching nurses and physicians the electrocardiogram when it was a new concept. Later She had worked in a private doctor's office and had recently retired.

"They are sort of sensitive," I said.

"I wonder if this is related to the fever you had." She was talking about the low-grade temperature I had experienced earlier that afternoon.

I said, "I don't know. I had a fever last night on the way over here."

"When did they appear?"

I explained that I had just noticed them at that moment, but my body aches and fever had begun the night before, on Good Friday, when I was driving the four hours from my home in Virginia to their home in West Virginia. During the trip, we broke down and had to have our conversion van fixed by a private repair garage owner who agreed to work late while Dee, my wife, and the two children ate dinner at a nearby restaurant. He was a good Christian man who was separated from his wife. He talked about letting things go that bothered him, which both age and practicing his faith in God helped him to accomplish. This had recently led him to reconcile with his wife.

I needed such a conversation at that time in my life. I was not sleeping well and was under a lot of stress. For one thing, I had read some things in my daughter's diary just two weeks earlier that were disturbing me greatly. She was a rebellious teenager with some psychotic behaviors that were making my wife, my son, and me miserable. She was doing everything opposite of the way she was brought up and had a secret life we were unaware she was living. She was very angry (she did things like kick in doors), which was apparently caused by events outside the family. Shortly thereafter, we got counseling for her and a medical check up and discovered she had Poly Cystic Ovary Syndrome (PCOS). Apparently, this caused her to have three times the testosterone level of a boy her age, which was the cause of her aggression.

Also, my wife and I were often working 12- to 15-hour days in the family seminar business. We had booked too many week-long training seminars that brought in speakers with personalities that were egotistical and uncaring. This caused personality conflicts in which we became referees instead of teachers and leaders in the holistic health movement. In addition, because of the strain, our interactions in the office were lacking the tact we usually employed. In general, the boundary between home and work was being blurred; we weren't maintaining the personal separation we each needed for our own peace of mind.

In an effort to reduce the stress, I had already started making some changes in our business. We eliminated the speakers who were focused on conflict and self-serving agendas. I cut back on travel and sent my wife, who enjoyed such events, to some conventions in my place. I resigned from a professional committee of national membership organizations that spent at least half of its meeting time bickering. But it wasn't enough, especially in combination with my stresses at home.

I knew about the correlation between stress and illness; I even taught other people about it in the seminars I led. I had written books about holistic health. But it was different when I was a participant, unconsciously engaged in the process. My stress was simply out of control.

In fact, I was feeling so much stress in my life after reading the diary that I told myself that life just wasn't worth living anymore. I was tired of the game of life. A death wish crossed my mind and I thought, "People who die are lucky, because the next world must be much better than this one."

Then one night a week later, shortly before our trip, I cursed life and then fell asleep. When I woke up on the sofa in front of the TV, I said to myself, "Uh-oh, I'm going to make myself sick." I dozed off again and then woke up with a hot feeling in my sternum, which I took to be indigestion.

So within a short period of time I had made a death wish, even though it was short-lived, and had given myself a self-hypnotic suggestion ("I'm going to make myself sick") when I was in a very suggestible state of mind. These two occurrences were probably just enough to give my body the negative message it needed to allow the disease to progress into a highly active state.

On Good Friday the flu-like symptoms hit me on the way to my parents' house. The day after Good Friday, my father and I went golfing. Since I practically grew up on the golf course we played, it was a relatively easy course for me to score well on. However, on that day, my game did not impress anybody. I felt depleted of energy, and as the low-grade fever began creeping up on me, my game fell apart. I was swinging wildly, hooking the ball way to the left, slicing it to the right, and so on—a golfer's worst nightmare.

On the way back from the golf course to my parents' house my father responded to my disappointment about my golf game by agreeing, "You didn't seem like yourself out there. What happened?"

By the time we returned, only a half-hour later, I was very tired and had a fever of about 100 degrees. I took a fever reducer and went to sleep on the couch in front of the TV, while my father catnapped in the recliner across the room. When I woke up, my father had already been awake for some time and kept asking me how I felt. I said I was better and kept chugging down liquids. Then we went into the kitchen for some pre-dinner wine and socializing. That was when my mother noticed the protrusion on my neck, as described earlier. It lay just above the collar of the low-cut T-shirt I was wearing.

That night I woke up about 3:00 in the morning drenched in sweat and thought I'd broken the fever of a 48-hour flu. But it was actually my first bout with night sweats. The next day, my little family of four left my parents' house, with me promising my parents I would see my doctor as soon as I could get an appointment.

Easter Sunday, we stopped at my wife's parents' house to have dinner and say hello. While we were there, I came down with a fever again, and broke it again with liquids and over-the-counter fever reducers. We went home later that night.

A Trip to the Doctor's Office

The next day, I went to my family physician's office for an appointment. They performed a complete physical examination, including blood tests.

Dr. Parks took one look at my neck, felt my lymph nodes, and said, "That's odd."

"What?"

"Those aren't supposed to be there."

I said, "What do you mean?"

He felt my nodes from the upper neck and jaw to the collarbone and pointed out that it was normal for lymph nodes to be slightly swollen in the neck area, but not that far down and inside the collar bone, and not that enlarged for an adult. He measured them, asked how I was feeling, ordered an X-ray, and took a blood sample.

Time for an X-ray, Time to Think

The next day, I went to the hospital and had a chest X-ray.

I was starting to get concerned, so that night I decided to conduct some research that might help me to heal cancer, should that be the case. Over the next several days, from approximately eight o'clock in the morning to about one or two in the afternoon, I started researching both traditional and alternative cancer therapies. I read about my symptoms: enlarged, rubbery lymph nodes; itching; night sweats; unexplained fever and/or weight loss. All of them fit me.

The books in my personal holistic health library contained literally dozens of alternative cancer therapies available in the United States and abroad. But as I navigated all these options, I began to get confused about what direction to take, should I have cancer. The therapies I came across included coffee enemas, colon cleansing (colonics), nutrition, diet, supplements, herbs, vaccines, and more.

I read about the value of stress reduction in cancer recovery, something that was an important factor to consider at this time in my life. I took time to look inward and reevaluate many things: how I interacted with the world, God's presence, my perceptions of the quality of my life, my role as a husband and the father of two teenagers, my role as the manager of a family business, the goals I'd not yet accomplished, the things in life I'd not yet experienced, and much more. I also decided to practice self-hypnosis and meditation every morning.

As a precaution, I began to create cancer-fighting imagery while I was in a state of self-hypnosis. I often combined self-hypnosis with transcendental meditation, in which I used imagery of a white light emanating from God and coming down through the left side of my body. Then I imagined great white sharks eating up my swollen lymph nodes.

I had already been exposed to the research done by O. Carl Simonton and Stephanie Matthews-Simonton, and had written a paper about Bernie Siegel's approach years ago, during my doctoral studies in hypnotherapy. I was aware of all the articles and books these people had published that showed a significant increase in recovery rates for those cancer patients who practiced tumor reduction imagery, using what was traditionally referred to as *visualization*. I committed myself to practicing imagery every morning (more on imagery in part two).

Late April 2003

While I was waiting for the results of the chest X-ray, my son came down with two of the exact same symptoms I had, fever and lethargy, so I took him to our pediatrician, who ordered a blood test. A few days later, I came home from work to find what sounded like a concerned message on my answering machine from Dr. Parks, our family doctor; he asked me to phone him. I called the office the next day, found that he wasn't in, then phoned radiology and requested a release of the radiologist's findings. At about noon I received the medical report, noticing that the signature on it was our neighbor's, Paul Faulkner, D.O., who was our local hospital's radiologist. Then I called my mother, who tried to interpret it with me over the phone. It mentioned a family history of Hodgkin's disease, but my mother and I were not able to accurately understand its implications. When Dr. Parks called later that day, he said that he didn't want to concern me but that there could be a problem that needed to be looked into. He set up an appointment for me to have a CT scan at the hospital the following week, and I was to see him the next day.

At my appointment, Dr. Parks, a short, stocky Italian with black wavy hair and an ethnic bluntness, explained the radiologist's findings. He saw a

STONEWALL JACKSON HOSPITAL
LEXINGTON, VA 24450

PATIENT LOCATION:OP

PATIENT NAME   :Chips, Allen   SERVICE DATE   :04/22/03
DATE OF BIRTH   :████████   PATIENT NUMBER   :10249522
PHONE NUMBER   :   MED REC NUMBER   :068073
ATTENDING PHYS   :████

EXAMINATION REQUESTED   CLINICAL HISTORY
   1. Chest PA & Lateral   Family history Hodgkin's

INDICATION: Left supraclavicular lymphadenopathy. Family history of
Hodgkin's disease.

Mediastinal widening is consistent with lymphadenopathy. No definite
hilar adenopathy, mass, infiltrate or pleural effusion. Lung vessels,
airway and cardiomediastinal silhouette are within normal limits.

IMPRESSION:
1. Mediastinal adenopathy is likely. CT suggested to further
evaluate.

PF:cs
D&T:04/22/03

_____████████, D.O.

mass between the heart and lungs, in what is called the mediastinum area, which could be consistent with Hodgkin's disease. I told him that I had started to use imagery and a few supplements to combat the potential problem and that it appeared that the nodes on the neck were shrinking.

He measured the larger one and said, "Well, it appears that this one is smaller."

He looked down at my chart and said, "The last time I measured it I wrote down 1.5 centimeters. It appears to be about one centimeter now. Hmmm." He peered over his reading glasses, feeling the nodes again.

At the end of the appointment, I expressed my concerns about possibly having the Hodgkin's gene. With his usual sense of humor he said, "Don't count yourself out yet," and recommended an oncologist named Dr. Fineman.

I asked if I would be better off going to the University of Virginia. He said, "If I had a problem, I would choose Fineman."

I agreed to do this and waited in his office until an appointment could be confirmed. Because his patient load was very high, I had to wait a week and a half to see him, even though Dr. Parks' office staff tried to get me scheduled sooner. I would later discover that Dr. Fineman had written three books on oncology that focused on patient education and spirituality, so he was quite popular and later closed his practice to new patients.

After receiving Dr. Parks' news, hoping it wasn't anything serious, I phoned my mother and one of my sisters, who were both nurses, and talked to them about the possibilities of a cancer diagnosis. In the meantime, I started to read about alternative cancer methods again in my spare time. Yet I felt like a small fish in a vast sea of unfamiliar waters, not knowing which approach was most effective and worried that if I did indeed have the big one, I might kill myself by spending too much time searching for the answer. It is well known that the sooner a person catches his or her cancer, the more likely it could be put into a solid remission.

End of April, 2003: Doctor Calls, Oncology Office Walls

Several days had passed when my son's doctor contacted us to let us know that according to my son's blood test he was recovering from mononucleosis. It appeared that I must also have had mono at the same time. This did not put our minds at ease, because I had read about the link between Hodgkin's lymphoma and the epstein-barr virus, the virus that causes mono.

In the meantime, my wife had been getting more and more angry over the past few weeks, which I knew was her way of rejecting something that she could not control in her life. Because I considered her to be my soul mate, it was easy for me to read her reactions to life's situations. But it was hard to see her with this non-nurturing emotion during my time of need. After much prodding, and a change in her emotions from anger to faith, she agreed to come with me to my appointment with Dr. Fineman.

We traveled into town from our home in the country, about 20 miles away, to an oncologist's sterile waiting room, with medical signs all over the counters and walls. One large sign asked patients to examine themselves for symptoms of potential anemia, which occasionally occurs with chemotherapy patients.

After filling out several pages of paperwork, which included federal regulations, patient history, etc., we were asked to move from the waiting room to a small treatment room. Dr. Fineman, a tall, thin man with black hair, dressed in white lab coat, came in about five minutes later and conducted an interview and performed physical examination.

He looked in the file and said, "Okay. Yes, those are unusual," as he felt the nodes on my neck.

I told him that I was doing imagery under self-hypnosis every day and that Dr. Parks had told me that the nodes on my neck might be shrinking.

He said, "If you want to go the alternative route, I would look up the NCCAM web site—the National Center for Complementary and Alternative Medicine. It's under the National Institutes of Health. It'll show you what studies are being offered for the type of cancer you may have. But I am heavily rooted in science. I need some scientific data to understand what we are dealing with. Right now we are just speculating. We don't even have a diagnosis yet."

My wife and I became fearful as he went on to list all the things I could have, from the most likely to the least likely.

"I would put Hodgkin's at the top of the list, then non-Hodgkin's lymphoma, then sarcoiditus [an illness similar to cancer], mono, and possibly testicular cancer."

The truth is, at that moment we didn't know how far down was "down" when it came to being in "deep doo-doo." By the end of the list, our heads were spinning. We began to daydream as the doctor's words became a mumble in the background. In my mind, I recalled how many times God had proved that he was part of my life, how he had touched me, and my family, in uncommon, paranormal ways in the past. I wondered if he was with us at this time in my life, somehow, somewhere.

I snapped out of my fog and interrupted, "I don't know, but I would say that God will heal me, if it's something serious."

The doctor paused, switched demeanors from a clinical to a more personal stance, and responded softly, "I think that God heals people in many ways, and chooses various means do it. For example, I believe that God works through me to heal cancer with chemotherapy." He looked at me for a response.

I said, "Oh yeah, I believe that, but I believe healing can also take place by direct divine intervention."

My wife came out of a daze and said, "Yeah, don't be surprised if a miracle takes place here," and a nervous smile came over her face.

"Again, I am a man of science; I'd like to look at hard data so we know what we're dealing with here. I think the next step is a biopsy."

He went on to explain how these were done. I was reluctant to have anyone cut into my body. I also asked about the theory behind biopsies, because I had read that cancer gets more aggressive from the biopsy itself. He explained that with most patients he hadn't noticed that, but with some it appeared that the cancer "got angry" afterward. It was unpredictable and each case was different. I was interested in more X-rays, and he said that he would have his office manager call my insurance to obtain preapproval for a CT scan, or CAT scan, as it is commonly called. The scan would show us more, because it takes internal pictures of the body. So we agreed to take this step first.

I walked down the hallway to the reception desk, which faced both the treatment rooms on one side and the waiting room on the other. There, the office manager and the nurse looked at my possible diagnosis, listed as Hodgkin's lymphoma, and asked me if I had any symptoms, like night sweats or fevers. I responded that this had occurred when I was sick a few weeks ago.

I was still in a daze when I finalized the CAT scan appointment, and when I came through the door to the waiting room I met my wife's red, weepy eyes. She was speechless, trying to hide her inner world, which was quickly crumbling.

I said, "Let's go," grabbed her hand, and helped her up from the row of chairs along the wall. We walked out into the hallway pressed the down button of the elevator. You could have cut the silence with a knife; we were both on the verge of tears.

After a long pause, she asked, "Did you set up the CAT scan?" as her eyes wandered up to meet mine.

"Yeah. Two days from now," I murmured.

We were whisked down to the ground floor. By the time we got to the car, we were discussing our faith in God again, our spirits lifting like a broken car being pumped up from the ground for repair. We were looking for the next tool to fix the problem. It was like a nightmare, except that there was no way to pinch myself and wake up. I mused that a human life span consisted of just one long dream, as I began to reflect on my birth, scenes from my life, and its potential end. Everything suddenly seemed temporary.

The Infamous Tunnel to My Inner Portrait

Two days later, I arrived at the hospital without my wife to have the CAT scan and went through the usual paperwork at the registrar's desk. It was becoming old hat. I answered several questions from the registrar, a friendly African American woman, and walked to the end of a wide hall, through large double doors labeled "X-ray," and sat in another waiting room for a while.

The X-ray tech called my name, and we entered a room with a table that moved people through what appeared to be a tunnel. The tech asked me to take my crucifix off my neck and explained that I was going to get hooked up to an I.V. injecting contrast, a material that would help illuminate the body's internal systems, such as organs, bones, and lymph nodes. I signed a release of liability for allergic reactions, was hooked up to an I.V., and heard instructions from a sterile, computerized voice.

"Breathe...inhale...hold your breath...exhale."

I felt a warm rush of heat throughout my body when the contrast was introduced into my veins. It tasted as if I were inhaling garlic fumes because the air from my lungs felt hot and spicy on the exhalation.

It was short. The X-ray tech tried to cheer me up by telling me not to worry about the results. She could read the concern on my face. She said that like most scans, it was probably just to rule out various problems. I then asked her if I could talk to Paul, my neighbor friend, who is the radiologist that reads the scans. Paul owned a 200-acre farm in the area and was heavily involved in naturopathic remedies, organic farming, and nutrition. I originally met him through my church.

She said that she would ask him, left the room, and returned to lead me to his office.

I walked into a room lit up with several X-rays on the walls and Paul extended his hand to meet mine. "Hello, Allen, how have you been feeling?"

"Okay, I suppose, except for a chronic fever that's lingered for about the last three weeks. My son and I seemed to have come down with mono at some point this spring, which sort of explains it, I guess."

Without giving much credence to what I said, he asked, "How's your energy level?"

"I guess it's been okay. I've been getting broken sleep because of my dust allergies in the winter. It usually puts me into asthmatic bronchitis."

Paul continued with a specific path of questioning. "What time of day or night have you been getting tired?

"Now that I think of it, I've been falling asleep around 9 o'clock every night, and lately I've been fighting to stay awake so that I can change my sleeping patterns and sleep all the way through the night."

He continued with a keener look on his face and a drop in his voice. "I don't think that that's what is causing your fatigue. Take a look at this."

Paul then led me into a small room with two chairs in front of a large, flat-screened computer monitor displaying my scan on it and said, "This is your scan."

"Oh, that was quick," I said as I rolled over the chair he pointed to and sat down.

He continued, "This is what we call the mediastinal area. It's a web of lymph nodes between your heart and lungs. There are many strings of these lymph nodes that run throughout your body, but the ones here seem to be enlarged."

"What do you mean by enlarged?" I asked.

He rotated the images of my chest cavity and zoomed in to get a close-up of the swollen nodes, which appeared to be in a semi-circle.

"These four nodes seem to be about 1.5 centimeters."

"What size are they supposed to be?"

"About .5 centimeters or less." He looked at me directly and said, "Out of all the things you could have, I would say you have the best one."

"What do you mean?"

"Well, I think you have Hodgkin's disease, which by today's standards is probably the best cancer to have, if you have to have one. But don't quote me on this; your oncologist is the one who diagnoses you. Have you gotten a biopsy done yet?"

STONEWALL JACKSON HOSPITAL
LEXINGTON, VA 24450

PATIENT LOCATION:OP

PATIENT NAME   :Chips, Allen   SERVICE DATE   :04/25/03
DATE OF BIRTH   :████████   PATIENT NUMBER   :10255156
PHONE NUMBER   :   MED REC NUMBER   :068073
ATTENDING PHYS   :████

EXAMINATION REQUESTED   CLINICAL HISTORY
   1. Chest CT   Mediastinal adenopathy on
                                         chest

INDICATION: Mediastinal widening on chest x-ray.

Mediastinal lymphadenopathy confirmed; multiple enlarged lymph nodes in
the pre aortic and paratracheal spaces averaging in the neighborhood of
1.0-1.5 cm. Question of thymic enlargement vs. adjacent
lymphadenopathy.

The lungs, airways, liver and adrenal glands are unremarkable. There
is a notch and focal calcification in the superior border of the spleen
that suggests the possibility of a prior laceration. The spleen is
mildly enlarged. The splenic index is 790; approximately twice normal
size.

IMPRESSION:
   1. Mediastinal lymphadenopathy.
   2. Splenomegaly? Spleen scar.

PF:cs
D:04/25/03
T:04/28/03

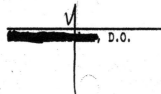

████████, D.O.

I told him no and he also recommended I get one done. Then we began to speak about the causative mind-body factors for contracting cancer, which he was aware of because he was also a natural health researcher.

He said, "Knowing a little about what you do for a living, I suppose you've already considered the conditions in your life that may have contributed to this problem."

"Yeah...I have," I said reluctantly.

"You know that there are many new treatments for this now." He went on to explain what he knew about laser radiology, which he'd read about in a medical journal recently. He also said that chemotherapy was more effective now, and if he had to choose a cancer, Hodgkin's disease was the one he would choose, because it's the one traditional medicine can most successfully put in remission. As a member of my church, he told me that he would pray for me, and I thanked him and left for home.

I called my oncologist, Dr. Fineman, who called me back and said that he recommended I get a biopsy through the local surgeon. I agreed. The surgeon worked me into his schedule within a couple of days.

May, 2003: Prayer, Meditation, and the Biopsy

I took my son with me. Outside the oncologist's office, I pulled out some water that I had brought back with me a couple of years earlier from Lourdes, France, just in case I, or someone else, needed a healing. With my son, I performed the ritual. Wash your face in front of a statue of Mary, then drink a little, and say a rosary with it. Having been brought up Catholic, it was an important ritual for me. The water had worked before, when I gave a small bottle to a legally blind woman, who drank some and miraculously recovered her sight. As a result, my faith was high for a potential cure or healing of some sort. My son and I then went inside and checked in, filling out the usual stack of paperwork.

The surgeon gave me a physical and said that the enlarged nodes he felt under my arms were characteristic of mono, and perhaps there was no reason for alarm. I was optimistic and lay down on the treatment table. He numbed me and then cut the largest lymph node out of the lower left side of my neck. He asked if I wanted to see it, and I agreed. It looked like an enlarged kidney bean. He then sliced it in half, and said, "Oh, look at that. You see all the white tissue in this?" I asked what that meant and he looked down, hesitated, and said, "We will just have to wait for the results." It was Monday, and they didn't expect the results until Friday.

The following Tuesday morning, I went into what I refer to as a "spirit guide meditation." I learned how to do this shortly after I took a self-hypnosis class and learned how to get myself into a deep meditative state, which improved my meditations.

In a spirit guide meditation, I try to quiet my mind and I ask my angels for a locution (a telepathic voice from God) that will shed some light on a problem or situation. Since I had learned self-hypnosis and practiced it for many years, I had learned to project my mind, or my spirit, into what I call the border area, a place where the heavenly light meets this world and where angel guides gather (explained in more detail in part two).

On that morning, I meditated on God's heavenly light and imagined it running through my body, relaxing my mind and body until I experienced a sense of peace. I then felt my mind drift upward toward the source of the light.

In the light, I felt a loving presence awaiting me, and I posed the question: "What am I facing?"

I quieted the chatter of my mind again and listened for a word, or string of words, or an image. And then the words came through: "Prognosis...major barrier...temporary hurtle...perseverance...to overcome."

It was not what I wanted to hear. I wanted to hear some comforting words of wisdom that indicated that I was not facing anything serious. I came out of the meditation and told my wife about it. As a result, we both expected to hear from the doctors later in the week that it was going to be a major health challenge. But we did feel a little more secure that the message indicated that I might get cured through perseverance—whatever that meant.

The next day, Wednesday morning, I entered into meditation again and asked God for a healing color. The color was a violet-purple that flooded my mind. It was a beautiful color. Then I began to do imagery that involved purple sharks moving through my bloodstream to the swollen lymph nodes on the left side of my body. I imagined hundreds of them, little tiny sharks eating away at the outside perimeters of the nodes.

Thursday morning, the phone rang. My wife answered and gave it to me. It was Dr. Fineman.

"Hello, Allen?"

"Yeah."

"It's Dr. Fineman. How are you doing?"

"Okay."

"Well, I've got some news for you on your biopsy and a diagnosis. I think it's really good news."

"Oh. Yeah?" I said with a lilt.

"It's Hodgkin's lymphoma."

It was not what I was hoping to hear.

"I feel it's good news because of the high success rate in putting it into remission."

My voice dropped as I fumbled with the words, "Uh, I was hoping it was going to be...better news than..."

"You stand a great chance with chemotherapy. You're young and in good health, and if my guess on your stage proves accurate (stage 2), you should arrive at a solid remission. In light of all the other things you could have come down with, I think this is pretty good news."

He explained that the next step was to get a second opinion and then go for staging—to find out if I was stage one, two, three, or four. He would set up a PET scan for next week. Then we hung up.

Positron Emission Tomography (PET) is a form of X-ray that illuminates cancer cells for the purpose of staging or tracking the progress of therapy. Radioactive intravenous glucose is administered so that cancerous tissues, which by nature have a high metabolic rate, consume more glucose and therefore exhibit a higher heat range than most other tissues in the body. These heat ranges are then measured by nuclear medicine specialists to determine the probable locations and activity levels of cancer cells.

I had been hoping for a simple mono or sarcoidosis diagnosis. I was also hoping for a miracle. Needless to say, it was a very emotional day for me and for my family.

My sister phoned me right after I hung up with my doctor; our phone calls often are intuitively timed. Upon hearing the news, she sounded a bit shocked, but then tried to boost my morale. She called all my siblings, bearing the bad news. She phoned my other sister, who was also a childhood companion. Both remained strong family supports to this day. I later heard, through my brother, that they were hit real hard by the news, even though they didn't sound like it over the phone. Apparently, it brought up some childhood wounds related to when my mother contracted the same disease and we didn't know whether or not she was going to come home from the hospital.

At that time, I was only ten and my sisters were in their teens. My mother was 41 years old. It triggered things in all of us, a nightmare come true. In 1972, my whole family—mother, father, two older sisters, and two older brothers— were devastated by my mother's cancer diagnosis. She was given six months to live. We all prayed our little heads off; then, when the diagnosis miraculously changed to Hodgkin's and she was put in remission by radiation therapy, we all felt blessed by God.

My mother lived into her seventies, but had two heart attacks from the radiation therapy's damage to her heart. Also probably as a result of radiation, when she was in her sixties she had a carcinoid in her colon that doctors at the Mayo clinic discovered. It was the beginning stages of colon cancer. A polypectomy was performed, which took care of the problem.

Needless to say, my mother's cancer changed our family forever. But now, the five of us (two brothers, two sisters, and I) were being forced to relive certain aspects of a past we would rather have forgotten.

Breaking the News

Thursday night, I sat the children down (a son age 14 and a daughter age 17) and told them I had some news for them that we needed to discuss. My sister's husband, who happened to be in town at that time and was a good support, was also there. By this time, I'd picked myself up from the floor and was able to pull it off with a reasonable amount of composure. At first, when I told them what the diagnosis was, they didn't take me seriously, because of my dry sense of humor that they'd become so accustomed to.

I told the kids that I was serious, no joking, and that I wouldn't joke about such a thing anyway. Then each person voiced their concerns in

BLUE RIDGE PATHOLOGISTS, P.C.
70 MEDICAL CENTER CIRCLE, SUITE 309
FISHERSVILLE, VA 22939

PHONE: (540)332-5885 Staunton
(540)932-5885 Waynesboro

FAX: (540)332-5888 Staunton
(540)932-5888 Waynesboro

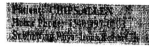

Chips, Allen

SURGICAL PATHOLOGY REPORT

Spec #: 03-SP3662

PATIENT INFORMATION:
PATIENT ADDRESS: P.O. BOX 249, GOS
OFFICE ACCT#:
COPY TO OTHER PHYS:
DATE OF SERVICE: 5/12/03
CLINICAL DX: LYMPH NODE

TISSUES:

Lymph node of neck, NOS - left

GROSS DESCRIPTION:
The specimen is submitted in one part in formalin labeled "lymph node of left side of neck" and consists of a circumscribed 1.9 x 1.6 x 1 cm ovoid lymph node with a homogeneous pale tan cut surface. Representative sections are taken and submitted in 2 boats. CRR/dgm

FINAL MICROSCOPIC DIAGNOSIS:
LYMPH NODE, LEFT CERVICAL AREA, BIOPSY: HODGKIN'S DISEASE, NODULAR SCLEROSING TYPE.

A second pathologist has reviewed these slides and agrees with the diagnosis.

Signed: ▆▆▆▆▆▆▆ M.D. 05/14/03

ALLEN CHIPS
31247

5-12-03

Is a 41 year old gentleman referred by Dr. ▆▆▆▆ and ▆▆▆ for lymph node biopsy in the left neck. He has some slightly rubbery adenopathy which appears to be freely movable. He also has epitrochlear adenopathy bilaterally and I am unable to feel a liver or spleen tip. Under local anesthesia an anterior cervical node on the left was excised, bivalved and submitted for histopathology. The wound was made hemastatic with fine ties and closed in two layers and he is instructed in wound care and will return on Friday for pathology report and suture removal.   ▆▆▆▆▆▆▆▆., M.D./ni

pc: Dr. ▆▆▆▆ and Dr.▆▆▆ with path report

succession. My daughter thought I was invincible because I was an alternative health professional. My sickness was hard to believe, as I was always proselytizing to family members about taking care of their health. My son wondered why God let it happen and my brother-in-law tried to answer his questions with theological answers. That night we prayed as a family, getting all of our concerns out on the table. My brother-in-law and I golfed the next day, which was a good escape for a short while.

Next, we needed to find out how bad was "bad." My submitting to a PET scan the following week would determine what stage the cancer was in. Stage one was easiest to put in remission. At the other end of the spectrum, stage four was the most difficult, with a person's statistical chances of survival being the lowest.

Chapter 2

Gathering Information

I called Dr. Fineman on Friday, the end of the first week of May. He recommended I get a second opinion. I made an appointment to see Dr. Hines, who was a teaching oncologist at the University of Virginia and had his own tumor review board.

My wife came with me. She had been reluctant to come because it meant taking another day off from the family business, which was beginning to suffer from our absence. Yet she understood how important it was and was glad she came. Dr. Hines was a good educator. He told us that the vast majority of people with Hodgkin's respond very well to chemotherapy. Four cytotoxic (cancer-killing) chemicals called ADBV (Adriamycin, DTIC, Bleomycin, and Velban) formed the treatment of choice, because they had a lower incidence of recurrence than other chemotherapies used for treating Hodgkin's.

However, ABDV did show a significant rate of lung and heart damage. Overall, though, these appeared to be pretty good odds. When I asked about radiation therapy, he adamantly stated, "Don't do radiation," explaining that with a blood disease like this radiation was likely to cause more complications, such as killing cancer cells in one area while facilitating growth in another part of the body where they may not have been detected. He also listed the side effects: future recurring cancers, and potential damage to the heart and other parts of the body, such as my mother sustained. And he showed me graphs of recurrence (the cancer coming back) statistics for chemotherapy and radiation.

When we asked him about how many treatments it would take, he said that research showed that it would take 12 cycles to put it in remission. It involved one treatment every two weeks for five and a half months, provided my blood counts were normal after each treatment. If not, it would take longer. He said that some people have no energy, while others have lots of energy and don't "miss a beat" in their everyday lives.

He was very positive about getting a solid remission, which helped my wife and me feel more at ease. He recommended that I do my chemo treatments at Dr. Fineman's office, since it was a standard formula that any oncologist would use for my condition, and it was also a local drive for me.

Early May, 2003: Another Damn CAT Scan

The next day, I was drinking some banana-flavored barium in preparation for another CAT scan, which would reveal if I had any other cancerous lymph nodes from the abdomen down. I was in a funk (a bad cancer patient mood) when I went in for this one. I was nervous, shaking, and uneasy about the turn of events in my life. And I was tired of being a pincushion.

9/08/1

STONEWALL JACKSON HOSPITAL
LEXINGTON, VA 24450

PATIENT LOCATION: OP

PATIENT NAME   :Chips, Allen
DATE OF BIRTH   :▓▓▓▓
PHONE NUMBER   :
ATTENDING PHYS   :Dr. ▓▓▓

SERVICE DATE   :5/21/03
PATIENT NUMBER   :10288561
MED REC NUMBER   :068073

EXAMINATION REQUESTED
  1. CT Abdomen & Pelvis

CLINICAL HISTORY
Lymphoma

INDICATION: Hodgkin's disease.

There is mild splenomegaly. Splenic index is about 1,000; spleen size
is about 3 times normal. There is a notch in the upper border, with
calcification with small cystic component that is suggestive of a
previous injury.

Two closely adjacent 1.5 cm cysts are found in the upper pole of the
left kidney. There is no evidence of other organ enlargement,
lymphadenopathy, or ascites in the abdomen or pelvis.

IMPRESSION:
  1. Splenomegaly. Benign left renal cysts. Otherwise normal.

PF:pf
D:5/21/03
T:5/22/03

▓▓▓▓▓▓▓, D.O.

DEPARTMENT OF RADIOLOGY
  RADIOLOGY RESULTS

10749   10/98

Then, just before the procedure, my needle stick was painful and bled a lot. It was either because I was so tense or because the vein was not properly harpooned, or both.

The X-ray technician said, "Oh, you're a bleeder."

"Not usually," I said, and I went through the tunnel, listening again to the sterile computer voice: "Breathe...inhale...hold your breath...exhale," as I was moved back and forth through the tunnel.

When it was over, I walked to the changing room as the technician brought over a few personal items I had left behind. I began to voice my concerns about chemotherapy.

"Just make sure you have the right attitude, that's the key," she said as she handed me my things from behind the white curtain.

"I know, people say this, but what is the right attitude?" I answered, my voice quivering. "I guess there are a lot of things I'm wondering about today. I think I'm in an off mood. I don't think I'm doing too well today."

"Do you need to talk to somebody?" she asked.

I was wondering if a person who has cancer should express their emotions when feeling down, or if they should avoid this by cheering themselves up and staying positive. Which one was more beneficial for recovery?

Because of my emotional instability right then, and because she was a compassionate professional, she gave me the phone number of the American Cancer Society and suggested that I contact them to talk with people who had recovered from my condition. She then asked me if I wanted to talk to my friend Paul, the radiologist, again.

When I saw Paul, he shook my hand and began to talk about some things about cancer treatment that he'd read in some journals. He said that modern technology was making cancer treatment more effective today. He had read about a new laser radiation that pinpointed tumors precisely, thus eliminating the damage that lasers could do to other parts of the body. Then he handed me an article he'd extracted from a medical journal he received. "I saved this for you and your wife, since I know she does this type of thing." It explained how cancer patients were getting great results with reiki therapy reducing the side effects of radiation and chemotherapy.

I reminded Paul that my wife, Dee, was a reiki master and teacher, because the article stated that reiki masters were now teaching nurses and oncology departments in a few select hospitals how to do the treatments on patients. Paul asked if she would be interested in teaching reiki in the hospital. We also discussed how Dee could be a wonderful resource for me. I explained that reiki was already helping in reducing my B-type symptoms.

B-type symptoms are thought by medical science to occur when cancer cells from blood diseases, such as Hodgkin's, are traveling in the blood and enter into another lymph node somewhere else in the lymph system. Such symptoms for most Hodgkin's patients often include flu-like symptoms such as low-grade fever and night sweats.

By using reiki, I would have more energy when I felt depleted and more relaxed when I was stressed. After that conversation, I tried to get Dee to implement a reiki treatment for me every week, and almost every day when I had B-type symptoms.

Reiki Therapy: A Message From Grandma

Later that day, I went home and Dee agreed to give me a reiki treatment, to try to balance my emotions. It was not her usual treatment this time, however. This treatment was more spiritual...

As I lay on our bed, I looked up and saw Dee. Her eyes were closed, the long red hair of an Irish girl flowed down her back, and her hands were positioned lightly on my chest. The master bedroom in our mountain home was surrounded by large pines, poplars, and small oak trees that could be seen from two large windows. A gentle breeze pushed through the leaves, orchestrating one of nature's random songs...

"Do you sense something?" I asked.

"Yes, I think it's your grandmother."

My grandmother was the strong, saintly matriarch in our family, who had transitioned to the next world just five years before.

"I sense it, too. I think she's laughing at me," I joked. I did not really feel that she was laughing at me; however, I did hear her chuckle with the sense of humor I was so accustomed to when she was in the living. Then, I heard her voice in my head.

"I think she said, 'Stop worrying.'"

Dee agreed. "Yes, she's saying that everything's going to be okay, and that she would be with you in this life and the one after. You are not alone."

This was important for me to hear, since at that time I was feeling alone. Later, after the treatment, I called my parents, who were worried about me.

"I wanted to tell you guys what happened this morning. Grandma showed up during a reiki treatment with Dee and told me to stop worrying."

"That's interesting. Your mother and I felt her presence here just before you called," my father said.

They proceeded to tell me how they had felt her presence that morning, which would not have been uncommon within a year after her passing, but was more so this many years later. My parents' faith in the afterlife has always been unshakable, because of the number of paranormal experiences they've had in their lifetimes. This was interesting, because they are both very objective in their approach to life. My mother was an experienced institutional nurse, and my father had been a chief internal auditor for the federal government dealing with embezzlement. Therefore, the information I received from them confirmed my grandmother's visit to me.

More Needles, X-rays, and Nutritional Research

A few days later, I traveled an hour and a half to get my PET scan done, because our local hospital did not have the budget to house this expensive device. When I arrived, I filled out the usual stack of admission papers, sat in a waiting room, and then was led down the elevator to a tractor trailer in the parking garage. This trailer had one seat for patients while they waited. A technician came and hooked me up to an IV. She talked to me while she put on radioactive deflection gloves and eye-wear, as she handled radioactive glucose under a shield and transferred it into a syringe. She looked like an astronaut and I felt like an abductee in an alien experiment.

The next step was tedious. I was wrapped in bed sheets with my arms at my side and told not to move for 45 minutes, as I went through yet another long dark tunnel. Shortly afterwards, I left the imaging resonance hospital. I did not know the results.

At this time, I was researching everything that I could get my hands on that explained my particular type of cancer. I would get up at six every morning and either surf the net or make phone calls until one or two o'clock in the afternoon. I was contacting patients who had lymphoma whom I'd heard about through friends and acquaintances, or I was talking to doctors or nurses at various cancer clinics. Once I started talking about my condition, I became a sponge for information, and I did not meet one person who was not willing to share information when I posed my investigative questions.

I remembered what Dr. Fineman advised…if I was going to do an alternative method, I should examine the clinical trials on the web site of the National Center for Complementary and Alternative Medicine, sponsored by the National Institutes of Health. On connecting to the site, I found several studies written in lay terms that were helpful in understanding which natural supplements would be most effective. When I phoned the NCCAM, an information specialist told me that they recently had seen significant results with mistletoe. I ordered several studies to be sent to me. About a week later I received a large packet of information, which included booklets on my form of cancer, the psychological impact, the traditional medical treatments, clinical trials, and more. The vast majority of information booklets revolved around traditional treatment.

It appeared that CoQ-10, a natural coenzyme that is created by our bodies, was found to be deficient in people with myeloma, lymphoma (which Hodgkin's falls under), and cancers of the breast, lung, prostate, pancreas, colon, kidney, and those of the head and neck. Three breast cancer studies were listed showing higher than normal recovery rates in those using a combination of traditional medical treatment, supplements, and CoQ-10. One woman even had full remission after cancer entered her liver. One study also showed that the chemotherapy drug doxorubicin had less of a negative effect on the heart when CoQ-10 was used. As a result, I started taking the highest dose of CoQ-10 that I could find on the store shelf (200mg/day), although the studies indicated 300mg/day for those with cancer.

I also read studies on shark cartilage. Apparently a myth had been born out the fact that sharks are immune to cancer. The studies at NIH showed that taking shark cartilage proved to have minimal to no effects for cancer patients. If anything, there was a placebo effect during the time this theory became popular wind. As a result, I stopped taking it.

I'd read that garlic was good for preventing cardiovascular diseases, but a high number of studies also showed it had a cancer preventive effect and tumor reduction actions. After reading this, I put myself on the highest supplemental doses of garlic extract and kyolic garlic (500 mg/day each). Also on the shopping list was a large jar of minced garlic, which we used on a regular basis in our food preparations.

Some NIH studies showed that several antioxidants were potentially deficient in people with a wide range of cancers, and this lack of antioxidants is probably linked to degradation of DNA, the code that protects us from this illness. After reading this, I started taking a one-a-day multivitamin that included antioxidant supplements. I also started taking vitamin E extract, which if taken in its natural form also provides some anti-wrinkle properties to the skin. The natural form is more effective for the body's assimilation.

Other research I ran across, such as a naturopathic medicine book titled *Encyclopedia of Natural Medicine* by Murray and Pizzorno, showed that by increasing the intake of antioxidants vitamins C and E, zinc, selenium, and beta-carotene, we can prevent thymus gland involution. The thymus, in combination with other organs, is responsible for maintaining our ever-so-intricate immune system. As it becomes less efficient, the body's ability to fight foreign invaders, such as cancer cells, is inhibited. By increasing specific nutrition-based antioxidants, we help various tissues and organs in our bodies to destroy our own cancer. Once I stumbled upon these naturopaths' findings, I began adjusting my supplemental intake to reflect them.

I thought back to a seminar I had conducted earlier in the year, when a participant came up to me and said that she thought I should get my thymus checked because my skin was off-color. I shrugged it off, thinking she was noticing the side effects of my wintertime asthma. I believe she may have been a medical intuit, but in any case she was accurate. I did not heed her advice and get myself checked out. If I had, perhaps I could have been treated for thymus involution, thus preventing the onset of mono and Hodgkin's a few months later. But some medical experts theorize that cancer incubates for one year before manifesting. I began to wonder: can cancer be corrected a year ahead, if a breakdown in the immune system is detected? If nutritional deficiencies were diagnosed early enough, could we prevent cancer? I concluded...probably.

The thymus gland's primary role in the immune system is something called cell mediated immunity. Its deterioration has been linked to infections of bacteria, yeast, fungi, parasites, and viruses, including the Epstein-Barr virus, which medical science now indicates is the precursor to Hodgkin's disease. Many books and articles from both traditional and alternative medicine have been published recently indicating a link between parasites and viruses, and cancer. The book *The Cure For All Cancers*, by Hulda Clark, claims there is a link between an intestinal parasitic infection and cancer, which to me further suggests the efficacy of colonics. However, she has been greatly criticized for gross generalizations, claiming that every person found with this intestinal fluke therefore has cancer. Supposedly when they rid themselves of the fluke, they are rid or their cancer.

Nonetheless, intestinal cleansing and detoxification are highly recommended by most naturopaths, and many cancer patients have derived great benefits from colonics and other intestinal cleansing therapies, which are organ cleansing and detoxification therapies. This whole concept makes sense, when we consider that certain organs regulate the immune system (more information on organ cleansing in the chapter on herbal medicines).

Researching Traditional Medicine

I phoned the oncology departments of two hospitals that appeared most often during my research, in order to look into options for radiation and chemotherapy: the Lombardi Cancer Center at Georgetown University, in Washington, DC, and the M.D. Anderson Cancer Center at the University of Texas in Houston.

The Anderson Cancer Center is a leading hospital in cancer research and traditional medical treatments. When I phoned them, they said that they were using ABDV for stage 2 Hodgkin's but with an additional antibody called Rituxan. This drug was approved by the FDA for CD-20 cells in cases of recurrence (Hodgkin's coming back again). These cells were the type of Hodgkin's lymphoma I had. The nurse on the phone claimed that they administered it with their ABDV for all Hodgkin's patients. However, even though I believed that pharmaceutical advancements would engineer a reliable cancer vaccine some day, and this treatment appeared to be along this track, I was not going to be able to travel to Houston every two weeks.

I also phoned the hospital in my region with the most advanced radiation therapy equipment, the Lombardi Cancer Center. They claimed that because of their extensive budget, they had the most state-of-the-art equipment of any hospital in the region; and it would probably be worth making an appointment with a radiation oncologist to discuss the newest radiation therapy for my condition. However, because of what it had done to my mother, and because it was against both of my oncologists' advice (who were hematologists—specializing in chemotherapy), I was reluctant to do radiation and decided against setting up the appointment.

In the meantime, the B-type symptoms (night sweats and fever) returned. They seemed to occur every two weeks and last for one week. Both of my oncologists said that this might indicate that the cancer was traveling through my blood to another lymph node somewhere else in my body. They also said that the B-type symptoms would stop after the first month or two of chemotherapy (approximately two treatments), as the therapy began to eliminate the cancer cells that were most susceptible. This was an attractive concept, to feel better quickly.

Yet, the idea that cancer is not cured by medicine and that it is only put in remission had me wondering. What caused recurrence? Was it the toxic chemicals of the chemotherapy, or was it because the immune system was still inadequate in its ability to fight off invading cancer cells? Dr. Hines at UVA told me that most chemotherapy studies showed some correlation between the type of chemotherapy used and the likelihood of recurrence. Some had a high recurrence between five and thirteen years after diagnosis. The risk of recurrence after radiation increases as patients get older. I was committed to the opinion that the immune system should be rebuilt to avoid a future recurrence, since cancer is a disease of the immune system. Yet the question was, "How would this be accomplished?" I'd really hoped for the long-term cure, a therapy that adjusted the immune system permanently, but where was it, or when would it be developed?

Late May, 2003: To Do Chemo, or Not to Do Chemo...

On the following Tuesday, when I returned for an appointment with my oncologist, Dr. Fineman, he informed me that he'd received the results of the PET scan. It showed that, at that time, I was stage two, meaning I had cancerous tumors in two areas of my body—the neck and between the heart and lungs. There was a high percentage of remission over 5 years (75–85%), and the protocol was chemotherapy. We discussed setting up an appointment to start chemo treatments, which included ABDV, but did not include Rituxan, since my insurance company was less likely to cover a non-FDA approved treatment for my condition. We talked about the heart and lung damage statistics, but Dr. Fineman didn't want to focus on this, and instead steered the conversation toward obtaining a remission and getting on with my life.

As I contemplated this, the discussion turned to my ability to run the family business. I told him that I wrote books on alternative health and led seminars approximately every month and that my energy level must be kept up to accomplish this. He informed me that I could try to do it, but that I may have to take nap breaks during the seminars, or find another way to make a living if I get too tired. Most people stop working altogether.

At that point, I was getting concerned. I asked him how to predict my energy level, and he said that I shouldn't count on having more than 75% of it for the first year, at most. Even after the chemotherapy stopped, it was going to take at least six more months to a year to get all my energy back (and for my immune system to normalize). Some people never get all their energy back, while the rare few don't seem to experience any lack of energy. Everybody responds differently.

Signing on the Dotted Line

I'd decided at that point, since I only made brief progress in shrinking my neck tumors, that I would do chemotherapy. I reluctantly signed a liability waiver so I could start treatments the third Tuesday in June, when I returned from a trip my wife and I had planned to Puerto Vallarta. Dr. Fineman said that the trip would be safe to take, because Hodgkin's was relatively curable, even if I should be stage three by that time. However, when I talked to Dr. Hines at UVA by phone a day later, he recommended against waiting any longer, implying that stage three Hodgkin's with B-type symptoms greatly reduces the chances for a solid remission.

```
C A R I L I O N   C R Y S T A L   S P R I N G   I M A G I N G

      P E T   I M A G I N G   S E R V I C E S   R E P O R T
                  Roanoke, Virginia 24033
M.D. COPY CRMH
NAME: CHIPS, ALLEN STANLEY        ROOM:             EXAM DATE: 05/19/2003
ADDR: PO BOX 249                  ADM#: 63956759     SERVICE: MRI
      GOSHEN, VA.  24439          MR #: 570290       PT TYPE: OA
AGE:  41   SEX:  M                DOB:               PH #:
ORD DR:                           DISCHARGE DATE:
ATT DR.:                          SS#:               CLINIC: PET
ADM. REASON: PET SCAN/LYMPHOMA
EXAMINATION(s):          RAD CODE(s)   RMH CODE(s)   RMS ORD#   INV#
   PET LYMPHOMA DIAGNOSIS    G0220       G0220        90001      3
```

PET LYMPHOMA DIAGNOSIS

CLINICAL: LYMPHOMA DIAG

REPORT:
15 mCi of FDG given intravenously. After about one hour delay,
images were obtained from the skull base through the pelvis.
Pathologic accumulation of FDG is seen in the mediastinum and
lower cervical region bilaterally. Lymphoma high in the
differential. No other abnormalities are noted.

IMPRESSION: (See Report Body)

                                    THIS REPORT IS FINAL
                                    AND ELECTRONICALLY SIGNED.

LEM   D: ( )
JOB#   T: 05/20/2003 01:04PM

PT. NAME: CHIPS, ALLEN STANLEY   (PET)   MR #: 570290
22-MAY-03   03:11:20   EXAM(s)DATE:05/19/2003
                                                    PAGE 1

I was very concerned at the prospect of chemotherapy, however, because I was not accustomed to taking drugs of any kind. I preferred to let my body heal itself when I got sick, by using natural remedies or simply rest, supplements, and fluids. I resorted to synthetic medicines only in emergencies. Loading up my veins with toxic chemicals was foreign to me, but I thought, what other options do I have while my family was pressing me to sprint for what they believed was most reliable?

When I got home, I told my wife about the chemo date I'd set, and she was glad to hear that my doctor thought it all right to take the trip after my next seminar, which was scheduled for the first of June at the Association for Research and Enlightenment (ARE) in Virginia Beach. Two days after the seminar we would leave for Puerto Vallarta for a week, and I would start treatment the day after our return.

Note: There is a difference between a cure for cancer and putting it in remission. Chemotherapies and radiation, which are scientifically documented as causing the return of the same or other cancers, put cancer in remission. Natural cures, which rebuild the immune system and allow your body to kill its own cancer, can be referred to as a cure, since the return rate is significantly lower. Regardless of the path taken, cancer survivors should use the word "cure" when referring to the cancer they had in the past, because this is the appropriate message to their bodies, when taking the mind-body connection into consideration.

Chapter 3

Researching Edgar Cayce and Harry Hoxsey

Because my eventual cure is based on the work of Edgar Cayce, we will look at the life of this great modern mystic and naturopath. It was he who founded the Association of Research and Enlightenment (ARE) in Virginia Beach, Virginia.

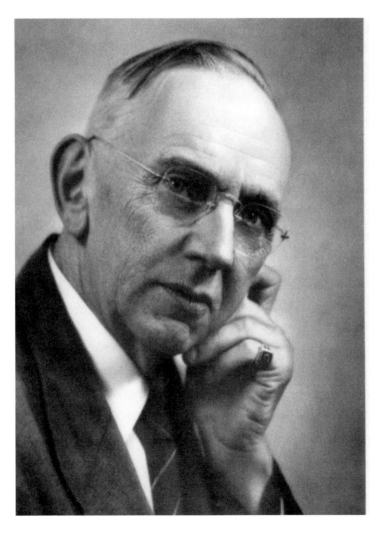

Edgar Cayce (1877-1945)

According to Sidney Kirkpatrick, who wrote *Edgar Cayce: An American Prophet*, Cayce remains the best-documented medical clairvoyant of the twentieth century. Because of his contributions to holistic health, he is often called the father of holistic medicine.

Thomas Sugrue's book, *There is a River: The Story of Edgar Cayce*, is possibly the best resource for a complete history and understanding of the work of Edgar Cayce. In order to give readers an understanding of my original attraction to the work of Edgar Cayce, which resulted in discovering natural cancer cures, I will briefly describe what he did, including his gifts of clairvoyance and healing.

When Edgar Cayce was a young boy, he was devoted to the Christian Bible. He read it from cover to cover every year, for each year of his life. When he was 12 years old, he went to his favorite place, a tree house located in the woods behind his house. While reading the story of Manoah in the Book of Judges for the 13th time, a woman appeared to him. He thought at first she was his mother, until he noticed that she had wings. She told him that his prayers had been answered and that whatever it was that he wanted most would be granted to him. He told the angel that he would like to be able to help people, especially children. Then the angel disappeared. Shortly thereafter, he fell asleep on a school book and the first recorded account of mental osmosis took place. On awakening, he was tested by his father, who found that Edgar knew every concept in the book. This was miraculous, because Edgar was a poor student, and it became the first event documenting his clairvoyance.

When Edgar was still a boy, he lost his voice. All his doctors' efforts to get his voice back failed, until a hypnotherapist came to work with him. Edgar's ability to speak was restored when the hypnotherapist asked him to come up with his own solution to the problem while he was in a state of hypnosis. With his parents' encouragement, he was then convinced that if he could help himself, he could also perform this service for others.

Years later, when Edgar Cayce was a young adult, another miracle was documented, an occasion in which Edgar used his gift to heal his son, Hugh Lynn Cayce. It involved the family-owned photography business, where his son burned his eyes from the flash powder used to illuminate photographs. The doctor told the family that the boy's eyes were burned so badly that he would never see again, and advised removing one eye. Aware of his father's gift, the boy begged his father to enter into a state of self-hypnosis and find a solution to the problem.

By this time, Edgar had used this method many times to help others, so he posed the question to his spiritual guidance and the answer came: "Apply tannic acid directly to the eyes." The physicians of that time thought this was ludicrous, that tannic acid was too strong to be put directly on the eyes and would cause more complications. Nonetheless, the remedy was applied and Hugh Lynn's sight was fully restored.

It wasn't long before the media became aware of numerous miracles resulting from Cayce doing this—a process that came to be called "readings." Many people came to him for advice on a variety of illnesses. Eventually, through the advice of the readings, the Cayce family moved from a small town in Hopkinsville, Kentucky, to Virginia Beach, Virginia. Cayce received funding from wealthy U.S. businessmen and the Cayce Hospital was built atop a large sand dune at the northern end of the beach. People would request readings from all over the world. Some of them visited the hospital, while others asked their questions in correspondence from thousands of miles away.

Edgar diagnosed people's problems with astounding accuracy, suggesting remedies that led to cures at an unusually high success rate. Eventually, his readings went from being health-related to being metaphysically oriented. They included spiritual insights into people's current life circumstances, soul journeys, and various prophecies for the future of our world. Many of these prophecies have been studied and judged 80–90 percent accurate, such as his prediction of the Great Depression.

How I became acquainted with the ARE

In the early 1980s I began reading many books on Cayce, hypnotherapy, and meditation. As mentioned in the introduction to this book, by the late 80s I had reached the end of the corporate ladder in pharmaceuticals and had decided to start a service-oriented career. This was when my training institute formed an alliance with the ARE and offered a wider array of professional hypnotherapy certification training programs.

I began meditating in the late 80s, and added some Edgar Cayce concepts—he was a strong advocate of meditation—in order to enrich my meditation. One day, while I was meditating, I asked where most of my life's purpose would be accomplished and the answer was "Virginia Beach." Shortly thereafter, a client in my private practice, who told me she was a clairvoyant, claimed she saw my picture in *Venture Inward* magazine, a publication of ARE Press. I was surprised, because I lived in Ohio at the time and had no intention of moving or of pursuing speaking engagements with the ARE. But in 1993 I went to teach a hypnotherapy class in Virginia Beach, as my guidance indicated, and at the end of the first course, I formed a relationship with the ARE. As a result, I began to teach hypnotherapy courses through their organization, as predicted. Over the next decade, as destiny would have it, I've accomplished most of my life's purpose in Virginia Beach.

I liked studying Cayce, because I could continue the religious practices I grew up with and was accustomed to, while increasing my knowledge of naturopathy, self-improvement, and spirituality. In fact, Cayce said more than once that the ARE was to be a resource of information and not a religion. People from all walks of life and various world religions have been known to study there. Cayce often stressed that being of service to others was one of the highest ideals one could attain. To this practice I have always aspired.

Although individualized readings were meant for the unique mental and physical conditions of his clients, some modern researchers have generalized that certain remedies that Cayce consistently prescribed for specific health conditions may still be effective for people with those illnesses today. This, in fact, was the motivation for my research trying to find an effective remedy for my cancer.

End of May, 2003: Off to Teach at the ARE

It was the last weekend in May, two days before my seminar would start at ARE, when I came down with B-type symptoms again. While driving to Virginia Beach, I was sick as a dog. I was sweating and had a fever, which consistently stayed around 100 degrees. The one tumor I had left on my neck was growing rapidly now. It had gone from the size of a pea in early May to the size of a large kidney bean and now it was fanning out at the base, solidly attaching to the side of my neck and forming the shape of a sideways mountain. This was the first time a tumor had gone from loose and moveable to attaching. I was concerned and still felt very sick, so I called a business associate, who agreed to take over my conference coordinating position, which left the majority of the teaching to him and two other instructors.

First of June, 2003: The Turning Point

I taught on Monday, the first day of a five-day seminar, and at the end of the day I announced to the group what my predicament was and that the other teachers could successfully complete the training program without me. The attendees were concerned but understood. Some students highly recommended the ARE Health and Rejuvenation Center, so I set up a lymph node cleansing appointment for the next day. The treatment consisted of one hour of lymph massage, one hour of acupressure with caster oil packs, and one and one-half hours of colonics, with breaks in between. I was slated for four and one-half hours of therapy. My primary objective was to get rid of the B-type symptoms I was experiencing so I could have a good time with my wife in Puerto Vallarta.

That night I hardly slept at all. I lay on my back with a washcloth on my face, popping Tylenol for the fever and trying to breathe. It felt like my chest was on fire and had a cinder block on it. I described it as a cross between walking pneumonia and the flu. I woke up after only a few hours of sleep, drenched in sweat but eager to try something new.

First was the lymph massage, which was a light stroking of the lymph node regions of the body in order to drain the toxins out of the lymph system. It was relaxing.

Next on the agenda was acupressure with caster oil packs; this was a process suggested by Edgar Cayce to pull toxins out of the body and stabilize the lymphatic system. During the treatment Kathy, my practitioner, said, "Wow, you're really moving a lot of energy." I was having breathing problems, was sweating profusely, and the pressure points in my inner forearms where she was pushing felt like a nail was being driven through them. The room became increasingly humid; we had to turn on the air conditioner to cool it off.

At the end of the treatment, she gave me a booklet titled *Cancer Medicine From Nature: The Herbal Cancer Formulas of Edgar Cayce and Harry Hoxsey,* by Robert Bloom. Kathy's gift would prove to lay the foundation of what would eventually lead to my recovery.

Next was the colonic, which was a process that involved the cleansing of the colon through water fill and extraction. Edgar Cayce recommended that these be done regularly to cleanse all the toxins out of the body. It was my first colonic, a peculiar experience but beneficial. My biggest fear was that my colonics practitioner would be somebody I knew. When the practitioner introduced herself and gave me some preparatory instructions, I thought she looked familiar. Sure enough, my fear came true. She began the process and told me that she was a former student of my hypnotherapy class! I thought, "Isn't life strange. It always manifests our fears in one way or another." Nonetheless, she had a professional presentation and an excellent way of putting her clients at ease, which is probably why she took the hypnotherapy class in the first place.

After the session, I felt lighter and very relaxed. That night I had the best night's sleep I'd had in several days, as all my symptoms were disappearing.

Even though the uncontrollable cells in my body had a mind of their own, my curiosity, stemming from the natural healing profession I was part of, resulted in an inner urge to dig deeper. I wanted to look at the resources that were available in the ARE Library to see what Edgar Cayce, the "sleeping prophet" had suggested for curing cancer. This step would prove to be the pivotal turning point in my quest for a natural cure for cancer.

Digging Deeper

It was early afternoon on a beautiful spring day. I stepped out onto the terrace in front of the old hospital building, which now housed the Health and Rejuvenation Center and had a breathtaking view of the Atlantic Ocean. From there, I walked down the familiar steps that connected the terrace to the parking lot. It was just a short walk across the parking lot to the larger, newer building, which housed the conference center where I was a frequent speaker. The conference center and book store were on the first floor, the library was located on the second floor, and the meditation room was on the third floor.

I thought back to a Cayce reading I had come across years before, which stated that there was a natural cure on the earth for every illness and disease on this planet. I thought that each remedy simply needed to be discovered. This resonated with me on a deeper philosophical level, because my thinking was that if God created the earth, then he would have created natural remedies for all its illnesses as well.

Edgar Cayce Reading 2396-2

"Yet the entity from that sojourn is a lover of nature, one that appreciates nature, the NATURAL sources; and that there is within the grasp of man all that in nature that is the counterpart of that in the mental and spiritual realms, and an antidote for EVERY poison, for every ill in the individual experience, if there will but be applied nature, natural sources."

The library was known to be the most comprehensive resource of alternative health. Upon entering, a very dedicated librarian steered me like a ship meandering through the oceans of all the naturopathic materials. She told me that she was familiar with both the Cayce and Hoxsey forms of herbal cancer treatment, and she also knew a local chiropractor who was using the method. She gave me the chiropractor's phone number. Then she gave me several books and videos that described the method, which emphasizes a combination of diet and herbs.

Cayce's Anti-cancer Herbs

I began by researching the Edgar Cayce readings and remedies using *The Complete Edgar Cayce Readings on CD-ROM*, by ARE Press, which contained all of the 14,000-plus readings in the library, as well as letters from his clients. I wanted to find any consistencies that existed from one case of cancer to the next that involved dietary and herbal recommendations.

First, I read a story about a woman who had cancer and was told by Cayce to do a grape fast. She wrote a letter back to him claiming that she ate grapes every day and had thereby cured herself of cancer. I later discovered the importance of grape juice for liver cleansing and boosting immune response.

Then I found a case where Cayce had recommended that a woman with breast cancer walk outdoors more in order to obtain more vitamin D from sunlight. He was way ahead of his time with this recommendation, because this link has only recently been discovered by conventional medicine and nutritional experts (more on this in the chapter on supplementation).

Soon, after examining several cases, I discovered a variety of herbs that Edgar Cayce recommended for various cancers, in addition to: electrical or vibrational treatments, oxygen therapy, spinal manipulations, castor oil packs, animated ash (an oxygenator), violet ray, ultraviolet ray, nutritional, attitudinal, and more. However, because I was more interested in discovering herbal compounds that were used successfully to treat cancer before the introduction of synthetic medicine, they became my primary focus.

The herbs used most often involved rectifying the conditions in the body that lead to cancerous conditions. These included: licorice, red clover, burdock root, stillingia root, berberis root, poke root, cascara sagrada, prickly ash bark, buckthorn bark, wild cherry bark, yellow dock root, elder berry/flower, sarsaparilla root, plantain, and an alkaline compound called potassium iodine, also known as potash.

I noted all of the Cayce anticancer herbal prescriptions, then went to the resource room and watched the videos on herbal cures that the librarian recommended. It was then that I was introduced to a popular alternative cancer therapy called Hoxsey therapy.

Harry Hoxsey and the Hoxsey Clinics

The next step would prove to be the most valuable naturopathic discovery in my recovery: researching the methods of Naturopathic Physician Harry Hoxsey.

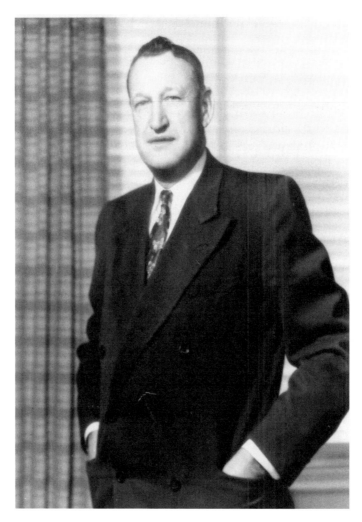

Harry Hoxsey (1901-1974)

At first, I watched a videotape titled *Hoxsey: Quacks Who Cure Cancer? How Healing Becomes a Crime.* It featured one of the most popular and controversial cancer treatment clinics in history, the Biomedical Center in Tijuana, Mexico. In 1983, a group of independent filmmakers began an extensive four-year investigation into this center's treatment programs. In September 1987, their accounts of healing led to an award-winning independent film that was featured at the prestigious Margaret Mead Film Festival in New York City. In his review of the film, *New York Times* film critic Vincent Canby praised it as "first rate reportage." Shortly thereafter, it was shown on the premium channel Cinemax and other broadcasting networks around the world.

This hour and twenty-minute film struck a chord within me. I started to realize that there may be a highly effective, alternative medicine therapy that was non-toxic and had a reliable track record of success. It was an all-natural treatment program that involved herbs. It did not involve surgery, chemotherapy, or radiation. The movie objectively examined the history of herbal medicine, the politics regarding the restrictive practice of medicine in the middle of the twentieth century, and the controversy over the effectiveness of orthodox cancer therapies. Most impressive were interviews with and stories about Hoxsey patients, who came from all over the world to get treatment from Hoxsey's clinics over the 80-plus years that the clinic had been in existence.

In fact, the Hoxsey family had been successfully treating cancer with herbs, discovered in North America, since the late 1800s. The story began on the Hoxsey farm in Illinois. One day, Harry Hoxsey's great-grandfather, John Hoxsey, a veterinarian, noticed the unusual behavior of a horse that was stricken with cancerous tumors. He was found straying from the rest of the herd to eat plants that were not normally part of a horse's diet. Soon the horse started to get well on its own. John Hoxsey noted which plants the horse was eating. After the horse fully recovered, he began experimenting with the same herbs on other animals with cancer and noticed an unusually high cure rate.

Soon thereafter, he began to experiment on people and noticed the same success rate, about 80 percent. Harry Hoxsey's father also treated many people with great results. On his deathbed, Harry's father gave him the formula and made him promise to take the herbal treatment program to the masses but to never turn away a patient because of finances. Harry accomplished this in 1924 when he set up the first clinic to treat humans in Dallas, Texas. By 1950, he operated the largest privately owned cancer clinic in America.

I found most interesting the period in the early- to mid-twentieth century, when naturopathic physicians were battling allopathic physicians over how to treat disease. It appeared that by the middle of the twentieth century, synthetic treatment modalities used by allopathic physicians started to supersede the naturopathic physician's legal right to practice. Allopathic physicians were allied with the American Medical Association (AMA) and the Food and Drug Administration (FDA), which at that time gained unprecedented legal control over the practice of medicine.

By the time Hoxsey therapy became popular, the allopaths dominated the practice of medicine through legislative efforts spearheaded by private interest groups. As a result of this situation, Dallas District Attorney Al Templeton arrested Harry Hoxsey approximately 100 times in two years. He was arrested so often that he carried a roll of hundred dollar bills in his pocket so he could bail himself out of jail. He was always out of jail in one or two days, since Templeton could never persuade any of Harry's patients to testify against him. Templeton wanted to put Hoxsey away for good, until his own brother secretly used the Hoxsey therapy. His cancer disappeared, and Templeton gave Hoxsey the credit. Templeton then became Hoxsey's lawyer and would prove to be one of his greatest advocates.

By 1962, Harry Hoxsey was treating 12,000 cases of cancer, solely with herbs, through 17 cancer treatment centers scattered throughout the United States. Dr. Fishbine, president of the AMA at the time, and a group of AMA doctors, tried to buy exclusive rights to the formula from Hoxsey. But Harry tried to rewrite the exclusivity clause of the contract so that every person would have access to the formula, regardless of ability to pay, which followed his father's wishes. Fishbine declined, and a 25-year battle ensued between Fishbine and Hoxsey.

Listed below are the original ingredients of the Hoxsey formula. This list was published in the June 12, 1964 issue of the *Journal of the American Medical Association* (JAMA) after an "investigation" into the Hoxsey Cancer Clinic of Dallas, Texas. Apparently at that time Dr. Harry Hoxsey was given restrictive orders to properly label the tonic for the purpose of shipping and commerce. A 16-ounce bottle of Hoxsey Tonic was analyzed by the AMA laboratories, which found that each 5-cc. quantity contained the following:

Potassium Iodine	150 mg.
Licorice	20 mg.
Red Clover	20 mg.
Burdock Root	10 mg.
Stillingia Root	10 mg.
Berberis Root	10 mg.
Poke Root	10 mg.
Cascara Sagrada	5 mg.
Prickly Ash Bark	5 mg.
Buckthorn Bark	20 mg.

Although his patients swore that Hoxsey had cured them of cancer, the AMA, which was trying at that time to discredit many natural healing modalities, publicly scrutinized Harry Hoxsey's methods. Fishbine succeeded in using the media to label Hoxsey a quack. In response, Hoxsey sued the AMA for libel and slander in an unprecedented court battle to prove the efficacy of Hoxsey therapy. Eventually, the conflict went as high as the U.S. Supreme Court, where hundreds of patients who had received a cure for their cancers appeared in testimony. As a result, Harry Hoxsey became the first person to sue the AMA and win. Near the end of the trial, Dr. Morris Fishbine admitted that his examination had proved that the Hoxsey method was curing cancer after all, but only with escharotics—the applying of herbal powders and salves to externally accessible tumors or external cancers just under the skin, thereby expressing them through the skin (more on this in future chapters and the photo gallery). However, he gave no credence to the herbal tonics that were ingested by patients for the treatment of internal cancers. Immediately after the case concluded in 1964, all 17 clinics were padlocked by the FDA for using unapproved medicines.

Mildred Nelson, who was Harry Hoxsey's head nurse at that time, agreed to move the primary Hoxsey Clinic from the home offices in Dallas, Texas, to Tijuana, Mexico, so they could legally continue to treat cancer with

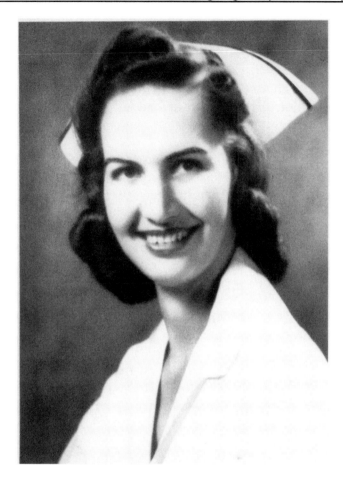

Mildred Nelson (1919-1999)

this non-invasive method. After the clinic relocated, Hoxsey was adamant about taking his name out of the title of the new clinic, so Mildred decided to call it the Biomedical Center.

Mildred had been a skeptic until her mother, Della, contracted terminal uterine cancer in the mid-1950s. When orthodox medicine gave up on her, she insisted on trying Hoxsey therapy. During this time, Mildred accepted employment at the clinic in order to expose Harry Hoxsey as a quack. But then her mother was cured and she became a staunch supporter, long-term employee, and then director. When the clinics were shut down in 1964, it was Mildred who took the Hoxsey clinics' work to Mexico. Harry Hoxsey died a decade later and Mildred carried on his mission until her death in 1999, due to stroke. Her mother had lived cancer-free until her death in 1997.

Mildred was an award-winning pioneer in cancer research, who was noted for the healing effects of her positive attitude, which instilled hope in her patients. When Mildred passed away, her sister Liz became the new director. Under her direction, the clinic now offers a fresh array of modern, natural treatment programs.

The second video I watched, which was a few years old, was called "Hoxsey's Biomedical Center: The Experience." It interviewed a medical staff that claimed an 80 percent success rate with the use of anti-cancer herbs, homeopathics, and an anti-cancer diet. Two of the doctors interviewed had been at the clinic for more than a decade; this was true for most of the staff. One doctor, Dr. Gutierrez, stated that he had left a traditional oncology clinic near Mexico City that treated children for leukemia, Hodgkin's disease, and other cancers.

Originally, he went to the Biomedical Center to disprove it, but after being convinced of its superior recovery rate compared to orthodox methods, he joined the medical staff there and had been there for 14 years. On the video, with an uncanny level of sincerity, he claimed that the orthodox treatment of cancer in his previous practice—radiation and chemotherapy—was not only "causing a lot of suffering to the children," but also was as life-threatening as the illness itself. In medical schools in Mexico City, he also took formal training in homeopathics and naturopathic medicine. When clinic director Mildred Nelson invited him for a visit in 1985, she offered him a position on staff and he had been there ever since. As of this writing, Dr. Gutierrez has been practicing at the clinic for more than twenty years.

It impressed me that the clinic's staff and patients' attitudes were so positive. There were many testimonials on the video. Patient after patient claimed that they'd been cured by the herbal methods, many for as long as twenty to forty years. One woman had breast cancer and I watched as the staff used the external herbal methods called "escharotics." I saw them pop out the dead tumor through the skin. Even Fishbine, the former president of the AMA, had admitted that escharotics proved effective.

I watched the story of another woman, who had mouth cancer. Her physicians in the United States had advised removing a significant portion of her face in order to get all of the cancer. She was told not to get cosmetic surgery done with the operation, because it would be much more costly and she would probably not live very long. The woman looked very much at peace with the escharotics that clinic staff applied to her face to kill the tumor and lift it to the surface. Afterwards, she had only a small hairline scar. Some patients on the video showed small indentations where large tumors had been removed.

Many people claimed success with the internal tonic as well. One patient was just a toddler when she contracted a large black tumor with hair, which spanned most of her back. Her parents took her to the clinic several years ago, and she was prescribed just a few drops of the black tonic (they also have a red tonic). The tumor was lifted from her back and she'd been cancer-free ever since. Pictures were shown of her in her teens. This was impressive, needless to say.

The film was narrated by its producer, Carol Main. She began the film by describing how she'd been cured by the Hoxsey method. She'd been diagnosed with pancreatic cancer and given only a few months to live. The doctors in the United States claimed that there was no viable treatment method that they could offer her, and sent her home to die. (I'd heard that pancreatic and liver cancers were among the quickest terminal cancers and that traditional medical treatment only shortened these people's lives.) She'd heard about the Hoxsey method from some friends, and she immediately booked a trip to the clinic. She claimed that she'd been cured, and I later found out that she'd been cancer-free for more than twenty years! I could hardly believe it, but I did, because something within me told me that it was true.

At the end of the video, I saw a man (whom I later found out was Bernie Main, Carol's husband) enjoying his custom automobile building hobby after recovering from lymphoma. His story began when he returned from a trip he took with his wife to Hawaii and could not speak. The doctors found malignant lymphatic tumors pressing against his larynx. Because his wife had been cured of pancreatic cancer, he chose to use only the methods of the Biomedical Center and he was cured. I started thinking, "Hey, lymphoma, that's what I've got. If he can be cured through this natural method, then so can I." I thought, "At least it's worth a try."

I watched again the segment on the video that described the diet and wrote down the things that a person with cancer should not consume and compared it to Cayce's alkaline diet. They were very similar. Then I watched the end of the video again. It showed Alaska—rivers, streams, fish, birds—and children. "There are many things here worth living for," the narrator said over beautiful scenes and pictures of young children. "Yeah," I thought, as I got teary-eyed. That's what *I* wanted to live for too. I loved nature and my family, and I wanted to see my children have children and have the opportunity to develop a relationship with my grandchildren, as the people on the video did. It struck a chord that rang true for me.

Locally, I could only find the anticancer herbs suspended in an alcohol base. I began taking a half teaspoon, four times a day, as recommended on the label of Cayce's herbal digestive tonic. In the meantime, I noticed an herbal tonic called "Hoxsey Formula" in one of the natural health catalogs that the librarian gave me. It was suspended in an alcohol base. I phoned the president of the company that distributed the tonic, someone I'd met at a natural health conference at the ARE in Virginia Beach several years earlier.

"Brian, this is Allen Chips. I met you at the Meridian Conference at ARE several years ago when you were promoting the wet cell (a battery recommended by Edgar Cayce to put the body's bioelectrical field in balance). I had a display table set up on hypnotherapy. I'm the one who teaches the hypnotherapy conferences there."

"Oh, yeah, I remember talking with you. What's up?"

"Well, quite a bit since then. It looks like you've really expanded your company's products since then too."

I asked about his growing into a mail order catalog company and then said, "I noticed that you sell a product called the Hoxey Formula, spelled without the 's.' Is it the exact same formula as the one that the Biomedical Center in Tijuana sells?"

"It's pretty close, but not exactly the same. Why do you ask?"

"Well, this spring I contracted Hodgkin's disease, and while I was researching some of the most common herbs recommended by Cayce to treat cancer, I saw your catalog listing this Hoxey formula for sale."

"You know Allen, if I had cancer I'd make a trip down to Tijuana to get the original formula and the medical care that you might need from the Hoxsey clinic. I'm not sure I would experiment with our tonic. I think I would go directly to the source."

"Well, I'm already scheduled for chemo on June 16th, since chemo for this type of thing has a respectable success rate. I just wanted to find out more about it and try it out. I'd heard that Barbara Steins, a local chiropractor, was going to the clinic in Tijuana and I also plan to call her to see what kind of results she is getting."

Brian was a no-nonsense kind of guy and I respected his opinion. I thanked him. He wished me good luck and I asked to be transferred to his customer service department. I ordered two 2-ounce bottles of the copycat "Hoxey Formula" with two-day shipping, so that when I got home on Friday, it would be there for me to take on my trip to Puerto Vallarta.

Later that day, I called Barbara, who was happy to talk to me...

"Hello, Barbara, this is Allen Chips. The librarian at the ARE library told me you were using the Hoxsey method and gave me your name and number."

"Yes. What can I help you with?"

I told her about my illness and that I was researching anti-cancer herbs, and inquired, "I was wondering what kind of results you've been getting."

"Oh, I can only say positive things about the Biomedical Center in Tijuana. I was diagnosed with breast cancer in September, with a tumor the size of a half-dollar, and now about six months later it's shrunk down to where it's barely detectable. It's about the size of a dime. And the people at the clinic are so positive, the doctors and the patients. It's such a positive place to visit. I just knew it was the right choice for me."

I was impressed that I was actually speaking with a living testimonial. We discussed the two independent films on Hoxsey therapy, the herbs that Cayce recommended and how they were similar to the Hoxsey herbs, and the Hoxsey diet.

"Oh, the patient video," she said. "I've watched it on a regular basis so that I can be sure I'm doing the diet right. Some people have a problem with the diet, but I don't because I've always been inclined toward eating health food, so it was easy for me to adjust to it."

She went on to describe the variables of the treatment program, and I questioned her about the individualized program that the oncologists in Tijuana recommended specifically for breast cancer. She told me about the supplements and two pharmaceutical agents she was prescribed by the clinic, in addition to the herbs. (I later researched the pharmaceutical agents and discovered that one was antiviral and the other was an antiparasitic; both were immune enhancers but neither was approved by the FDA.)

I told her that I was just experimenting with the herbal approach and that I was scheduled for chemotherapy in the middle of the month. I explained that I had made progress already using certain supplements and talked about the effectiveness of using imagery and self-hypnosis.

She complemented me on my research and methods, and I told her how humbling it was to be an alternative health professional who contracted this illness. She talked to me briefly about her lifestyle changes and how she had different approaches now to her private practice and her free time. I told her that I was reassessing my lifestyle as well. We both agreed that there was a higher purpose for our experiencing such a life-threatening illness.

She wished me well, saying, "With your background in alternative health, you should do well with this sort of thing. You're going to be fine."

At this stage, I was preoccupied with the large tumor protruding from my neck and I hoped to find these herbs as quickly as possible. I was very interested in experimenting even though I was committed to my June 16th chemo date. My thinking was that if these herbs could shrink the tumor that I could see and feel on my neck, then the others between my heart and lungs would recede, and perhaps I could cancel chemotherapy.

I went directly to the largest health food store in Virginia Beach to buy any of the herbs that I could find. When I got there, I could not find potassium iodine but did find one-ounce tinctures of licorice, red clover, and burdock root. The only place I could find Cayce's wild cherry bark and yellow dock root was in Cayce's Formula 545: Herbal Digestive Tonic. In addition, I bought an eight-ounce bottle of elderberry extract. I took my discoveries back to my hotel room, where I mixed them together in an eight-ounce bottle, as follows:

Formula 545	4 ounces
Licorice Extract	1 ounce
Red Clover	1 ounce
Burdock Root	1 ounce
Elderberry Extract	1 ounce

That evening, I lounged in my hotel room reading books on the herbs and Hoxsey therapy. As I thought back to the Hoxsey videos, I began to ponder the effect that medical politics of the middle twentieth century had had in reducing the credibility and widespread use of naturopathic medicines. If this method had such a high success rate, and Barbara's testimonial and the video testimonials were authentic, could it be that there was a highly effective, natural, nontoxic herbal medicine that was scarcely available today strictly because of medical politics? Could it be that there was an effort by corporate America and the AMA to monopolize the health care industry when they patented and restricted the use of medicine in the 1950s and 60s—and that this continues to make Hoxsey therapy illegal even today? Naturopathic methods didn't really start to come back into popularity until the 1980s and 90s, and even then it was under the strict scrutiny of federal and state authorities. Because of public demand, we have many alternatives available today through the practice of various natural health providers, but how restricted are they still? How far do money and greed really reach in dictating the American public's health care options?

Hoxsey therapy appeared to be very affordable, as traditional cancer therapies are progressively becoming unaffordable, even for insured Americans. I'd heard stories of insurance companies' benefits not covering all of a cancer patient's medical bills. I recalled a conversation with my health insurance representative a year earlier, when I first applied, about a "cancer benefit." I could have added it to my self-employed catastrophic plan. The agent recommended it, because of the many bankruptcies of, and hospital lawsuits won against, cancer patients and their surviving family members. He showed me newspaper articles of real cases where people lost their homes. I never thought cancer would happen to me, and if it did, I thought, "By that time America will have corrected her errors; after all, we do have the most advanced medical system in the world. Surely, the best government, 'of the people, by the people, for the people.' At that time, I was wondering where the national health plan was that everybody said they wanted, which eventually got swept under the rug at capitol hill.

I didn't take the cancer benefit. I later discovered that I had a $4,500 deductible and a 20 percent co pay if I went outside the provider network, and a $3,500 deductible if I stayed in the network. I'd already reached my deductible with one PET scan, which was used to stage my cancer.

I thought back to the 1980s, when I switched from a career in pharmaceuticals to become a hypnotherapist, and how my friends and family thought I was crazy because of the income I sacrificed. The health care industry referred to my practice as "alternative health." By the mid-1990s the health care industry tried to change the term "alternative health" to "complementary health," in an attempt to meet public demand. Around the mid-90s both terms— "alternative and complementary health care"—stuck. During the process, the National Institutes of Health developed a research arm titled the National Center for Complementary and Alternative Medicine (NCCAM). I began to wonder if the NIH had performed research on the Hoxsey Method, and if they had would they accurately report its efficacy as a cancer therapy.

I was fortunate to find a paper published by Mary Ann Richardson, Dr. Ph. in the *Journal of Alternative and Complementary Medicine* (v. 7, No. 1, 2001, pp. 19-32) a researcher from NCCAM who investigated the two most popular alternative cancer clinics, the Biomedical Center and the Livingston Foundation Medical Center, which specialized in cancer vaccines and an anticancer diet. Her conclusion in this feasibility study follows:

"Historical, widespread use of clinics, such as these with anecdotal reports of extraordinary survival, merit perceptive, systematic monitoring of patient outcomes. For data to be meaningful, however, disease status must be pathologically confirmed and patient follow-up improved."

At this point, I was primarily concerned with what would save my life. I thought about how I had more to do here on earth before I wanted to leave...writing, teaching, learning, places to see, and time with my family. The next chapter looks at whether my independent research and a self-implemented, herbal remedy worked on *my own* cancer.

Chapter 4

Let the Races Begin

Early June 2003: Escaping, Planning, and the Little Miracle

My seminar had ended, we'd packed up all of our materials, and on the trip home I'd begun to feel I had more energy. My sleep was getting better, I could breathe more easily, and my night sweats were diminishing. I got home and immediately packed up for a week-long vacation, adding the pseudo-Hoxsey tonic and the Cayce herbs to my suitcase. The next morning, I took both herbal concoctions and we flew to Puerto Vallarta. After we were settled into our hotel, we were invited to a timeshare presentation at Rancho Banderas in neighboring Puerto Nuevo. The next day we took the tour and fell in love with this gold-rated, five-star resort. We thought it would provide a higher quality of life on my recovery, so, uncharacteristically for us, we bought into it.

Making a purchase like that was something we normally would have never considered, but my wife and I were thinking that life was short, so we might as well pull our nest egg out of savings and do it now. Major health issues tend to change people's perspective on life, and they start to think about living in the "now," rather than waiting to live it up some day during a retirement that may never arrive.

The salesperson for the resort got us the presidential suite for the week when he discovered I had cancer and it was our anniversary, because his heart went out to us. We abandoned the hotel and moved into a two-bedroom villa that provided the quaintest getaway we'd ever had. The pool cascaded over the rocky cliffs that stepped down toward the ocean. The restaurant was located on a round rock cliff that protruded over the ocean. While we ate, we could see iguanas and butterflies just a few feet away in the cliff-side foliage. Just beyond was a 150-foot drop to the ocean and a breeze that harmonized with the sound of waves crashing on the coast. It was breathtaking.

We engaged in a variety of activities, including sailing, snorkeling, and horseback riding on the beach. I meditated every morning on our balcony, which resembled old-time Mexico, with its bold pillars, white stone trim, and a southern Pacific exposure. My meditations included white light and tumor reduction imagery. It was a great spot for meditation. During the trip, I implemented a version of the Cayce alkaline diet and the Cayce-Hoxsey alcohol-suspended, herbal compounds.

Every day I woke up dreading the chemo date, because I'd never put toxic chemicals into my body before. I hardly ever used synthetic medicines when I was sick, because I researched and used effective natural remedies instead. I was hoping something would start happening soon. Maybe the tumor on my neck would start shrinking. It was a daily anxiety, kept at bay by starting meditation with passages from a book called *The Lord's Answer to Your Every Need*. I read segments that addressed the emotion or mood I woke up with that day. It quoted Scripture passages that answered the mood fairly accurately, which seemed to give me a sense of faith and inner strength.

On Tuesday, June 9, when I woke up I called to Dee. "Dee, come here and feel the lump on my neck. Does it seem to be shrinking a bit, or am I just imagining it?"

"Well, yeah, maybe a little."

"Are you sure I'm not making it up?"

"No. It seems like it's getting smaller to me, too."

I asked her the same thing Wednesday morning. By Thursday, it appeared to have gotten even smaller. That afternoon, after swimming in the third-level pool, I got out to lie under a large umbrella and drink the fresh-squeezed pineapple juice, which was very tasty there. I turned my head to look at something when I felt as if a rubber band snapped against my neck. I said, "Ouch" and then felt the lump on my neck. It had detached itself and was now moveable. I was amazed.

"Hey, Dee, feel this. Doesn't it feel like its moveable and smaller now?" I asked, attempting a reality check.

"Yeah, it does" she said with a crinkled brow as she felt it. Then she committed to the obvious: "It really seems like the herbs are working."

By the end of the week, the tumor appeared to have shrunk down to the size of a small pea. I was elated. We got home on Sunday, June 15, and I spent some time pacing the floor. I didn't know what to do. I was trying to decide whether or not to keep my chemo appointment, so I called the oncologist's office and briefly explained my dilemma. The nurse was very nice and said I should come into the office (where the chemo room was located), since my oncologist would need to talk to me either way, whether I took the chemo or not. So I drove into town.

When I got there, I was taken to an examination room, where I waited to see Dr. Fineman. While I was there, I spent a few minutes drawing the different stages that the tumors on my neck had gone through over the past two weeks. After about ten minutes, Dr. Fineman walked in, noticed the drawings, and asked, "What are these?"

I pointed to the drawings to illustrate the tumor's stages as it had shrunk. He said, "Really? Let me see." He set his jaw, squinted, and examined all the lymph nodes around my neck and jaw line with his fingertips.

When he felt the left side, I asked, "Don't you think it's smaller? I mean, it used to be the size of a large kidney bean, and now it's the size of a pea."

He said, "Pea? I think it's more like the size of a BB. That's remarkable. What happened?"

I told him about the supplements, the herbal tonic I created, and the imagery I was using, and he said he hoped I documented it all so it would be clear as to what caused which results. I asked him if it was true that cancer goes either one way or the other; it's either growing or shrinking. He agreed that this was correct. He said that perhaps this was some sort of miracle and asked me if I heard the voice of God. I responded that I felt I may have experienced a form of divine intervention. I told him about a dream I had after asking God for a healing color, the color I could use most effectively in my mediations, and that's when I saw a purple bird on our bird feeder.

He said, "You are the most exceptional patient in the history of my practice." He suggested we cancel the chemotherapy scheduled for that day, and we walked to the nurses' station. He turned to me and suggested I get a CT scan. I agreed. Then he asked his nurse to call it into the hospital. He then said to them, "It looks like Mr. Chips will not be needing chemotherapy today," and walked down the hall. They looked a little surprised. Tears welled up in my eyes with the realization that I had just begun to win the war taking place in my body.

Third Week of June, 2003: Winning the First Battle

I received a fax of the results of my CT scan, but Paul, my friend the radiologist, wasn't in when I called the radiology department. Paul's partner, the other DO who shared the position, was there and he explained the scan to me in layman's terms.

"Essentially what I am saying is that the tumors in your mediastinum (between the heart and lungs) are sagging. It's as if they were plump cherries on a cherry tree and now they're drying out, like prunes. Somehow, they are beginning to go the other direction. Are you doing chemo?" I said no and briefly told him about the herbal medicines. He said that my tumors were "hollowing," which was a good sign, and that they may have shrunk by about 5%. He said that though the progress was not greatly significant yet, he thought the whole concept was fascinating and he would help me in any way he could.

The next day I was due to see Dr. Fineman again. During a long ride through Goshen Pass, a beautiful river gorge on the way into town, I pondered how God was creating some miracles in my life. I signed in at the front desk and went back into the examination room. Shortly thereafter, he stepped in. We discussed the CT scan, and he said that his interpretation of the radiologist's report was that my tumors were hollowing, as if the blood supply was getting cut off. He led me across the hall to a room where my scans were up on the lighted wall and proceeded to point out the lymph nodes in the mediastinum. There were about five tumors between my heart and lungs.

"You see this?" he said, pointing to one of the larger tumors with a pencil. "See this blood supply right here? This is a small vein that feeds the tumor. You see how the inside lining of the tumor has darkened?"

"Yeah," I responded as I peered into the inner maze of my chest cavity.

"Before, they were brighter, which showed how well they were lined and fed with small capillaries, allowing them to grow. But you can see that the inside capillaries are dying off in these, causing the darker appearance. This is what the radiologist referred to as 'hollowing.' I think it's amazing. Whatever you are doing seems to be working, be it alternative medicine, God, or whatever."

STONEWALL JACKSON HOSPITAL
LEXINGTON, VA 24450

1002c

PATIENT LOCATION: OP

PATIENT NAME   :Chips, Allen
DATE OF BIRTH   :▮▮▮▮
PHONE NUMBER   :
ATTENDING PHYS   :Dr. ▮▮▮▮

SERVICE DATE   :6/23/03
PATIENT NUMBER   :10329084
MED REC NUMBER   :068073

EXAMINATION REQUESTED
  1. CT Chest with IV Enhancement

CLINICAL HISTORY
Lymphoma

Study performed utilizing 5 mm helical study from the thoracic inlet through the spleen; comparing to a most recent study chest 4/25/03 and of the abdomen of 5/21/03.

INDICATION: History of Hodgkin's lymphoma; patient receiving non-standard therapy with blood thinners, purifiers, and herbal therapy.

FINDINGS: No size measurement change can be stated regarding the anterior and mediastinal adenopathy with conglomerate nodes most prevalent in the mid to anterior mediastinum in the aortopulmonary window, extending into the anterior mediastinum to the level of the sternal notch. I have been informed by the patient that a cervical lymph node has decreased in size; this is not observed; he has received 3 weeks of therapy.

The only observation is that while the size of the anterior and middle mediastinal lymph nodes has not measurably change they appear somewhat more inhomogeneous and there margins somewhat less defined which can be a supportive finding in early increase in volume of disease.

This is in part speculative and cannot be stated as clear measurable evidence of resolving disease.

The lesion within the spleen which includes an approximately 1.8 cm cystic focus cephalad and probably within a calcified focus measuring 6 mm is unchanged and is unlikely to be of any significance; this is most likely a benign finding; the spleen is slightly prominent at 13 cm cephalocaudal diameter and unchanged. There are incidental small 1 to 2 cm cyst in the upper pole posteriorly at the left kidney.

IMPRESSION:
  1. Slight decrease in homogenaity and margin definition of prominent anterior and middle mediastinal adenopathy; no other change observed; no size (diameter) change in any single focal lymph node or conglomerate group of lymph nodes; see details above.
  2. Splenic findings unchanged; unlikely to represent lymphoma.
  3. Cysts incidental upper pole left kidney.

DEPARTMENT OF RADIOLOGY
RADIOLOGY RESULTS

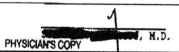

, M.D.

PHYSICIAN'S COPY

10749   10/98

I tried to discuss the herbs, diet, and supplements I was using, but he stated flatly, "I don't know anything about alternative medicine. You're on your own in that arena."

I went on to question him about when the B-type symptoms (night sweats, fever, burning chest, breathing problems, loss of energy) might subside, when a patient succeeds with chemotherapy. He responded that they subside within 30 to 60 days. Yet B-type symptoms often indicate that the cancer is traveling through the blood to another lymph node. He said that he wanted a hematology blood test next month, and monthly thereafter, in addition to monthly check-ups, to be able to safeguard against any of the organs being infected with Hodgkin's, in which case I would need chemo right away. He also said that I could probably experiment like this for another six months or so without getting into serious trouble, since in the past he had cured Hodgkin's patients who were stage three, possibly four, with ABDV chemo.

He found my case fascinating. We discussed the disadvantages of doing regular CT or PET scans, because of exposure to radiation. Dr. Fineman rated each form of X-ray, chest X-rays, CT scans, and PET scans. CT scans had by far the most radiation, chest X-rays had less, and the lowest dose of radiation came from PET scans. He also reminded me that my insurance probably had annual limits on the number of CT or PET scans it would allow, due to their cost: over a thousand dollars for a CT scan and almost four thousand for a PET scan.

Fourth Week of June: Two Steps Forward and One Back

Immediately after the appointment, I was feeling a fever coming on. I wondered if it was the radiation from the CT scan. I phoned Paul, my neighbor and radiologist, and told him that I was having B-type symptoms again. I asked him about the radiation exposure from a CT scan. He claimed that it was such a minute level from each test that he did not feel just one test was adding significant risk. I wondered *how much* radiation was considered to be *too much*.

The B-type symptoms lasted a week. I became concerned, so I contacted the Biomedical Center and asked to speak to Dr. Gutierrez, the physician I saw on the videos, to discuss the herbs I was using. I also wanted to know why they recommended against consuming alcohol, pork, tomatoes, or vinegar. He asked if I was a patient at BMC, and I responded, not yet. He briefly explained that cancer is stifled in an alkaline environment, and that the diet helps turn body fluids alkaline. He also said that alcohol, even at minute levels, such as that used in normal herbal tinctures, reduces the potency of the herbs.

I explained that my CT scan showed the tumors hollowing but that I was still experiencing B-type symptoms approximately every three weeks. He explained that it would generally take only two to three months to discover if the more potent herbal compounds, combined with specific supplements designed for Hodgkin's lymphoma, were being effective, at which time a follow-up visit with new X-rays was recommended to measure my progress. He also said that comparing the clinic's findings with my traditional medical doctors' findings was permissible, if I wished and the U.S. doctors were willing.

Later in the week, I called Baar Products and got the contact information for the company that manufactured their Hoxsey formula. They were located in Taos, New Mexico. The person on the phone said that they had many requests for the Hoxsey herbs. I told her that the medical doctor at the Hoxsey clinic had informed me that using potassium iodine suspension, instead of alcohol, made the herbs more potent; and I asked if they could manufacture them this way. She responded that it was too expensive, because the manufacturing process with potassium iodine was too volatile. The solutions often caught fire or exploded as they were heated if they didn't maintain a specific temperature when going into suspension. After hanging up the phone, I resigned myself to continuing the Hoxsey formula that was similar in ingredients but suspended in alcohol.

July 2003: Dreams, Trials, and Tribulations

I visited with relatives on the Fourth of July—who months later told me my color was not good. Apparently my complexion demonstrated a grayish color, but my relatives didn't want to tell me this, fearing it could affect my attitude.

In late July, I phoned my oncologist, who recommended a chest X-ray. It showed that nothing had changed.

I phoned Paul and told him, "The June scan and the July chest X-ray seem to show no change one way or another. It appears that the herbs I'm using are stifling it, but not killing it."

Paul responded, "Yeah; it seems that you're just treading water."

"With the B-type symptoms I've been experiencing lately, indicating that cells may be traveling in the blood, I'm wondering if I should get some more potent herbs, or maybe do chemotherapy."

Paul was impressed with the results I was getting, as the tumors ceased from growing or multiplying. He and the other radiologist had discussed my case and were very interested in what I was doing, but they also felt that chemotherapy surely was going to kill the cancer. Even with its risks of recurrence and organ damage, they felt it was my best chance.

The third week in July, my wife and I went to Baltimore with my two children for an extended weekend as part of my daughter's college search. At that time, the B-type symptoms had returned full force and I was getting concerned. I was very sick at the hotel. The lymph nodes on my neck seemed to be swelling and I was worried that the Hodgkin's cells were spreading, so I asked God for a definitive dream to tell me what I should do.

That night I had a very clear dream. I dreamt that I was at a stock car race, with many contestants revving their engines. I asked the master of ceremonies, who was a tall dark-haired woman, where my car was. She gave me a car with three large dark-skinned men in it, one in the front seat and two in the back. I got in the driver's seat and began to accelerate around the track for a trial run. On the first lap, I realized that with these three 250 to 300-pound passengers, my acceleration was stunted. I could not go fast enough. I complained and the guy in the front passenger seat started to struggle with me

STONEWALL JACKSON HOSPITAL
LEXINGTON, VA 24450

PATIENT LOCATION: OP

PATIENT NAME   :Chips, Allen
DATE OF BIRTH   :███████
PHONE NUMBER   :███████
ATTENDING PHYS   :Dr. ████

SERVICE DATE   :7/21/03
PATIENT NUMBER   :10364297
MED REC NUMBER   :068073

EXAMINATION REQUESTED
  1. Chest

CLINICAL HISTORY
Lymphoma

INDICATION: Lymphoma, mediastinal widening persists.

Essentially unchanged from 4/22/03. Lung parenchyma, pleural cavity
and bony structures are within normal limits. Heart size remains
normal.

IMPRESSION:
  1. Persistent mediastinal widening without interval change.

PF:pf
D&T:7/22/03

████ ███████, D.O.

for control of the steering wheel. I insisted on driving. He insisted on driving. When we got back to the MC I complained that I was overloaded, but she said that I needed the assistance. Then, while I tried to argue with her, she started the race. I knew I couldn't win. Then I woke up.

I thought long and hard about the meaning behind the dream. I interpreted the dream to mean that the MC was my oncologist urging me to start chemotherapy. I wondered, "Is this a sign from God that I needed to win the race with chemo, because it's a faster cure?"

My family was begging me to stop experimenting and trust our traditional medical system, claiming that traditional medical science was better researched, regardless of potential conspiracies to cover up natural cures. After much outside pressure from concerned loved ones, I decided I should consider chemotherapy. But I planned to practice a form of imagery that a fellow hypnotherapist used to help chemotherapy patients reduce side effects. The imagery was a good concept. I was to imagine that the intravenous drugs were like rain falling on my cancer cells, but the good cells in my body had umbrellas opened over them to deflect the chemo drugs. I practiced the imagery under self-hypnosis and then went to my oncologist for my appointment on the last Tuesday of July.

To Do Chemo or Not To Do Chemo: That is the Question.

Dr. Fineman asked how I was doing, and I told him that I was scared. I didn't want to continue experimenting. I just wanted to get it all over with through chemotherapy; quick and easy. He asked why. I told him that the nodes on my neck had briefly swelled up again and then went back down, but that I was concerned about the B-type symptoms meaning a possible spread of cancer. He reminded me that the CT scans looked like everything was starting to go in the other direction.

"You are doing well on your own. Are you sure you want to do this?" he asked me.

I told him about the dream and my interpretation of it, to which he responded by saying, "I'm not sure about your interpretation, but I will do whatever you want. It's your choice."

He seemed to be a little disappointed in one sense, because he thought that what I was doing was "neat," but his responsibilities as a physician outweighed his curiosities, and he scheduled my first chemotherapy treatment for two days later.

Black Thursday: Intravenous Nuclear Waste Causes Crash

It was the last Thursday of July. My mind was racing, but I was sure I would be the exceptional patient. I believed I would come through chemo unscathed by using a positive attitude and protective imagery techniques. I joked with the nurses to stay upbeat. The large windows of the treatment room offered a grand view of the Blue Ridge Mountains behind the hospital parking lot. I drank lots of fluids. During the Bleomycin drip, I started breaking out in hives and the nurses were very concerned that I might stop breathing, so they gave me an antihistamine. My physician was called at home, and he told the nurses that I was having an allergic reaction and to keep the epinephrine nearby, just in case. Then I was given medicine for nausea to take home with me.

On the way home, an hour and a half drive by myself, I was getting extremely sick. After I got home, I phoned the doctor on call at the hospital to explain my symptoms, because they were getting more severe. I had sores breaking out in my mouth; I was dry heaving, constipated, and having difficulty breathing. Sometimes I felt my heart skipping a beat. The only advice from the doctor on call was that the side effects were probably psychosomatic, due to my reading about them in the literature I had received earlier in the day. I told him I hadn't read it. He encouraged me to create a positive attitude and ended the conversation.

When I lay down that night, I could not sleep because every time I started to fall asleep, I would stop breathing and then wake up trying to catch my breath. The next day I contacted Dr. Fineman, and he said that this is just the way it is, and that I had to accept it and get through it. By that time the bone marrow activation medicine kicked in, which was designed to raise my white blood cell count and fight potential infections. I could not sit down without my whole pelvic region feeling as if it were being squeezed in a vise. I tried to lie on my back or stomach and learned to tolerate the extreme pain and nausea. But the worst side effect involved my short-term memory.

I couldn't remember what I said from one moment to the next. I later found out that this was a side effect of the intravenous steroids. After discussing this with a physician friend from college, I discovered that the personalities of people who take chemo over a long period of time are often altered. Unfortunately, without the steroids, the body may reject the toxic chemicals used to kill the new cells forming in the body. This new cell formation includes cancer cells, so the body must be brought to the brink of death to kill most cancers.

On Sunday, I made it to church. As I wobbled my way through the front door, my minister noticed my pale color and asked, "What happened to you?" I told him that I took a treatment of chemotherapy. With a look of concern, he responded, "Well, maybe you needed to take it to find out that it is something you should never do again."

I heard the Holy Spirit talking through him. During the service, I almost fainted, nearly falling over the balcony railing. Immediately after the service was over, I checked myself into the emergency room. Blood tests showed I was slightly anemic and the ER physician told me not to drive. By then, my biggest concern was that my brain was impaired. I couldn't think straight. My wife drove me home, about a twenty-mile trek on country roads.

Dee and I reflected on our minister's statement. Generally, he was not for or against traditional or alternative medicine therapies. He didn't know anything about alternative medicine, and very little about traditional cancer treatments. Yet to us his message seemed to be a sign from God.

A few days later, I balanced the checkbook of our family business, where I was working part-time because I felt wiped out. My wife was very concerned when she asked me if I balanced the checkbook and I told her "No, not yet." The truth was that I had done it, but my brain was fried and I couldn't remember doing it.

On discovering this a few days later, we were both concerned, because my mind is the most valuable asset I had. It was not uncommon for me to remember people's name, and other facts about them years later, just from one-time conversations. Participants in my training seminars were in awe over my ability to memorize thirty or forty names in the first few hours. I often spit out statistical data quoted from texts and articles better than most public speakers I'd studied. My writing abilities—I'd written hundreds of articles and several books—stem from a sharp mind, a sharp mind now in jeopardy of becoming severely dulled.

The next key question was, "How does my family feel about this?" My parents, two brothers, and two sisters are from the traditional medical model. Almost all of them are medical professionals or have had formal medical education. Most had pushed hard for me to stop experimenting and start chemo, because they loved me and this was all they knew—traditional medical science. However, after I put out an e-mail that sounded like half my head was gone, they started to worry. They called and noticed that I wasn't myself. At the end of the week, my wife told me that she couldn't bear to see me do twelve treatments like this over the next six months, as it would probably permanently cripple or kill me. I agreed.

First of August, 2003: Dream Reinterpretation and Logic

Dee and I discussed the spiritual message that came through our pastor. We also talked about how the dream might have suggested something different. As we discussed it, I began to feel as if we were no longer guessing at an interpretation. It became clear as a bell. I was to go to the Biomedical Center and let the dark-skinned Mexican staff drive my car, my physical vehicle, letting them be at the helm of my race for life. We concluded that my local oncologist's doubts about my initial interpretation of the dream, that it meant I should start chemo, was accurate. Perhaps the dark-skinned people represented the dark— i.e., black—tonic that was part of the clinic's regimen (for more about the tonic, see later chapters). Perhaps somebody else needed to navigate the healing process for me from here.

I phoned Barbara again (the breast cancer patient from Virginia Beach) to talk about my inclination to move from self-treating to submitting to the guidance and direction of the BMC. She told me that her most recent test results from her local doctor indicated the solid remission of her breast cancer. She also discussed how her supplements were prescribed for the specific type of cancer she had and reminded that they included an antiviral medicine and an antiparasitic medicine (I looked up both on the Internet later; neither was available in the United States).

She was very supportive of my decision. The last words she said to me etched themselves in my mind. "You can't beat eighty years and eighty percent success."

Then I contacted Carol Main, the videographer and coproducer of *The Experience*. We talked about her bout with pancreatic cancer. She reminded me that her doctor in Alaska had given her only a few months to live, telling her there was no cure for her type of cancer. When she found out about the BMC, the staff there told her that the sooner they saw her, the better the odds were of saving her life.

She said, "I booked my flight the second I got off the phone."

She cautioned me to stay with the diet. She speculated that for people who did, the success rate was higher than eighty percent. She said how much better it was to give up all the foods not on the diet and stay above ground.

"Do everything the doctors tell you," she advised, and with a stern demeanor added, "I had some friends who did not follow the diet and they wound up six feet under."

It was a sobering conversation, considering that I was only following a portion of the diet recommended on her video. I was primarily using the Cayce diet (which I later discovered provided less alkalinity), and I was not well educated in nutrition at the time. Carol also told me that the doctors at BMC put her on a rare cactus extract, in addition to the black tonic, in order to cure her pancreatic cancer.

I contacted Dr. Gutierrez at the clinic a second time to discuss the treatment program they offered. He was very patient with me. We discussed the various supplements that were prescribed for each individual, which depended on the type of cancer he or she had. I also asked him about the antiviral/antiparasitic medicines Barbara was on (mentioning her as an anonymous breast cancer patient). He said that one medicine had shown great results in boosting the immune system and was manufactured by Mexican pharmaceuticals; the other was from Europe, where it was used for parasitic conditions. I was impressed with his expertise, so I told him I would probably see him soon.

I was pleased with how Dr. Gutierrez gave me the time I needed to comprehend the benefits of becoming a patient at the clinic. He patiently and fully answered all my questions and concerns about the therapy, even before I became a patient and invested the minimal fees required. Then I asked to be transferred to the office manager for more information.

She said that no appointment was necessary, just some preparatory steps, including fasting and showing up by 9:00 on a weekday morning. That would be a full day, involving a checkup and a team approach to diagnostics, natural prescriptive recommendations, and education. The manager thoroughly explained what was involved in the first visit and requested that I fax a copy of my medical diagnosis. In return, she would fax the new patient information papers to me. I was impressed at how they screened their patients for a medical diagnosis.

We discussed which hotels in the San Diego area, near the Mexican border, provided the free shuttle service to the clinic, and whether I wanted to bring my X-rays, scans, and blood tests, or have them done there. I asked for phone numbers for some people who had lymphoma and were cured with Hoxsey therapy. She agreed to fax these. She told me that the new patient information forms would likely contain everything else I needed to know to arrange my first visit.

After I faxed my diagnosis, I received a return fax with all the information I requested. I was impressed by the professional, cooperative approach of the clinic. I looked up more information on the clinic in other books and found research showing that the Hoxsey Clinic (the BMC) was the oldest, least expensive, and most reputable alternative cancer therapy clinic in operation today. It sees the highest number of cancer patients of any alternative medicine cancer clinic in the world.

I discussed with Dee how life would not be worth living if I had to continue chemotherapy. She agreed. That day, I vowed never to do chemotherapy again. The herbs would either save my life or end it. My life would depend on the success of Hoxsey therapy from here on. I called (on a day when my oncologist was on a fishing trip) and canceled my next chemo treatment, which was set for Tuesday, August 8th. When I got off the phone, I booked an airline ticket to San Diego for August 9th. August 10th would be the day I entered the Biomedical Center in Tijuana, Mexico.

Chapter 5

Off To Tijuana

August 2003: "Go West, Young Man."

The first week of August, I pulled out the Biomedical Clinic's patient video again and examined the map at the end that had directions to the clinic. I copied the map and decided that I would rent a car. My other option would have been to take a taxi to the Best Western Americana in San Ysidro, California, located approximately 20 miles from the San Diego airport, stay there overnight, and then take the complimentary shuttle to the clinic the next morning.

I packed up all my X-rays, CT scans, PET reports, and blood tests and flew to San Diego. When I got to the hotel, which was only a few miles from the border, I confirmed the discount clinic rate that I was quoted over the phone, then asked if there were other people checked into the hotel who were also going to the Biomedical Center. The staff responded that there were a few other popular cancer clinics in addition to the BMC, so some of the other guests might be going to them. That night, I fasted from midnight on, just as the new patient information instructed.

The next morning, I drove over the border but got lost for a while, because General Fererra, the street the clinic was on, was not marked. I felt fortunate to have found the clinic at all, not only because of the lack of street signs but also because none of the locals knew where the clinic was. I speak basic Spanish, so I was able to communicate with people, but it became apparent how much better off patients are when they take group shuttles with a guide.

At the top of the hill, I noticed two large gates on the left side of the road. I pulled into the second gate, recognizing the large tropical bird cage from the video. It was located in the middle of the parking circle. I am a bird lover, so this was another sign from the holy spirit that I was in the right place.

After confirming that the long-term parking was next door, I parked and entered through two twelve-foot doors into a beautiful three-level marble building of several thousand square feet. It overlooked the Tijuana Valley. The large windows in the bright and cheerful waiting room, which led to a large sunny deck, had an awesome view.

I filled out my paperwork and handed it to the receptionist, along with my X-rays, scans, and medical reports that I had brought with me. Then I was directed to the nurses' station for blood pressure and weight measurements.

From there, I went down the hall to the lab, where I was told to change into a long gray gown. In the changing room, I put my personal belongings into a locker with a wrist key chain, and then was handed a specimen cup for a urine sample.

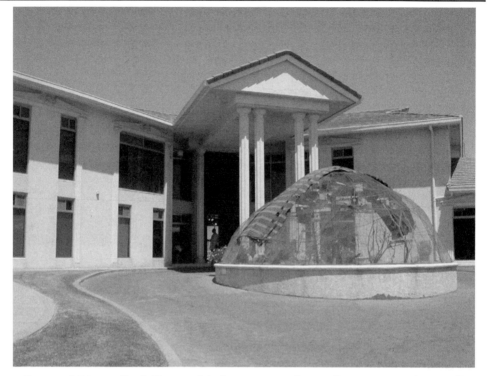

Front of Biomedical Center, bird sanctuary, horseshoe patient drop-off

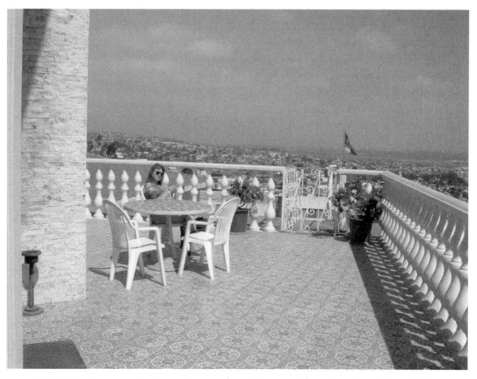

BMC's balcony during a trip when Dee, author's wife, joined him

Thereafter, I was told to wait in the waiting room. There were about a dozen other patients there, so I began to join in their conversations, which were very positive and motivational—unlike the depressing, sterile waiting rooms in the States, where people are suffering greatly. People encouraged each other, shared recipes, and talked about the success stories of friends and relatives who had been cured at the clinic.

One woman I met was very talkative and positive. She lived in an area between Los Angeles and San Francisco. She had been coming to the clinic for about nine months for breast cancer therapy, and the cancer was headed into remission.

I also met a man who had been treated previously by the BMC for skin cancer, and was back again to use the escharotics. He described how the salve was put on the skin just covering the tumor and the tumor would die and then be extracted—just as the AMA admitted in 1964 in court when asked if the external salves were curing cancer. I was amazed that I was meeting somebody who had undergone Hoxsey therapy more than a decade ago.

I met a writer and his wife. His wife had breast cancer and had tried chemotherapy and surgery, but her cancer had returned and they opted to do only Hoxsey therapy this time. She started on the tonic about three months ago and said that her medical tests were showing marked improvement.

I began to catch the positive attitude I'd seen on the video as I leafed through the large visitor's registry on the table in the corner of the waiting room. I was shocked by what I saw. The testimonials read:

"...was in stage four of prostate cancer and have been cured now for seven years."

"The doctors in Canada don't know how I'm getting better, they just know it's happening. I am so grateful to the doctors here at the Biomedical Center..."

"My mother's cancer had metastasized and she had several brain tumors. We figured we had nothing to lose by coming here. That was six months ago and now all of her tumors are gone and she feels healthy again. Thank you and thank God for saving my mother's life. We are all so impressed with the treatment program here that we are returning with our mother so that all of us can take preventative doses of the tonic ourselves. My three sisters...."(See more in Appendix A.)

I looked to see if any of the pages had been removed, as a result of the clinic pulling negative comments. Being in the literary business, I know what missing pages from a binding look like. But they were all intact. As I read through dozens of pages, I only found one negative comment out of over a hundred (see Appendix A). I was happy to be there and I became more certain about putting my life in their hands—which to me were also God's hands.

My name was called from the reception room in the front of the building. The first doctor I saw was Dr. Gutierrez. He gave me a physical and noticed that my organs were slightly enlarged, just as the radiologist in the States recognized. But my blood test looked good, so Dr. Gutierrez predicted the

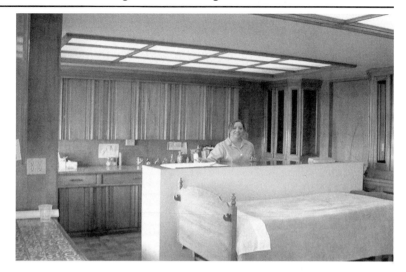

Nurses'
Station

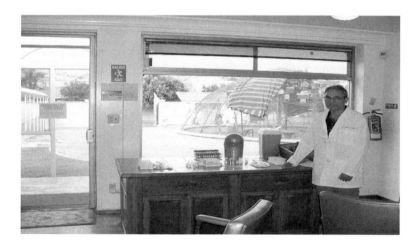

Lab

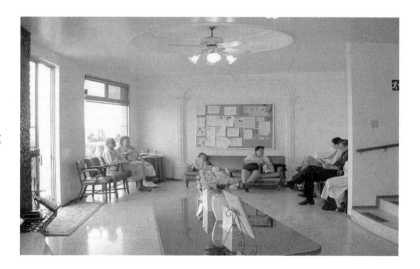

Waiting
Room

Hodgkin's cells had not yet spread to my organs. He did say that it was important to have regular blood tests and to pay attention to my color. If I lost my color it could be a sign that the Hodgkin's had spread to my organs and I would need another treatment of chemotherapy. I told him that I had endured one chemo treatment and vowed never to do it again.

I was surprised he advocated chemotherapy as an option, since I'd read that, according to the Hoxsey approach, chemotherapy and radiation reduced the immune system's ability to fight the intruding cancer cells on its own, the premise of the Hoxsey system. When I asked about it, he said that doctors in the States administer excessive amounts of chemotherapy, because they do not have any other means of treatment (other than chemotherapy, surgery, and radiation). Using toxic levels of chemotherapy was not necessary.

In some cases, when a patient is stage four, the BMC administers a mild form of chemotherapy, to get the cancer to move from an "active state" (progressing) to an "inactive state" (regressing), as they were called. However, most cancers responded to herbal medicine and dietary therapy. He said that their program, even with occasional chemo, still would not make a patient sicker or kill them, unlike traditional medical treatments. Dr. Gutierrez also confirmed what my traditional medical oncologist had said, which was that one chemo treatment may have helped me, but would not cure my particular type of cancer.

He then led me to the X-ray room, where he, Dr. Rodriguez (the radiologist), and I discussed my scans and X-rays.

The X-rays took up an entire wall and were organized by date. I was able to examine how my cancerous lymph nodes progressed between May and June. But what scared me the most was that my liver and pancreas were obviously enlarged. The physicians were also concerned about this, which demonstrated that my disease was progressing. Dr. Trujillo, the internist, came into the room and confirmed that one treatment of traditional ABDV chemotherapy would not cure Hodgkin's, and I needed to be closely monitored.

The four doctors who met regarding my case agreed that I should watch my color and get regular check-ups to make sure that my liver and spleen did not continue to enlarge, an indication that the cancer was spreading and taking over. A grayish color was one sign of this. It was a sobering conversation, and I could see the concern on their faces.

I was impressed by the doctors' compassion. I felt that they truly had a personal desire to help me get better. I was also impressed that, for the first time, it was really explained to me, in complete detail, what was on the X-rays. I learned more about my disease in one day at the clinic than I did in four months of traditional medical care with five different doctors and three different hospitals in the States. I had received all of this information within the first three hours I entered the BMC.

After that, I was told that it was customary to see patients a second time after lunch, so I was released to eat brunch at the restaurant, which served food that was safe for patients who were prescribed the Hoxsey diet. I went down to the other side of the horseshoe driveway into the restaurant, and examined the menu.

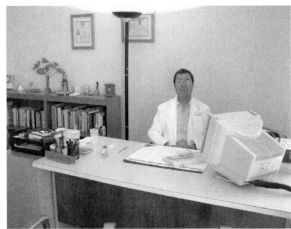

Dr. Gutierrez

Dr. Rodriguez
and the Author

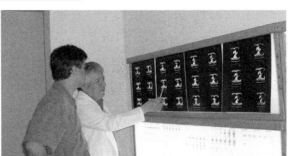

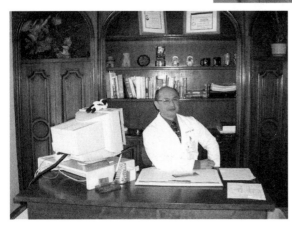

Dr. Trujillo

Dr. Percioli

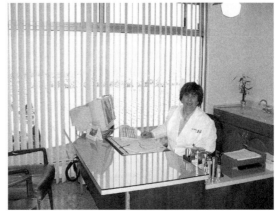

A lover of Mexican food, I was like a kid in a candy store. I ordered the vegetable omelet with the red and green spicy sauces, and the whole-grain pancakes with all-natural maple syrup. The entire breakfast, with beverage, cost around six and a half dollars. When I got up to pay, I saw that there was no cashier, only a cash drawer against the wall behind me with a sign discussing payment. Most of the change was in U.S. dollars, and it was entirely on the honor system.

When I returned to see Dr. Gutierrez after lunch, he gave me an extensive consultation on the treatment program, the supplements, and the diet, all of which were uniquely designed for the form of cancer I had. First, he told me that the doctors had met and discussed my case and decided that the "black tonic" was best. I heard that and it was like a bell went off in my head and a choir started singing hymns, as I immediately thought of my dream and the dark-skinned race car drivers. It all made sense. Let them take over driving me to the finish line. The doctor explained how to mix up the black tonic for the correct dosage: add two ounces of concentrated tonic to 14 ounces of spring or well water, and take one teaspoon four times a day with food. Never take it on an empty stomach. Do this for one month, then increase the dose to two tablespoons.

I asked what the difference was between the red and the black tonics, and he said that a couple of herbs are left out for people who have stomach problems from the black tonic. We agreed that since I was already taking similar alcohol-based herbs, I could start with a dose of two teaspoons four times a day. (I later calculated that 25 drops of concentrate from a tincture dropper, which was more mobile than a spoon, was equal to two teaspoons of the diluted mixture; so I received approval to use 25 drops of concentrate in tea, spring water, or juice, four times a day.)

Dr. Gutierrez gave me an article on the benefits of using raw sugar rather than processed sugar, and an article on artemisinin, a Chinese medicinal herb used to treat malaria that was now showing dramatic capabilities in curing various cancers, including lymphoma. He also prescribed coral calcium and gave me a pamphlet describing its health benefits. He approved all the supplements that I had researched and was already taking, and we briefly discussed the benefits of using vitamin Ester-C and yew tree needle capsules. I also got a prescription for Chinese herbal medicine "for lymphoma." (When I returned home, I was to order the Chinese medicines.)

He agreed I should stay on 200 mg. of CoQ-10, vitamin E with B-6 and B-12, and a multivitamin. All these could be purchased at Wal-Mart, if I wished, as mass-marketed vitamins were increasing in quality. Then there was a very long consultation on what the Hoxsey diet consisted of and its benefits to a body with a compromised immune system. (Refer to the chapter on diet and the chapter on supplements and Chinese medicines for more detailed information on the above.)

I also received lifestyle counseling. I aired all my stresses and we discussed each one—what could be done to reduce or eliminate them, or what perceptions could be adopted to better tolerate them. As we shall see, an overload of stress causes body fluids to become acidic; therefore, stress

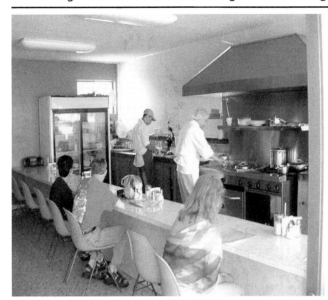
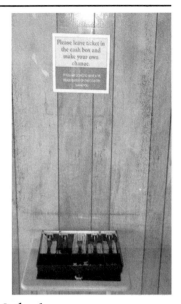

Restaurant and its Payment Method

Pharmacy
and the
Black
Hoxsey
Tonic

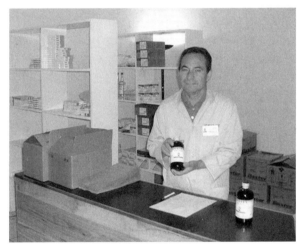

Aida
in patient
admissions

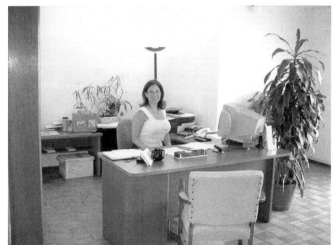

management becomes an important factor in the natural healing approach. I told him about my daily practices of self-hypnosis and meditation, which he received with a high level of approval. (Refer to the mind-body chapter for a discussion of the exact tools that proved beneficial for my recovery.)

I asked Dr. Gutierrez when he wanted me to return, and he said it is traditionally three months after the first visit, and then six months after the second. Patients visit twice a year, every six months, until they are stable, which is generally three to five years. Thereafter, check-ups are recommended once a year. He said that if I had any further questions I could phone or e-mail him.

I was amazed at the amount of time we had spent together for the purpose of patient education. I shook Dr. Gutierrez's hand and went upstairs to billing, where I bought the lifetime supply of the tonic, in consideration of my genetics (my mother had Hodgkin's and later a colon carcinoid; one grandfather died of colon cancer; the other grandfather died of myeloma). Besides, I knew this would work. I found the entire system to be very affordable. I walked down the hallway from there and picked up a six-month supply of the tonic from the on-site pharmacy. I was told to keep it refrigerated when I got home to avoid spoilage, because potassium iodide-based herbal tonics require refrigeration, while alcohol-based herbal medicines do not.

I was bid farewell in the usual way—a hug—by Aida, who handled patient admissions in the front office. I left, realizing that in the past four months, not one person from the traditional medical community in the States had delivered that important hug that said, "Everything is going to be okay."

Chapter 6

A Happy Ending

Mid-August 2003: Home Sweet Home

On returning home, I contacted Allergy Research Group/NutriCology Innovative Nutrition, and ordered the herb sweet wormwood, highly concentrated and manufactured as artemisinin. I also phoned Spring Wind Herbs, a Chinese medicine pharmacy that sells powdered herbs for lymphoma. They would not take the order until my prescription arrived from the Biomedical Center. When I received the powdered tea, it was in a large bottle labeled "Lymphoma-RX. I drank the tea twice a day, and at the same time took the artemisinin capsules. The consultant at Spring Wind Herbs said that Chinese medicines were most effective when taken on an empty stomach. The literature I received on the artemisinin, also a Chinese herbal medicine, concurred.

As soon as I started taking the original black tonic, (the Hoxsey formula with the potassium iodine I brought back from Tijuana), I experienced what naturopaths refer to as a period of purification or cleansing. This is a process that often involves the digestive tract. I was also warned by Dr. Gutierrez of such side effects. In fact, some Hoxsey patients experience such intolerable gastrointestinal side effects that they are subsequently put on the red tonic instead. The process of purification I'd experienced on the black tonic was similar to the one I experienced when I was taking the alcohol-based, Cayce-Hoxsey compound in early June, only much more intense. This time, it lasted two and one-half months. To avoid dehydration, I consumed a lot of liquids.

I felt quite certain that my system was cleansing itself of candidiasis— a condition of intestinal yeast overgrowth. This condition often precedes cancer. I was probably experiencing these side effects from taking a more potent berberis root compound, in a potassium iodide suspension (in the Hoxsey tonic), as opposed to the alcohol-suspended berberis I had used earlier. However, it is important to note that the discomfort from the side effects of the herbal medicine was significantly more tolerable than the single chemotherapy treatment I had tried earlier.

I contacted the clinic about the cleansing process and they asked if I felt I could tolerate it. I affirmed that I could, because I wanted to take the tonic with the highest number of herbal compounds in it. As Dr. Gutierrez had stated during my first visit, the black tonic created a slightly higher chance for a cure if I could handle it (wasn't consistently nauseated, etc.). I found I was able to work full-time, conduct normal family activities, such as errands with the kids, and exercise at the local health club. I lived a relatively normal life.

The most difficult aspect of the treatment was getting used to the diet. I became ravenous for certain foods I had to eliminate, until I found a comparable replacement food for each one. In other words, chocolate had to be organic. Coffee creamers had to contain evaporated cane juice instead of sugar. No more caffeine, only naturally decaffeinated coffees and teas. Vinegar was difficult to eliminate, but lemon juice was a good substitute in salad dressings and condiments. There were many other adjustments that took about two months to successfully accomplish. (More about this in the chapter on diet.)

By the end of the third week in August, I was due to see Ben Fineman, my local oncologist who, on seeing me, apologized for being on vacation when I made an independent decision to walk away from my next chemo treatment.

He entered the room, closed the door behind him, leaned the back of his hip against the counter with his arms folded, glanced down and then up to meet my eyes with a solemn look of concern, and said, "You know that one treatment won't do it, don't you? It might knock it down, but it won't cure it."

I explained how hard the one treatment was on me and that my mind was my most valuable possession, one I simply couldn't allow to waste away. In addition, I told him that if I had to undergo six months of it, I wouldn't be able to work, would have to give up the two businesses I ran (a seminar business and an independent press), which I'd worked for 15 years to build up to where they were, and my wife, who worked with me, and a few contract employees, would have to find jobs.

"It's going to take at least five treatments to have even a remote chance using chemotherapy. Maybe there's some way we can figure out what will make it tolerable," he said as he put his hand on his chin and gazed at me.

"Do you think the dosage was too high?" I asked.

"No." He looked down at my chart.

"Well, maybe there's a lighter dosage..."

"No," he interrupted. "That's the correct dosage." He said it with commitment, as if he didn't want to be questioned by a rookie. "That was correct for your weight, so that's what it will take."

"Well, I can't do it anymore," I said as my lips tightened.

He pushed a form across the table that had an "x" next to a signature line. Above it was today's date and the words "Refused Treatment." I looked up at him and said, "I don't really think that's necessary, Ben, do you? I'll take responsibility for my choices."

He pulled the paper back, glanced down, back up, looked me in the eyes, put his hand on my shoulder, dropped his voice and said, "You know I want this to work for you, don't you?"

"I know you do" I said as my voice also dropped. We both knew this was literally a life or death situation. To me, this was it. Either the alternative medicine did the trick or I was history. That was my decision.

With chemotherapy, B-type symptoms would subside after 30–60 days of treatment, indicating remission. He and the oncologist at UVA both said that remission might be possible after just six treatments (or three months) but it was a long shot. The full six-month regimen should be followed. If a cancer free remission wasn't accomplished, I would need another six months of chemotherapy.

I assumed that remission through using herbal medicines would be signaled by my B-type symptoms subsiding, just as in the case of chemotherapy. If the night sweats, fevers, lethargy, and burning sensations in the chest subsided after 30-60 days, then I could be certain that I was making major progress.

Dr. Fineman agreed to continue to chart my progress through X-rays and monthly blood tests, and we parted ways until my next visit in October. As we parted, there was a feeling of my sailing off into a vast ocean in a ship of which I'd just become captain. I was not entirely sure what storms I would navigate or where I would end up.

One thing I was certain of was that I was due to have B-type symptoms by the third week in August, if cancer cells were still traveling through my bloodstream to populate my body. According to past experience, it was like clockwork—sick every three weeks for a week. But that day never came. The end of July marked the last time I have ever experienced B-type symptoms.

Late August 2003: Family Psychosomatics Begin

In the meantime, my wife's and my daughter's health were becoming affected through a psychosomatic connection to the events that were happening in our lives. Dee's blood pressure was significantly elevated and my daughter was having irregular menstrual cycles with sharp pains in her ovaries. I began to research natural methods for lowering blood pressure, and we scheduled an appointment for my daughter with an gynecologist in our preferred physician network. We were lucky and got an appointment the following month. Dee's blood pressure measured 176 over 105 one day, and stayed consistently high in subsequent readings. A normal reading is somewhere in the neighborhood of 130 over 80. This put her on the charts between "moderately high" and "severe."

Upon hearing this news, some members of our extended family were concerned about the potential for stroke and suggested a visit to a traditional medical doctor for drug therapy. I pressured my wife to learn to take care of this hereditary condition, which was exacerbated by my medical condition. We were reluctant to use pharmaceuticals, because the drugs for high blood pressure consisted of diuretics, beta-blockers, calcium channel blockers, or ACE inhibitors, all of which have side effects, and many of which offer only moderate help. She asked about a drugless therapy based on naturopathic research that I would personally conduct, and I agreed.

I researched herbs and supplements, and found the following to be effective: potassium, vitamin B complex, hawthorn berry, omega three fatty acids (fish oil and flax seed oil), coral calcium, ester C, and an antioxidant blend.

In addition, she agreed to change her diet and exercise more; we noticed results immediately. Within a month, her blood pressure was back in the normal range. Not only was the natural remedy effective in reducing the symptoms: later tests showed that her cardiovascular system was clear of excess plaque and cholesterol.

September 2003: More Testimonials; Daughter's Test Results

I contacted again one of the people who had given a testimonial about the Biomedical Clinic. It was a woman who had struggled with stage four lymphoma, and when traditional medicine gave up on her she went to the BMC and obtained a cure. Because of her gratitude, she agreed to let Aida give out her name and phone number to people who had lymphoma.

"Hello, Linda, this is Allen Chips. I contacted you in August, when I was considering going to the Biomedical Center."

"Oh yeah, how are you doing?" she cheerfully questioned.

"I've been on the black tonic and some Chinese medicines for the past month, and it seems to be working. I haven't had the B-type symptoms since the end of July, and according to my traditional medicine oncologist, this is a sign of going into remission."

"Oh, that sounds so good, Allen. I talk to many people who get help there, and I am sure I've told you my story already about how I was helped, haven't I?"

"Yes, I talked to you about your situation and it helped convince me that it [going to the BMC] was the right decision."

"How have you been feeling?" she inquired.

"I feel great. Besides some gastrointestinal side effects that Dr. Gutierrez warned me about, which are very tolerable, it appears that I am doing well."

"How is your energy level?" she asked hesitantly.

"You know, that's what I've noticed the most—that my energy level has snapped back to normal."

"Oh, that is a very good sign, Allen. It is the first indicator that you are getting well."

"Yeah, because I used to be tired all the time, having to take naps in the afternoon, going to bed early, fevers, and night sweats. But I haven't experienced any of that for a couple of months now."

"That is such good news, Allen. God and the Biomedical Clinic are blessing you. You know I've kept you in my prayers."

"I really appreciate that. I'm sure that it helped."

"I pray for all the people that I talk to through the BMC. God does answer prayers, you know. I am living proof of this."

I interjected, "I believe that God answers prayers sometimes through other people, like you, rather than through a direct intervention, and those are the people who guide you into the right direction."

I thanked Linda for sharing and for her encouragement again, we talked a little bit about the diet and supplements, and then said good-bye. I felt like a dark cloud was drifting away from a stormy sky and the sun's rays were beginning to peek out. It felt warm, like after a storm.

As for my daughter, her appointment with the gynecologist confirmed cysts on her ovaries, by way of ultrasound, and she agreed to take hormone supplementation therapy, or birth control pills, in order to rid herself of the symptoms. She was told that Poly Cystic Ovary Syndrome (PCOS) was a lifelong, incurable condition. Therefore, she would have to stay on hormone therapy the rest of her life. This was also supported by the literature we received from the doctor's office.

She was relieved in one sense, as her blood tests revealed three times the normal testosterone levels of a teenage boy her age. This explained her extremely aggressive behavior over the past couple of years, which was very hard on the entire family. We were all relieved to think that this vexation to the spirit was going to subside. However, with all the bad publicity hormone replacement therapy was getting, particularly the dramatically increased risk of various cancers, we were concerned. I began to keep my ears and eyes open for alternatives.

Around that time, my daughter also totaled our truck on a mountainous curve and ended up with neck pain. So she went to a neurologist and told him my burgeoning success story. His response was, "Tell your father to stay away from Tijuana. Those clinics in Tijuana just kill people." It was then that I realized that I needed to circulate a copy of the independent award-winning film, "Quacks Who Cure," to all the doctors in our community who saw members of our family. I was out to pierce the veil of their ignorance so they could begin to comprehend the truth behind big corporate medical politics, and open their minds to the efficacy of natural cancer cures.

I dropped off the video with my family doctor and told him he could keep it. Because of his reaction afterwards (acting as if I were from Mars), we never spoke again. I noticed that some physicians were highly inquisitive, while some simply felt I was challenging their authority. Some have told me they are afraid of potential legal problems, or of losing their medical license, for advocating the use of natural medicines. It was then that I realized that there was a great division in the traditional medical field over the use of alternative medicine, and I would need to be careful about which doctors I could talk to and see for my own health conditions. My wife and I decided to use physicians who were either knowledgeable of, or at least amenable to, alternative and complementary medicine.

October 2003: Signs of a Solid Remission

It was time for some scans again. I phoned my doctor and his office manager to set up one PET scan and one CT scan.

The first step was to get a CT scan, so it could be compared to the PET scan for a more accurate read. I entered the hospital at a time when my neighbor Paul was working in the radiology department. I had the scan and waited to see if Paul could see me. He invited me into his office. The first thing he asked me was, "How's your energy level?"

"Good. I think I'm turning the corner."

"I understand that you left treatment."

"Yep. I couldn't take the chemo. It wasn't for me."

"Well, we've kept you in our prayers."

STONEWALL JACKSON HOSPITAL
LEXINGTON, VA 24450

PATIENT LOCATION: OP

PATIENT NAME   :Chips, Allen
DATE OF BIRTH   :███████
PHONE NUMBER   :
ATTENDING PHYS   :Dr. ███████

SERVICE DATE   :10/27/03
PATIENT NUMBER   :10489144
MED REC NUMBER   :068073

EXAMINATION REQUESTED
    1. CT Chest
    2. Abdomen & Pelvis CT

CLINICAL HISTORY
Lymphoma

INDICATION: Lymphoma.

CT Chest

Comparison to 6/23/03.

There is resolution of most of the lymphadenopathy of the superior
mediastinum noted on the previous scan. A few small nodes about 1-1.5
cm remain in the preaortic space which appear confluent in several of
which are centrally lucent indicating necrobiosis.

No additional lymph node enlargement, infiltrates, effusions, etc.
Otherwise normal findings.

IMPRESSION:
    1. Significantly improved superior mediastinal lymphadenopathy
       comparing 6/23/03.

Abdomen & Pelvis CT

Comparison 5/21/03.

Unchanged 1.3 cm cyst upper pole of left kidney. Continued normal
appearance of the abdomen and pelvis with no evidence of organomegaly,
lymphadenopathy or ascites.

IMPRESSION:
    1. Normal except for a small unchanged left renal cyst.

PF:pf
D:10/28/03 @ 0947
T:10/28/03 @ 1118

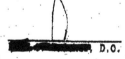 , D.O.

"Well, let's take a look" he said and we went into the computer imaging room. I took a seat next to him as he brought up the scans on his computer screen. "Wow" he said in a distracted voice as he peered into the pictures of my mediastinal area.

"What?" I queried as I swallowed nervously.

"These look necrotized," he said excitedly and shocked.

"Necrotized?"

"It means dead. The tumors appear to be all necrotic."

"Sounds like great news to me," I said with a sigh of relief.

Paul owned land about five miles over the next mountain from where I lived and he was involved in organic farming. He asked what kind of anti-cancer diet I was on. I told him that it involved the elimination of certain preservatives, the addition of several supplements, and the elimination of alcohol, processed sugar, flour, tomatoes, and pork.

"Ah, pork. I could have guessed."

"Why? What have you discovered about pork?"

"Pork cells look a lot like cancer cells under a microscope."

"Hmm. That's interesting. So the Jews were right. It's not good for you." I chuckled. "You know, the primary objective behind the diet I'm on is to create an alkaline environment in my body, because according to Cayce and Hoxsey, cancer cannot grow in an alkaline environment."

Paul was familiar with both of these naturopaths' health diets. We discussed anticancer diets further, talking about the volatility of tomatoes, on which I was currently doing research (discussed further in the chapter on diet). I was invited again to his organic farm to pick fresh herbs. Then I thanked Paul for his kind support and prayers and then departed.

Walking out of the hospital, I was floating on cloud nine. This was the first piece of real evidence indicating that I was beating this thing. Next was the PET scan, which my local oncologist claimed was the most accurate. The PET scan is accurately read with a CT scan, so the first step had been accomplished.

November 2003: More Tests, A Longer Road; More on PCOS

The PET scan was to be done in Roanoke a week later, at the beginning of November. After going through the tunnel again for about an hour, I asked the PET scan technician to show me the scans on the computer. She indicated that it was something that she was not permitted to do, but under the circumstances (my alternative medicine journey), she would show me the results, making sure I understood that she was not officially authorized to read them. She did inform me that her understanding was that heat ranges measured in my body should not be over 2.0. Anything above this limit indicated hypermetabolic activity (double dividing cancer cells). The area between my heart and lungs read 2.67, indicating some minute cancer cell activity.

The radiologist's report later concluded, "Two hypermetabolic foci remain in the region of the anterior mediastinum left of mid line consistent with residual disease. Overall, marked improvement compared to the previous

CARILION CRYSTAL SPRING IMAGING

PET IMAGING SERVICES REPORT
Roanoke, Virginia 24033

NAME: CHIPS, ALLEN STANLEY   ROOM: EXAM DATE: 11/03/2003
ADDR: PO BOX 249   ADM#: 64908445   SERVICE: MRI
      GOSHEN, VA. 24439   MR #: 570290   PT TYPE: OA
AGE: 41   SEX: M   DOB: PH #:
ORD DR: DISCHARGE DATE:
ATT DR.   SS#:   CLINIC: OPT
ADM. REASON: PET SCAN/HODGKINS LYMPHOMA

EXAMINATION(s):   RAD CODE(s)   RMH CODE(s)   RMS ORD#   INV#
   PET LYMPHOMA RESTAGING   G0222   G0222   90003   2

PET LYMPHOMA RESTAGING

CLINICAL: HODGKINS NO CURRENT THERAPY RESUME CHEMO OR NOT

REPORT: PET scan for re-staging lymphoma. Approximately 11 mCi
of FDG given intravenously. After about one hour delay, images
were obtained from the neck through the pelvis. Comparison is
made to previous PET scan from May 2003.

Marked interval improvement compared to the previous study.
Resolution of pathologic foci of hypermetabolism in the neck.
Resolution of most of the abnormalities in the mediastinum. There
are still two hypermetabolic foci in the region of the anterior
mediastinum to the left of mid line consistent with residual
disease.

No other suspicious abnormalities are noted.

IMPRESSION: Two hypermetabolic foci remain in the region of the
anterior mediastinum left of mid line consistent with residual
disease. Overall, marked improvement compared to the previous
study.

                              THIS REPORT IS FINAL
                              AND ELECTRONICALLY SIGNED.

                              _____ MD

LEM   D: ( )
JOB#   T: 11/03/2003 08:20PM

PT. NAME: CHIPS, ALLEN STANLEY   (PET)   MR #: 570290
9-NOV-03 14:43:31   EXAM(s)DATE:11/03/2003

study." I will never forget the "clinical" segment of the report, which stated, "Hodgkin's. No current therapy. Resume chemo or not...?" It seemed to indicate confusion on the part of this M.D. as to why I was getting better. I simply chuckled.

I made an appointment to see Doctor Fineman. He walked into the treatment room with a smile.

"How's it going?"

I declared, "I feel great. What do the scans say?"

"It appears that all your affected lymph nodes are necrotic, and the ones in your neck are no longer active, which is really good news, but there are two nodes still active between your heart and lungs" he said.

"Oh, well, if I recall, you said that cancer either goes one way or another...it's either growing or receding, right?

"Yes."

He went on to say that he would normally recommend that a patient doing traditional medicine do another round of chemotherapy, or at least do it until there were no active cancer cells left. Then he said that I was outside of the box.

"Okay, then, it appears that everything is still receding from my using the herbs, supplements, diet, and imagery, right?"

He concluded with a puzzled yet optimistic expression, "I don't know what you are doing, but just keep doing it, because it appears to be working."

As I left his office, Doctor Fineman agreed to watch a video on the approach I was using, so the next day, on my way to the airport for another visit to Tijuana, I dropped off the *Quacks Who Cure* video. I then checked out my CT scans from the local hospital and flew to the San Diego airport.

Instead of renting a car from the airport this time, I'd decided to take one of the free shuttles that come over from Tijuana to make rounds to the San Ysidro hotels. Their passengers are mostly patients, and mostly cancer patients hoping for a cure that America, Canada, and Eastern Europe could not provide.

I took the early morning shuttle to make sure I was at the BMC before 9:00 am. The BMC is adamant about patients being there by 9:00 am so that all patients who arrive that day can be seen by the various members of their medical team. The medical staff stays as long as necessary to see all the patients who check in each day and like to be done by mid-afternoon.

On the shuttle, I met a woman and her husband. They had seen videos on the Biomedical Center, done an Internet search, and had thought they'd found the Hoxsey Clinic. Unfortunately, it was another clinic in Tijuana that advertised itself as the originators of the Hoxsey therapy. Apparently, the woman had paid it much more than the BMC program and was not happy with the initial results, particularly when she found out the doctor was an impostor. She demanded a full refund, and it wasn't until she threatened to sue the clinic for false claims that her demands were satisfied. She was very religious, claiming the BMC cured her stage four cancer within the miracles God provides. She and her husband owned and operated a business in Florida.

I also met a person from Sarasota, Florida, who'd had metastasized melanoma and been given one month to live. After traditional cancer therapy failed, he committed himself to the BMC. That had been several years ago. He had the glowing smile of one who enjoyed the fact that he'd been given a second chance at life. The shuttle dropped people off at a few other health clinics in Tijuana, and although all the passengers were Americans that day, Canadians, Australians, and New Zealanders are often seen frequenting the Tijuana health clinics as well.

When I got to the BMC, I received the usual warm hug from Aida, the office manager, and then I was called to see Dr. Trujillo, the internist. Although his specialty includes the natural chemotherapy program offered for people with well-advanced cancers, he also implemented and monitored the herbs, supplements, and diet. The BMC policy involved rotating patients among all their doctors, so there is a variety of opinion on the prescribed programs for each patient, which naturally leads to a more effective group approach.
Dr. Trujillo examined my CT scans, and then I went back to his office.

He stated, "Mr. Chips, we are very surprised with your quick progress. The tumors in your chest are so small! We were talking about it together and thought that your rapid progress could be due to the addition of the Chinese medicines."

"What did you see?"

"Your lymph nodes are small and dark," as he held up his fingers showing a gap of about .5 centimeters, indicating necrosis. This is very, very good," he said with a South American lilt in his voice.

"Great! Just out of curiosity, how long does it usually take to get to this point?"

"Oh, well you know that varies, depending on the patient and the type of cancer."

"Yes, but for Hodgkin's lymphoma, does it normally take a year or two to get to this level?"

He nodded his head in agreement, got up from his desk and began to move toward the exam table, beckoning me to move to the table. "It can, Mr. Chips, it certainly can in some cases. So let's have a look at you over here."

He felt my organs and lymph nodes and said, "Everything seems to be looking good. How have you been feeling?"

I told him about my high level of energy. He was very encouraging about my progress and stated that I must still continue the diet and herbs as prescribed for the first five years.

While I was at lunch, a shuttle driver by the name of Daniel ate next to me. I asked him how long he'd been driving the shuttle, and he responded, "Fifteen years." Just like the staff at BMC, he was a permanent fixture. I was impressed with this continuity, and prodded further to discover why he'd been driving people back and forth from the San Diego airport for so many years.

He told me that had it not been for the BMC, he wouldn't have a son today; his son was now in his twenties. His wife developed PCOS twenty-two years earlier. She went on the tonic and diet for six months, the cysts disappeared, and she bore a son. This impressed him so much that he kept coming back to the clinic and saw hundreds of people, mostly cancer patients, getting cured. He decided that this was God's work and has committed himself to helping the clinic ever since. Daniel was a Jehovah's Witness and added that spin to the conversation, mentioning that the *Watch Tower*, a popular Jehovah's Witness publication, had printed articles about the BMC in the past, which led to many people coming to the BMC for help.

After making sure it was just six months of tonic (1 teaspoon 4 times a day) and the normal Hoxsey diet that led to a permanent cure for his wife's PCOS, I thanked him and set out for home with a plan to make my daughter the center of another live biochemical research project. When I arrived home, my daughter became interested in trying Hoxsey therapy, so I gave her a dosage of just 2/5 the normal adult dosage of the tonic, which I based on her weight. She took this instead of hormone therapy, as a New Year's resolution. She was also to start the Hoxsey diet then, and to continue with six months of the treatment. I also put her on extra burdock root, evening primrose oil, and a multivitamin.

May 2004: The Scare of My Life; Lifestyles; An End to PCOS

It was time for my six-month X-ray. I saw my local oncologist, who referred me for a PET scan. It showed heat where the radioactive glucose had been absorbed into areas of my neck, chest, and bowels. This generally indicates the cancer is spreading or has metastasized. It was terrible news the day that Dr. Fineman phoned my wife at the office. I had just come back to the office from a mail run. As I walked across the front yard to the second building on our 30-acre mountain retreat, where our office was located, I was confronted with my wife bearing the news.

"What's wrong?" I asked, my smile fading in response to her expression.

"Your doctor just called."

"So what did he say?"

"It's not good news."

"What?" I noticed she had been crying.

"He said that your PET scan showed that your cancer has probably spread."

"What? That's hard to believe. I don't have B-type symptoms anymore and my energy level is back. I haven't felt better in years!" I was beside myself.

"I'm just telling you what he said. You'd better call him," she said, her voice shaking.

I immediately called him but he wasn't in the office, so I left a desperate message with his office manager. He contacted me about a half-hour later.

"Allen, this is Doctor Fineman."

"Yes, I was wondering about the PET scan result."

"Well, I wish I had better news for you. The PET showed some higher than normal heat ranges in three different areas, the chest, neck, and lower bowels."

"Jeeze, you've got to be kidding me. I *feel* good though."

"It appears that the PET is indicating Hodgkin's in three areas, which means you could be stage three now."

CARILION RYSTAL SPRING MAGING

PET IMAGING SERVICES REPORT
Roanoke, Virginia 24033

NAME: CHIPS, ALLEN STANLEY
ADDR: PO BOX 249
      GOSHEN, VA. 24439
AGE: 42 SEX: M
ORD DR: ████████████
ATT DR. ████████████
ADM. REASON: PET TUMOR METABOLISM

ROOM:
ADM#: 65953226
MR #: 570290
DOB: ████████
DISCHARGE DATE:
SS#: ████████

EXAM DATE: 05/03/2004
SERVICE: MRI
PT TYPE: OA
PH #: ████████████

CLINIC: PET

EXAMINATION(s):   RAD CODE(s)   RMH CODE(s)   RMS ORD#   INV#
  PET LYMPHOMA RESTAGING   G0222   G0222   90004   3
==
  PET LYMPHOMA RESTAGING

      CLINICAL: LYMPHOMA RESTAGE \

      REPORT: PET scan for re-staging lymphoma:

      Approximately 18 mCi of FDG given intravenously. After about one
      hour delay, images were obtained from the neck through the
      pelvis.

      Comparison is made to previous PET scan from 2003.

      Hypermetabolic foci are again identified in the anterior
      mediastinum to the left of midline. This finding is consistent
      with residual active disease. New from the previous study there
      is asymmetric increased accumulation of FDG just caudal to the
      skull base, to the right of midline. Potential etiologies include
      asymmetric tonsillar activity. CT or MRI of the skull base and
      neck recommended for further evaluation.

      Also new from the previous study there is a focus of increased
      accumulation of FDG in the pelvis, to the right of midline.
      Potential etiologies include prominent physiologic bowel uptake,
      mass cannot be excluded. CT of the abdomen and pelvis with IV and
      oral contrast recommended for further evaluation.

      No other suspicious abnormalities are noted.

      IMPRESSION: New abnormalities compared to previous study warrant
      further evaluation as discussed in the report.

                                        THIS REPORT IS FINAL
                                        AND ELECTRONICALLY SIGNED.

                                        ████████████ III M

JAW
JOB# \

D: (\ )
T: 05/03/2004 04:45PM

PT. NAME: CHIPS, ALLEN STANLEY   (PET)   MR #: 570290
  4-MAY-04 15:43:18   EXAM(s)DATE:05/03/2004
                                                         PAGE 1
                                              ** TOTAL PAGE.002 **

Dr. Fineman did a bit of stress management to calm me down, and also some spiritual support, which I didn't even comprehend because of my state of mind. I told him I wanted a CT scan immediately, which he agreed to order when we got off the phone. I hung up the phone and immediately contacted Dr. Gutierrez.

"Hello, Dr. Gutierrez, this is Allen Chips again, one of your patients at BMC."

"Yes, Allen. What can I do for you?"

"I just got my PET scan results today, and my traditional medicine oncologist here said that I could be stage three."

"If I recall, you were doing pretty well the last time I saw you," he said.

"Well, the PET showed that I had heat ranges slightly higher than normal in three areas, the neck, mediastinum, and the bowels."

He began to ask specific questions. "How have you been feeling?"

"I've been feeling well. My energy level has been high."

"Have you had any sinus problems or a sore throat?"

"You know, now that you mention it, my allergies have been acting up and I've had some post-nasal drip with some soreness on the right side, where they said the heat range was elevated."

"And your bowel area could just be a sign of an infection."

"That would make sense, since I have had some diarrhea lately with some soreness down there."

Dr. Gutierrez went on to describe how I might still have some minor hypermetabolic activity in my mediastinal area (between my heart and lungs), but it wasn't anything to worry about because things were regressing rapidly, indicating a level of success typical of a cure. I felt much better after talking to him, but was anxious to have another CT scan. I phoned Paul at home.

"Paul, this is Allen Chips."

"Yes, Allen. How are things?"

"I don't know, as of late." I proceeded to explain my PET scan results and both of my oncologists' interpretations.

He said, "The CT scan will be able to show us much more than the PET. It's like taking an internal picture of your body, so we will be able to see a lot more of what's going on in there." He said that if I got worked in for a scan tomorrow, he would be working in radiology and would be able to show me the results.

That night I gave everything over to God. I gave him permission to subject me to anything that my family and I needed to experience in this life, as well as the next life.

The next morning, the hospital called me with an appointment time that day late in the afternoon. I drove to the hospital, and was scanned by the compassionate young woman who had offered me hope when I was feeling down before. She said, "I suppose you want to see your friend again. Do you want me to see if he's available?" I told her that Paul was expecting me.

Paul came out to the waiting room and escorted me back to his office with his normal friendly demeanor, adding something about my being in his prayers as he thought about how I abandoned traditional treatment. I thanked him.

"Okay, here it comes," he said with a tight jaw as we sat down in front of the large two-page computer screen and my scans started to appear under his mouse cursor. "I see further resolution here."

"What do you mean by that?"

"In layman's terms, your lymph nodes appear to be just about normal size in the mediastinum. It looks normal to me."

I let out my breath with a sigh of relief as I watched him surf through another picture, and asked, "What about the bowel area?"

"That's what I'm looking at now," he said distractedly. "Nope, nothing there. Everything appears to be normal."

"Are you sure?"

"It must have been something else that the PET was showing, because I don't see anything here. What did the PET show as the other hot area?"

"The back right side of the neck."

Paul scanned through the neck area and found nothing. I was relieved, to say the least. Paul asked me a few questions about the herbs in the black tonic, so I listed them off the top of my head. We discussed the Chinese medicine I was taking as a powdered tea and the sweet wormwood (artemasia) capsules, which he was familiar with. According to his research, long-term use of artemisia was controversial, but most studies indicated that it was relatively safe.

The next day, I was back on the road. I was headed for the Roanoke Regional Airport to go to Tijuana again, this time with Dee accompanying me. The airport is about an hour and a half drive from our home, which is just west of the Blue Ridge Parkway on the side of a mountain in the Allegheny mountain range. In the car, I phoned Dr. Fineman at his Roanoke clinic.

"Hello, Ben, this is Allen Chips again."

"Yes, Allen."

"I just wanted to ask if you received my CT scan results."

"Yes, I have."

"Paul said that he didn't see anything in the bowels or neck."

"I know. I read the results. It appears that you are fine."

"Well, I really prayed last night and just put it in God's hands. I thought, 'There's nothing that I can do if this system I am on is not working, even though I've researched it so thoroughly. So if God wants to allow me to suffer for some reason, I will just have to let go and let God.'"

"I wouldn't think God wants anybody to suffer."

"I know, but I am just saying that I am doing the best that I know how to beat this thing, so God is either with me on it or I will have to release everything to him if he's not and trust."

"Well, it looks like you don't have to worry about any of that now."

"What do you think happened with the PET scan?"

"The PET was wrong."

"I wonder how that could have been the case."

STONEWALL JACKSON HOSPITAL
LEXINGTON, VA 24450

PATIENT LOCATION: OP

PATIENT NAME :Chips, Allen   SERVICE DATE   :5/6/04
DATE OF BIRTH :▒▒▒▒▒   PATIENT NUMBER:10750974
ATTENDING PHYS:▒▒▒▒   MED REC NUMBER:068073

EXAMINATION REQUESTED: CLINICAL HISTORY:
1. CT of the Neck   Hodgkin's
2. CT of the Chest
3. Abdomen & Pelvic CT

CT of the Neck

INDICATION: Hodgkin's disease.

There are no priors available to compare. There is no evidence of
mass, lymphadenopathy, asymmetry or other finding. There is uniform
vascular enhancement.

IMPRESSION:
1. Normal CT of the neck.

CT of the chest

Comparing 10/27/03.

There is continued resolution of lymphadenopathy of the mediastinum.
There is persisting soft tissue density in the preaortic space and
several areas of necrosis unchanged in size; aggregate transverse
measurement about 2.5 cm.

IMPRESSION:
1. Continuing improvement of superior mediastinal adenopathy without
   other finding or significant interval change.

Abdomen & Pelvic CT

Unchanged comparing 10/27/03. Small left renal cyst. Otherwise normal.

IMPRESSION:
1. No interval change or significant abnormal finding.

PF:tl
D:5/6/04 @ 1241   ▓▓▓▓▓▓▓, D.O.
T:5/6/04 @ 1352

"The PET measures heat ranges and with you just being slightly above normal in those other two areas, it could have been fecal material, or something like that. Either way, you are amazingly doing quite well."

"Yeah...thank God for that," I said, lowering my voice.

"There is nobody doing anything remotely similar to what you are doing in my practice. But hey, if it's working, more power to you. Just keep it up."

It was nice to have Dr. Fineman's spiritual, moral, and clinical support, particularly through regular blood tests and scans. I had talked to many Hoxsey patients who did not have the support of their traditional medicine physicians. Some patients have told me stories of how many of their doctors had refused to see them as long as they were doing Hoxsey therapy.

My wife and I were very excited about attending the clinic together this time, so when we got to the San Diego airport, we rented a car and drove to Rosarito Beach, Mexico, which is located about 20 miles west of Tijuana. Aida, the BMC office manager had advised against it; she felt that the U.S. side was safer. However, I'd talked to a friend of mine, also an author on holistic health, who grew up in Southern California and said that it was a fun place to go when he was younger. In addition, I'd booked a very economical bonus week in Rosarito through one of our time share memberships.

It was a cute little villa located right on the beach. It proved to be a nice anniversary getaway, and the lobster was a real bargain—twelve dollars for a superb three-course dinner, including steamed vegetables, beverage, and a dessert with natural sugar ingredients. The cliff-side restaurant overlooking the rocky Pacific coastline at sunset was impressive.

On Monday, I saw Dr. Percioli. They refer to her as the Lady Doctor. She has a reputation of being very direct with patients, which some patients need in order to face their disease from a holistic perspective and take responsibility for their treatment program and take better care for themselves. This time, my wife came back to her office with me.

She stood up from her desk and approached the doorway as we crossed the threshold, extended her hand and said, "I am Doctor Terese, Mr. Chips."

"Hello. This is my wife. Is it okay that she came in with me?"

"Yes, of course. Sit down", she said matter-of-factly, as she pointed to two chairs across from her desk.

She sat down and said, "So, Mr. Chips, tell me about everything that you are taking."

"You mean all of the supplements and Chinese medicines?"

"Yes. Let's go through each one."

I listed everything, and she diligently took notes. When I got to the artemisinin caps, she jotted down some notes and said, "I want you to stop taking the artemisinin."

"Really, how come?"

"It is a new medicine and we don't know at what level it becomes toxic, so I want you to go off it for the next three months. Then after three months you may resume it again at your current dosage."

I questioned her judgment, asking about her research, but she held firm to the lack of data on artemisinin, and sternly said she was making the decision based on what she thought was best for her patients. She said that it was non-negotiable. From there I led the conversation to some lifestyle questions about whether to move from our current home, which has a pesticide plant only five miles away, to the ocean, where I felt healthier and could breathe easier. She agreed that a move would be a good idea when I was ready to do so, because of the studies I'd found correlating the use of pesticides and the rise in the incidence of lymphoma. In addition, we talked about my work environment and career goals.

I asked about my need for rest, which is part of the Hoxsey program, and the stress level in having my wife work with me. Particularly when I needed to rest, Dee would sometimes phone me at home while I was napping in order to motivate me to come back to the office. Dr. Percioli was very careful not to get caught in the middle of this dispute and showed an uncanny ability to unite my wife and me in creating ways to communicate better to avoid such conflicts in the future.

I asked about my writing career, which was my passion, and the implementation of the on-line university I was spearheading for holistic health and alternative medicine degrees, which was very labor intensive. The university was taking an immense amount of energy. I was wondering if I should continue. In addition, I told her of my third book project (this book), which she had heard about. Her response was direct and profoundly beneficial and really hit home.

"Mr. Chips, each soul has a purpose on the earth while they are here, a unique purpose that only God and they know about. Each must do soul searching and use their intuition to understand that purpose as they go through life. In using intuition, the person may better match their purpose with their passion. Your intuition and your passion, when in alignment, is the deciding factor for your making your decisions with what you want to do with your life. Therefore, my advice for you is to use your intuition, pray, meditate, and then follow your passion...the passion that sustains you...that nourishes your soul."

I was misty-eyed, choked-up, and speechless. I had surfaced from the depths of a potentially terminal illness and was seeking answers, and finding them, at least in the abstract. I gazed off for a moment.

"Does that ring true for you, Mr. Chips?"

Reorienting myself, I responded, "Yes, yes it does."

I ended up making the decision to do both. I'd worked too hard to let the university go. There were too many people waiting to enroll in its programs, and I knew that the mental health therapists and naturopaths who wanted to study under our unique degree programs would learn about treatment programs that were unique to the fields of transpersonal psychology and natural health. And this would provide a real service to society. In addition, I kept alive my passion to write and added a goal: to pick up again and write a novel I'd started a year earlier. It was a mind-body science thriller about the consciousness of earth, which, entwined with prophecy, resulted in a global transformation. My writing was my passion, while alternative health education was my purpose. The details of how to meet the labor demands of both of them would be confronted later.

On the way out of the clinic, I ran into Dr. Trujillo, who told me that my CT scans looked a little better than the last one, and that I have what they refer to as "non-active lymphoma." It was important to stay on the diet and herbs to make sure that all the Hodgkin's cells would be eliminated. I told him that he could count on it. I then found Dr. Gutierrez and quickly asked him about taking a break from the artemisinin. He concurred with Dr. Percioli that it was indeed a good idea to be on the safe side. I also thanked him for responding to my e-mail a couple of weeks earlier, when I inquired about a potential legal conflict involving my daughter. His e-mailed response, involved a beautiful metaphor about ships bumping into one another in a vast ocean, and how life was short, so we should exercise the philosophy of "letting go." The advice was so pertinent for cancer survivors, I decided to publish in the chapter, The Holistic Approach.

We drove back to our cute little beach bungalow in Rosarito, Mexico. On the way, we saw a large billboard with a picture of the newly elected local government official claiming that all corruption had been eliminated and that tourism was welcome. And we discovered that Aida was correct: the Tijuana area has "policia corrupcione problemas." Almost exactly like what had happened to me in Cancun just ten years before, the police singled us out in traffic with an erroneous traffic violation in order to obtain the usual twenty-dollar tip. I was disappointed to learn that Tijuana had not been cleaned up yet, as was the case in other parts of Mexico, such as Puerto Vallarta. I was unpleasantly surprised to hear that same line again, "I am doing you a favor. If you pay twenty dollars now, it will be much less expensive than going downtown and paying the ticket."

I would take a rental car over the border only one more time, which proved to be the last time after having a third, identical experience in downtown Tijuana in December of 2004. That time I stuck out like a sore thumb with a rented convertible sports car. The truth of the matter is that Mexico is still a very poor country compared to the United States, and people in service positions, such as the police, would barely eke out a living without receiving these illegal tips. As a result of these kinds of experiences, the clinic advises patients to take the clinic shuttles. The local Mexican people, and the authorities, rely on these groups to contribute to their local economy; therefore, they are generally never bothered.

My daughter had been on the program, with my supplements, for five months now for her PCOS condition. The cysts had disappeared, never to return, even though she'd been caught by her father cheating on the diet (chocolates with processed sugar) on a few occasions.

Late June, 2004: A Friend in Need is a Friend Indeed

I walked into my office and my wife greeted me. She then replayed a message for me from Dr. Jans, an alternative health professional who teaches meditation and clinical hypnotherapy courses at our annual convention, where many alternative health professionals give workshops and presentations. In the message, he explained with a cordial Indian accent that he had cancer and could not teach at this year's conference. He sounded concerned.

I phoned him back and discovered that a malignant tumor had been discovered in his lung this spring. He was not a smoker, although his father had been one when he was growing up. Shortly after it was discovered, it grew to four centimeters, at which time Dr. Jans did radiation and chemotherapy. It shrank to 2.5 centimeters, but by June it was growing more aggressively than before, and it began to approach 6 centimeters. He was so winded it was difficult for him to climb a flight of stairs.

He apologized for not being able to make our September event, and it was evident that he wasn't sure he would survive that long. His doctor was not responding to his and his family's phone calls trying to request another CT scan or more therapy (I later asked my mother about this and she said that many physicians do not respond to patients who are on their way out.)

I told Dr. Jans my story, and the stories of others I'd talked with who were successful with the Hoxsey method. He responded that he had tried a traditional and alternative medicine treatment program in Chicago, which was too expensive and turned out to be ineffective. I told him it was different using the herbal medicines and nutritional concepts of the mystic Edgar Cayce and the naturopath Harry Hoxsey, and I told him about the 80-year reputation of the clinic. Finally he implied that in a last-ditch effort he would try the program.

A few days later he was bound for San Diego, destination Tijuana, Mexico. On his return in early July, he called me and said the oncologists at BMC put him on a cancer vaccine, which was used as a nasal spray and was not approved in the United States. He was also prescribed the black tonic and the Hoxsey diet. Within a month, his lung capacity and energy level had returned, and two months later he was in full swing teaching at our conference.

(A year later, he credited his recovery from lung cancer to the Hoxsey system. I questioned the doctors at the clinic, who said that their success rate for lung cancer is higher than 80 percent, perhaps as high as 90 percent, because of the addition of the cancer vaccine.)

November 2004: A Clean Bill of Health

I was faithful about getting the once-a-month blood test ordered by my local oncologist, and decided that it was time to see him again, particularly since in the summer he'd suggested seeing me. There in the treatment room, I laid out all my supplements on the table, so he could see what I was taking and for what purpose.

Entering the room with my health file in hand he said, "Mr. Allen Chips...so, how are you doing lately?"

"I feel good, real good. In fact, if there was a problem, I would have to say that I work too many long hours and then have to catch up on my sleep because I feel tired."

"Well, I don't think working too hard and being tired is a red flag in this case. We're not going to concern ourselves about that." He smiled, stepped back, looked me up and down, and said, "Look at you. You look great. I mean just look at you. Your color is good, you are obviously in great shape."

"Yeah, I lost weight from this all-natural diet and continue to work out at the Y on a regular basis. I really feel great."

"I look at you, then I look at your file. It says, 'Allen Chips...Hodgkin's Lymphoma,' and I look at Allen Chips, and Allen Chips should be dead. It's been a year and a half already."

He was obviously happy for me. I received a brief physical and we talked about my blood test indicating that everything was normal. We talked about a final CT scan or PET scan, and he said that I didn't need to prove that I was done with this chapter of my life. And besides, he said that when X-rays hit the DNA just right, it will "screw you up," causing various illnesses or potentially the recurrence of cancer.

He recommended against it, saying, "Why put yourself through it when you don't need to? I can see you for a check up in six months, but you're virtually done with this stuff."

I asked him if he wanted to go out to lunch to learn more about what I did to get well after my six-month check-up at the clinic, and he agreed, but joked about how much he liked red meat, so the restaurant would have to serve ribs or steak.

December 2004: More Testimonials; More Good News

I tried to go to the BMC just before Thanksgiving, but the airlines were quite busy because of the holidays, and I could not locate a frequent flier ticket on one of the airlines where I'd built up enough miles for an award ticket. As a result, I booked my flight for the middle of December, when I could also locate a bonus week at a timeshare resort in Palm Desert, California.

In mid-December, I flew into San Diego, which I was so familiar with, rented a car, and went to a writing retreat there at Palm Desert. While I was there I met a woman who had several family members with cancer who were cured by the clinic. A genetic predisposition to cancer, but all were cured. It was impressive. Her husband, brother, sister in-law, grandmother—all cured strictly using Hoxsey therapy.

At the health food store where she worked, she would invite people with cancer to shuttle to the BMC in her van from Palm Springs. She received no compensation, just gratification from all the success stories. As she told of more than a hundred people who'd received treatment there, and claimed that only two had been lost, an elderly man came up to our table where we were having lunch. He smiled and said, "Still clean and clear" when he saw the two of us speaking about Hoxsey therapy.

By the end of the week, I'd given my typing fingers a rest, and went for my six-month follow-up visit. Over the border I went, in a rental car this time. When I got to the clinic, it was slightly past nine, and the staff was worried that I might not get in to see the doctors. However, they managed to work me in, since the patient load was light that day.

Dr. Trujillo saw me and ordered a chest X-ray. He said that it was such a low dose X-ray, as compared to a CT or PET scan, that it would be harmless, so I agreed.

After the X-ray, I ate lunch at the BMC cafeteria and then went back to see Dr. Trujillo again. He said that the chest was clear, but warned that I would need to stay on the diet, tonic, and herbs, just to make sure there was no recurrence. He said that we must keep the immune system up. We talked about the benefits of juicing in the mornings, to maintain the integrity of my immune system. I was experiencing a solid recovery.

I went back to Palm Desert to research and write more on the book. During that week, I phoned dozens of Hoxsey patients. Most recounted impressive recoveries, but one woman with ovarian cancer admitted to cheating on the diet, eating out at a lot of Chinese restaurants, where the food traditionally contains toxins, such as monosodium glutamate (MSG), and sodium benzoate (a preservative in soy sauce). She had a return of her cancer in the fourth year of treatment and the physicians at BMC were permitting her to have some radiation therapy through her traditional medicine oncologists in the States. This confirmed the importance of continuing the Hoxsey diet for a period of five years.

At the same time, I was amazed at how many people I interviewed in the southern California region who had used Hoxsey therapy and were free of cancer for many years. Many of them just kept smiling during our discussions, a smile that was becoming very familiar to me.

October 2005: My One Year Checkup

It was time for my annual check-up with Dr. Fineman in Roanoke, Virginia. By that time, for health reasons, my wife, son, and I had moved to North Carolina to our beach house. My daughter was attending a college in the mountains of Virginia.

"So, how are we feeling lately?" Dr. Fineman asked with a keen look of interest as he walked into the white-walled, sterile examination room.

I sat on the edge of the table, the paper beneath me crinkling as I repositioned myself. "I still feel good."

He reached up and felt my neck immediately. "Any swollen lymph nodes anywhere?"

"Not that I notice."

He sat down to make notes and said, "This is so cool. I'm just amazed."

"You think I'm in the clear."

"It looks that way to me," he said with a lilt, raising his eyebrows.

"Cancer either grows or it's in remission, right?"

"You should be dead by now. You would be if what you are doing wasn't working."

"Do you recommend any tests?" I asked.

"Your guess is as good as mine on that one. I mean, I'll do whatever you want."

I asked about a blood test, and he said that wouldn't tell us anything. A CT scan had the most radiation, so we both agreed not to do any more of these. The PET scan was the most definitive, according to Dr. Fineman, but the most costly; and because I'd had a bad reading in the past that showed hot spots that didn't exist, I declined. The traditional chest X-ray was the most economical and would show a mass between the heart and lungs, should there be a return of Hodgkin's disease, so we agreed that I would wait and do a chest X-ray at the BMC in Tijuana that month.

The visit ended with my describing the herbal medicines and how I had discovered Park Davis & Company's formula. It was documented as using almost identical herbs for cancer treatment in 1890. He asked me if I documented this in my book. I did.

A few weeks later, Dr. Jans phoned me and told me that his physician had informed him that he didn't have any other chemotherapies to offer him, so he had decided to use Hoxsey therapy. We decided to go to the BMC together at the end of the month.

Once we got on the shuttle, we heard numerous testimonials of Hoxsey cures from other patients. We met a woman and her husband, who told us their story.

Appearing to be somewhere in her seventies, she explained that her oncologist wanted to remove both breasts and perform chemotherapy treatments. She said, "There's no way I was going to let them cut both my breasts off. And I wasn't going to die barfing my guts up from those poisons [chemotherapies] they give you. I saw what it did to others, and I decided I wasn't going to die like that. And now look at me, do I look sick?"

I confirmed that she certainly did not look unhealthy at all. She was a vibrant, energetic woman with a contagious positive attitude and the familiar Hoxsey smile. As I questioned her, I found that she'd become a patient at the BMC a year ago, after being diagnosed through a needle biopsy. She was fortunate to have found a conventional physician in California who was willing to monitor her results, as she used only the Hoxsey system of therapy. She had several active breast tumors when she was first diagnosed, which had recently tested negative for cancer.

On our arrival at the clinic, we registered and then went to the waiting room. There were about a dozen people there. A large white-haired man who appeared to be in his late fifties shared several stories with a room full of eager listeners. With an upbeat voice, he explained how the red salve was used on his face at the BMC to extract a cancerous tumor.

"You see this little dimple here?" pointing to an indentation slightly smaller than a dime on his forehead. "When I first got cancer, I had a tumor there with tentacles that grew all the way down into my jaw. The doctors in the states would have had to take my whole face off in hopes to get it all."

I prodded for further information about the appearance of the cancer at the time of extraction, and the methods used.

"It was like a scab growing on the surface of the skin. After a week on the red salve and a week on the yellow powder, they pulled it out, and boy did it hurt, so they had to give me painkillers. But by the time they extracted it, it was all dead in there. It looked like black spider webs as it was pulled out of my forehead here and one [tentacle] came out of my jaw all the way down here," he exclaimed as he pointed to the right side of his jaw.

As many times as I'd heard stories about the escharotics treatments, I was still astonished. I asked if he was also prescribed the diet or the internal tonic, as the rest of us in the waiting room apparently had.

"Oh, yeah. They put me on the internal tonic and the diet for about six months. Now I am just using the red salve for this small one this time," as he pointed to another spot on his head.

I asked how he'd heard about the clinic.

"There was an old woman in Phoenix who lives down the street who'd had cancer twenty-some years ago. She still praises the clinic because she's still cancer-free after all these years. Then six years ago, when my brother had metastasized prostate cancer with a PSA of 1800, I asked her about the Hoxsey treatment. When the cancer spread to his bones, I came to visit him, and you couldn't even touch his bed railing without him yelling out in excruciating pain. I brought his X-rays to show the doctors here and see if there was anything they could do; and they gave me a bottle of the black tonic to give to him. Within nine days, he was out of bed and had no more pain. The doctors in the States said that he would never recover his bone density, but the doctors here said he would, using certain supplements—and by God he did. He regained all of his bone density through the nutrition and supplements they recommended here. After I saw all this, and then contracted skin cancer, I came here myself and experienced nothing less than miracles here. It's just amazing."

The man had the smile I've described many times, as he went on to tell other stories to the group of Hoxsey patients crowded around, dressed in gray or blue examination robes. Many of them were with their family members in plain clothes.

The man had another story. During his visit a year ago, he saw a man in the waiting room who had a large tumor on the top of his head. Six months later he encountered the same man; both of them were there for their six-month check-ups. He noticed that the tumor was completely gone and the man was on the road to recovery. Many of the people in the waiting room assumed that a combination of external and internal treatments was used. Apparently, witnessing cases such as these was not uncommon.

One woman said that when she'd been there in the late 1970s and even up to the late 90s, you couldn't find a seat in the waiting room (approximately 70 feet by 40 feet), and the line of people waiting for the lab extended all the way to the waiting room (about 80 feet long). I explained that I was told during my recent interviews with the staff at the BMC that after the terrorist attacks of September 11, 2001, the number of patients dropped, due to people's reluctance to fly.

Next, Dr. Jans and I had our doctor's appointments. My blood test showed I needed more protein, preferably by consuming more lentils and beans. My sodium and chloride levels were in the normal range (too high leads to an acidic condition), and my urine test showed high alkalinity levels (7.5), which was a favorable condition. My X-ray, also taken at the clinic, showed that the

Bio Medical Center S.A de C.V.

Ave. General Ferreira #3170 Col. Madero Sur C.P. 22150, Tijuana B.C México. Tel : 684-9011 Fax : 684-9744
RFC: BMC 971022-2K5

Nombre : CHIPS ALLEN

Doctor: Dr. Ruben Trujillo

Estudios: Lab Rutina

Edad : 43

Sexo: Masculino

No. Lab : 8645

Fecha Rep: 10/31/05

Impresión: 10/31/05 12:06:17 PM

BIOMETRIA HEMATICA

Prueba	Dentro Rango	Fuera Rango	Valores Normales
Leucoc	6.3		4.4 - 11.0 x 10³
Eritroc	5.39		4.4 - 5.7 x 10⁶
HB	16.2		13.3 - 17.5 g/dl
HCTO	45.8		40 - 53 %
MCV	85		80 - 97 ft
MCH	30.1		27 - 31 g/dl
MCHC	35.4		32 - 35.4 g/dl
RDW	13.4		11.6 - 14.8 %
PLQ	185		150 - 400 x 10³
Eosino.	5		0 - 6 %
Baso	0		0 - 2 %
Bandas	1		0 - 4 %
Segmen	57		47 - 73 %
Linf.	28		16 - 45 %
Monoc.		8	1 - 7 %
Neutrof.	58		47 - 73 %
VSG	9		0 - 16

Observaciones

QUIMICA SANGUINEA

Prueba	Dentro Rango	Fuera Rango	Valores Normales
F. Alc.	66		36 - 141 U/L
F. Acid.	4.4		0 - 5.1 U/L
Colest.	182		< 200 mg/dl
Trigl.	77		35 - 160 mg/dl
Glucosa	79		70 - 110 mg/dl
BUN	16		5 - 25 mg/dl
Creatinina	1.5		0.9 - 1.5 mg/dl
BUN/Crea	10		6.0 - 25.0
Ac. Urico		3.1	3.7 - 7.7 mg/dl
Sodio	141		136 - 146 mmol/L
Potasio	4.6		3.5 - 5.2 mmol/L
Cloro	101		98 - 107 mmol/L
CO2	30		22 - 32 mmol/L
Anion Gap	14		9.0 - 18.0
Calcio	8.9		8.5 - 10.5 mg/dl
Fósforo	3.1		2.5 - 4.8 mg/dl
Magn.	2.2		1.8 - 2.9 mg/dl
Hierro	124		70 - 180 mcg/dl
UIBC	116		70 - 420 mcg/dl
TIBC		240	250 - 450 mcg/dl
% Sat	52		12 - 57 %
Proteinas	7.0		6 - 8.3 g/dl
Albumina	4.9		3.5 - 5.5 mg/dl
Globulina		2.1	2.2 - 4.2 g/dl
Rel .A/G		2.3	0.8 - 2.0
Bilir. Total	0.7		0.2 - 1.0 mg/dl
AST	19		6 - 38 U/L
ALT	23		0 - 35 U/L
LDH	133		71 - 195 U/L
GGTP		10	11 - 50 U/L
HDL-Col.	40		27 - 75 mg/dl
LDL-Col.	127		90 - 215 mg/dl
Ind. Riesgo		4.6	<4 baj, 4-4.9 med >4.9 alto

Observaciones

URIANALISIS

Prueba	Dentro Rango	Fuera Rango	Valores Normales
Densidad	1.015		1.005 - 1.030
*pH		7.5	5.0 - 7.0
Albumina	0		0
Glucosa	0		0
Cetona	0		0
Bilirrubi	0		0
Hb.	0		0
Nitritos	NEG		NEG
Urobili.	0		0 - 1 U/dl
Estearasa	NEG		NEG
Color	AMARILLO		
Aspecto	TRANSPARENTE		

ANALISIS MICROSCOPICO

Prueba	Dentro Rango	Fuera Rango	Valores Normales
Cel. Epit.	-		/Campo
Cel. Ren.	-		/Campo
Leuc.	0 - 1		/Campo
Eritroc.			/Campo
Bacterias			
Levad.			
Filam.			

Observaciones

Melanina		NEG

Q.F.B. E. Berenice Pocoroba U.
Ced. Prof. 2974808

lymph structure in my chest was clear for the second year in a row, which confirmed a strong recovery.

Dr. Jans went for his appointment, which also showed that he was free from his cancer now, going on one and one-half years. Shortly thereafter, we collected our CT scans and took a shuttle to the natural pharmacy. During the shuttle ride back to the hotel in San Ysidro, California, Dr. Jans said that he felt that the United States was ripe for a clinic like this. He claimed that there were so many naturopathic and homeopathic physicians in business today that the AMA and FDA couldn't possibly shut them all down. There were too many, and public demand for such a clinic was at an all-time high. He suggested that the BMC set up a branch in the States somewhere. I agreed.

A Summary of My Success

In the first month of my illness, in May 2003, my family doctor noticed that the larger tumor on my neck had shrunk from 1.5 centimeters to about one centimeter. I believe that it was a result of a combination of the imagery I was using and some of the supplements I began. These alone were obviously not enough to put my cancer in remission, as I was not using any blood purifiers, nor was I on an alkaline diet.

In June 2003, when the large tumor on my neck shrank and snapped free from my neck, I believe it was due to the introduction of the Hoxsey and Cayce herbs to my system. I also believe that the Cayce diet assisted in moving my body fluids into an alkaline state much of the time, which is when the CT scans showed the first sign of progress. However, again, I do not feel it was enough to put my cancer in an inactive state.

In July 2003, when I took the chemotherapy treatment, I believe that my oncologist was correct when he said that one treatment might knock it down, but wouldn't cure it. I was glad to make a little jump on progress, but I suffered short-term memory loss for several years thereafter. The only people who recognized this were those who were close to me. Eventually, it became just a minor variable, and by the time I was fully engaged in writing this book, two years later, I noticed that my short-term memory capabilities were back to normal, but memories of things that occurred in the six months after the chemo were still hazy.

In August 2003, when I started the more potent Hoxsey herbs, the Chinese medicines, and the more strict Hoxsey alkaline diet, I experienced a lot of digestive cleansing. This was the only time that I started to feel completely healthy again, and my B-type symptoms never returned, which according to my traditional oncologist was a sign of my entering into remission.

My November 2003 CT scans showed the definitive progress of the Hoxsey therapy. My traditional oncologist said that the tumors would return if I didn't do at least six of twelve chemotherapy treatments, and at that there was only a remote chance of a cure. The November CT proved that the naturopathic system worked.

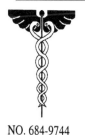

BIO MEDICAL CENTER

JUAREZ

22150

AVE. GENERAL FERREIRA #3170, COL.

TIJUANA, BAJA CALIFORNIA, MÉXICO

PHONE NO. (01152664) 684-9011 FAX

NO. 684-9744

Ysidro,   Ca.   92143

Billing Address: P.O. Box 433654, San

E-mail address: bmed@bc.cablemas.com

RADIOLOGICAL REPORT

PACIENT: CHIPS ALLEN
ESTUDY: CHEST AND ABDOMEN X-RAY
DATE: 10/31/2005.

CHEST X-RAY PA. AND LAT. VIEW. - The morphology of the thorax is normal to phenotype and with interphases of soft tissue well defined and preserved.
The bone structure has normal mineralitation with/out evidence of lesions.

The cardiovascular morphology and the cardiac index are normal, The mediastinum shows a centrally located trachea and without widening.

The lungs are well pneumatized without lesions of the parenchyma.   The pulmonary vascularity is normal. - There are no nodules or tumors.
The pleura's and hemi diaphragms are normal.

ABDOMEN, X-RAY. - There are not hepatomegally and esplenomegally, the stomach, colon and mesentery are unremarkable, the inter face of the retro peritoneum are normal, the pelvic cavity are unremarkable.
The bone structure has normal characteristics.

IMPRESSION:

CHEST AND ABDOMEN X-RAY BASICALLY IN NORMAL LIMITIS.

Dr. Arturo Rodriguez Ceceña

Certified Radiologist (License number 3394759)

My May and November 2004, CT scans showed my lymph nodes to be within normal range, and that is when I was out of the woods, figuratively speaking, according to my traditional medicine oncologist.

The chest X-rays of 2005 further document how everything is back to normal. And my conventional oncologist assured me that the most recent tests and physicals, and the number of years that have passed, indicate a solid remission. I didn't continue CT or PET scans thereafter, due to inherent risk factors (radiation, recurrence, etc.).

The need to stay on the system throughout the five-year period was recommended by the team of doctors at the BMC, so that is what I am doing. And now I am a testimonial, along with thousands of other people. I am alive and well and able to tell people about this amazing natural system of recovery—a therapy that won't make you more sick, kill or disfigure you, or give you more cancers in the future.

Part Two

The Reasoning behind Things

"In the future, doctors and medicine will no longer
be needed to heal the sick." Thomas Jefferson

Chapter 7

Common Causes and Traditional Therapies

Cancer has been recorded as far back as four thousand years ago in Egypt and India. Hippocrates created tag names for the disease, referring to it as *karkino* or *karninoma*, which led to its current label, *carcinoma*. In 131–200 AD, Galen, a physician, first gave it the term "cancer," a word that described its similarities to crab's feet.

Cancer Statistics

Three million people in the United States have cancer, and one in three, or approximately 33 percent, will die from it. This is one person every minute. Although the mortality rate specifically from cancer (not including deaths caused from traditional medicine's side effects) has declined over the past few years, the incidence of cancer has dramatically increased. At the current rate, it has been documented that one out of every two men and one out of every three women will develop some form of cancer. In the year 2000 in the United States, there were 1.2 million new cases of cancer out of an estimated 10 million cases worldwide, which indicates the severity of our problem in America. In 1999, more than 560,000 lives were lost to cancer, making it the second leading cause of death in the U.S., according to *Food, Nutrition and the Prevention of Cancer: A Global Perspective,* published by the American Institute for Cancer Research.

At the turn of the twentieth century, the five leading causes of death in the United States were:
1. Pneumonia and influenza
2. Tuberculosis
3. Diarrhea
4. Heart disease
5. Stroke

Cancer didn't even make the list. We must ask why, because something has changed in the world in which we live to change the diseases that we humans contract today. We will need to explore the causes of cancer relative to diet, lifestyle, and other factors, as we proceed through this chapter to gain a greater understanding of its natural cure.

Today, arterial sclerosis (heart disease, stroke, etc.) is the leading cause of death, and cancer is second on the list. Consider the sedentary lifestyle of most Americans, the poor dietary habits, mass-produced and processed foods, and the increased amount of stress in today's society, and the increased incidence of cancer makes perfect sense. Some statistics project that at the current rising rate of cancer, in the next twenty years one in two persons will contract the disease.

The Causes

There are more than 100 varieties of cancer, some with a higher fatality rate than others. Most types of cancer fall into four categories:

1. Carcinomas, which involve the skin, mucous membranes, glands, and internal organs;
2. Leukemias, which involve cancers of blood-forming tissues;
3. Sarcomas, which affect muscles, connective tissue, and bones; and
4. Lymphomas, which involve the lymphatic system.

All are on the rise. We must ask ourselves, particularly we Americans, the sobering question, "Why?" This question should not be answered with speculation or opinion. The U.S. government should conduct a comparative, geographically-based population study that gives us definitive answers about why so many Americans, and other industrialized, left brain-dominant cultures similar to ours, are so rapidly contracting, and dying from, this disease. Until that day, here are some things I've discovered on my journey.

The Underlying Causes of Cancer

Alternative and traditional health researchers are discovering more and more links between cancer and viruses, bacteria, parasites, and other microorganisms. For example, a few years ago there was an outbreak of mononucleosis in Africa, which led to an outbreak of Hodgkin's lymphoma in many of those same individuals. In addition, studies show that people who have had the hepatitis B or C virus statistically have an increased risk of contracting liver cancer.

It was remarkable how Harry Hoxsey was way ahead of his time in the 1950s, when he reported his theory (in his autobiography, *You Don't Have To Die*, reprinted by Transpersonal Publishing) that viruses cause cancer. As indicated in my chapter on the Cayce/Hoxsey herbs, it is clear that the compounds found in the various herbal medicines used at the BMC rid the body of several infectious microorganisms, including yeast, viruses, and bacteria, proving the efficacy of treating cancer with living, antimicrobial herbal compounds.

Now, if we accept that our immune systems are becoming compromised because of various forms of infections, we must ask why. We must take a broader view of ourselves and the world in which we live, through what I refer to as the "causative triangle," shown below.

Causative Triangle

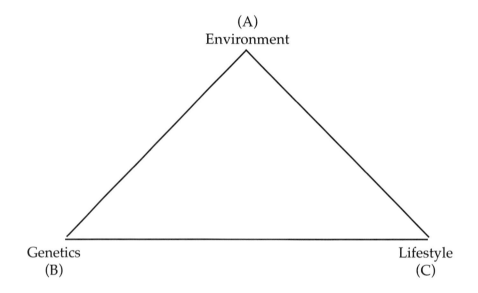

A. Environment—includes air and water pollution, farming practices and nutrition, electromagnetics, radiation, microwaves, and traditional medical practices and therapies

B. Genetics—includes hereditary factors from our ancestors who have contracted various forms of cancer.

C. Lifestyle—includes stress factors, such as relationships at home or at work, work habits, diet and exercise, and other habits, such as smoking or drinking.

Environment

Air

Air pollution is at an all-time high. A visit to the North Pole in the summer proves this. The ozone layer is at such a dangerous level of deficiency that we now must take a boat there, rather than walk across a layer of ice. Fluorocarbons from fossil fuels have eaten a hole in the ozone layer, which was put here by God or Mother Nature as a balance for keeping various light rays from dangerously penetrating our bodies. The haze we see over most cities, or even over beautiful mountain ranges, is not clouds or morning mist anymore, but smog from factories and cars. When the air quality index is yellow or red, there are more pollutants in the air, and experts say that people with respiratory diseases should not go outside during red days. As our immune systems fight these air pollutants, it struggles to maintain enough energy to fight other foreign invaders, such as cancer cells.

While the World Health Organization engages in an international effort to promote pollution control systems, our government has currently pulled its support from the energy summit in Kyoto, Japan, whose intention is to police and curb international industrial pollution. However, former president Bill Clinton has announced a world organization he's forming that involves many world leaders taking action against pollution. With more political efforts such as these, perhaps there's still hope that our government may make a difference before more people find the planet uninhabitable.

Not only has the incidence of cancer been rising with time, but so has the incidence of respiratory diseases such as asthma. In 2005, the American Lung Association declared asthma to be an epidemic that affects 24 million people. As one of the most common respiratory diseases today, it also has an ever-increasing fatality rate. More people die from asthma every year. The majority of fatalities are people over age 60, who tend to be undiagnosed asthmatics. Now we must watch the air quality index on the news, or in the newspaper, to see if it is safe to spend time outside. Research released in 2005 also shows that people suffering from respiratory diseases, particularly asthma, have a much higher incidence of cancer.

There is a wide variety of construction materials in homes and buildings that have been proven to cause cancer. This includes not just the well-known asbestos, but also the commonly-used fiberglass insulation, the urethane gases that emanate from carpeting, foam pads, and pillows, and even arsenic in treated lumber, as it comes into contact with the skin. In many cases, internal air pollution is as much a hazard as what comes from our factories.

One consideration for the cancer patient, or for those concerned with cancer prevention, is the ozonating air purifiers designed for inside the home. I examined all the models on the market that could remove dust particles less than one micron. I prefer the ionic breeze models. Their filters are metal grids that do not need replacing. The manufacturer will sell refurbished models via mail order at half the cost for those who are budget-minded. The ozone creates negative ions, similar to those produced with rain, which cause dust particles to cling to one another and fall to the floor. The unit also filters smoke, animal dander, and more. The germicidal model kills airborne microbes, such as bacteria, viruses, and mold spores.

I also have a top-of-the-line hepa vacuum. It has such a draw on it that it sometimes lifts the carpet as it passes over it, pulling much of the dust in the carpet out, and, I believe, some of the urethane gases. I like the Dyson model but had used the more economical Eureka hepa vac models with good success over the years. However, I have been gradually replacing my carpeting with wood flooring, since carpeting puts off dust. Also, I use electrostatic and extra-fine filters, which are very beneficial for use with forced air heaters and air conditioners. Many pull out dust particles of less than one micron, which is what tends to collect in our sinuses and lungs.

For fumigation efforts, it is a good idea to crack windows and doors whenever possible, particularly in the winter or hot summers, and certainly in a new house or a house that has new furniture or floors. Recently, some home builders have been offering to blow newspaper fiber into walls, in place of fiberglass insulation. This appears to be a good idea, provided the fiber isn't treated with any harmful chemicals. All alternatives to cancer-causing substances should be explored, and many do not cost any more than traditional materials.

Water

Water contamination is no surprise to anyone, as purified and spring water products have become a big business. A gallon of water at a convenience store costs approximately eight dollars when bought by the quart; this is almost two to three times higher than a gallon of gasoline.

There are few people who would dispute that our water quality is on the down-slide, and there are plenty of studies that show this fact. The causes? Factories, machines, construction, and large-scale commercial farming. Until we find alternative energy sources, or have better pollution controls, unfortunately for all of us living on this planet the incidence of respiratory diseases, cancer, and other illnesses will continue to rise.

Between public outcries and the Safe Drinking Water act of 1972, the federal government continually revises its standards to reflect the awareness of changes in our drinking water. In many areas, arsenic contamination has reached epidemic proportions, due to the real estate boom spurring new construction that uses arsenic-treated lumber.

Arsenic as a micromineral is actually good for our health in the minuscule quantities naturally found in water, but in higher quantities it's highly toxic. Years ago, the federal arsenic level was set at 50 parts per billion. Now, according to the federal government, if the arsenic level is more than 10 parts per billion at any water treatment site, it is dangerous to public health. As a result, federal law mandated that starting in the beginning of 2006, state laws must conform to these federal regulations. More commonly, wells in the western United States contain dangerous levels of arsenic.

Another carcinogenic by-product of water treatment, trihalomethane (THM), occurs when water treatment facilities have a high amount of bacteria in their water sources. In these cases, authorities add higher levels of chlorine, which mixes with organics, such as salts or chlorides, bacteria, and minerals, and creates dangerous levels of trihalomethane.

To avoid this, many treatment facilities are switching to sodium hyperchlorite, due to strict federal safety regulations governing the use of chlorine gas. Chlorine gas often boosts one of the four trihalomethane compounds in water treatment facilities above federal limits. Limits in most states, as set by the federal government, were 80 parts per billion for each individual treatment facility at the beginning of 2006. It is my understanding that because of the chlorine versus sodium hyperchlorite dilemma, many water treatment facilities are struggling with staying within state regulations. In fact, in some states, such as my new home state of North Carolina, treatment facilities are required by state laws to send out letters to each citizen in any affected community warning of levels that are above the federal limits.

There are other chlorine treatment by-products, such as haleocedic acid, which have recently been revised to limits of 60 parts per billion. The longer chlorinated water sits before being used, the more likely it will contain higher levels of carcinogenic chlorinated organic by-products. It is my understanding that the common carbon filter attached to most refrigerator ice machines and water dispensers pulls chlorination out of potable water, reducing these carcinogenic chlorine by-products.

In addition, the federal government is also looking into regulating other minerals besides arsenic, such as Boron, at community reverse osmosis (RO) plants. Until more solutions are found at water treatment facilities, under-the-sink RO units and carbon filters may be the best answer for home owners seeking to purify their drinking water.

Another solution involves buying spring water, but bacteria levels may also be an issue if the water is not consumed in a timely manner. However, most spring water is highly healthy, due to the high number of microminerals it contains, which we tend to lack in our foods because of over farming our soils. Home RO units seem to offer good protection when using tap water, but tend to extract all the minerals. Distilled water is also very pure, yet it too lacks minerals, many of which may be deficient in the cancer patient's body. Therefore, the best solution seems to be untreated well water, or spring water (that has been tested for safety), or taking micromineral and macromineral supplements, in addition to purified water (more on such supplements in a subsequent chapter).

Industrial Farming

By now, everyone is familiar with the detrimental effects of PCBs and their ability to create cancer in animals and humans. Polychlorinated Biphenyls are a mixture of chemicals which are no longer produced in the United States, but are still found in the environment. When it comes to industrial farming and mass food production, the wide use of other, similar pesticides is sad.

When I first contracted cancer, I had a discussion with another author in the field of alternative health, who had recently survived prostate cancer. Our conversation turned to the environment, and he said that there were many new Christmas tree farms cropping up in the southwestern tip of Virginia, where he lived, and he believed that the increased use of pesticides by these farms was causing many members of his community to contract cancer. Just prior to that discussion, I had been exploring the web site of the American Cancer Society, which stated there was a link between the widespread use of pesticides and the increased incidence of lymphoma. Lymphoma, the most common form of cancer, has been on the rise for a number of years.

Coincidentally, I discovered that there was a pesticide plant near my home town, and many days I could smell the pollution from it as it crossed our mountains. I also discovered that exposed insulation was shown to cause cancers. The insulation in the ceiling of our basement was exposed for the first two years we lived in our house, and we covered it all only a few months before I contracted cancer. People were saying my color was off—yellow— long before I was diagnosed, however, which falls into line with theories that it takes a year or so for an individual to contract cancer. So if we have cancer, we must look at what our environmental factors were one to two years before we are diagnosed with it, in order to pinpoint those factors that may have triggered our disease. By eliminating these factors, we further ensure a long-term recovery.

Electromagnetic Radiation (EMR)

The Biomedical Center generally counsels their patients on their environment during their wonderfully thorough interviews, which is something that traditional medicine doesn't do, or simply doesn't have the time to do. The physicians at BMC have noted several environmental factors to avoid. One of these factors is, of course, microwave ovens.

In fact, Russian scientists found microwave ovens so dangerous that the Russian government outlawed their use.

Microwave ovens tend to leak dangerous micro waves through their housing. Furthermore, micro waves have been known to remain in the food they cook. Worse yet, these ovens change the molecular structure of food. Microwaves work by dismantling the atomic structure of the food and, by doing so, they activate the atoms so they bounce off each other so rapidly that they create heat. For this reason, the BMC recommends against the use of microwave ovens because the nutritional value of microwaved foods is inferior to other forms of cooking and food preparation. For this reason, I have replaced the microwave oven in our home with a deluxe convection/toaster oven.

It is a known fact that cell phones, which also emit micro waves (this is why they get hot after continued use), cause cancerous brain tumors. As a result, brain cancer is reported by the BMC to be on the rise, as evidenced by the higher number of patients who check into the clinic with this disease. I remember a young man in his twenties, whom I met in the waiting room of the BMC, who checked into the clinic with a malignant brain tumor. He claimed it was due to his cell phone, which he used several hours a day as he traveled to various construction sites in his job as a builder.

I also have an acquaintance who had a daughter who used a cell phone for hours each day. The daughter recently passed away after a course of traditional medical treatment for a malignant brain tumor. The tumor was discovered just past the ear that she commonly pressed her cell phone to. The best way to avoid this hazard is to invest in a headset and talk on a cell phone while it is placed away from the body.

Areas with powerful electrical fields are very dangerous to our health. In fact, all electrical devices—shavers, hair dryers, stoves, washing machines—emit a field of electromagnetic radiation that may be hazardous to our health with regular use, particularly if the devices touch our bodies. We can't avoid all electrical devices but we can limit our exposure to them and protect ourselves against them when we need to use them.

As documented through Kurlian photography, each living thing has an aura surrounding it, which can be visible when photographed. A bioelectromagnetic field surrounds each of us. When this field is disturbed by electromagnetic devices, it may contribute to disease. The connection between high intensity wires and cancer is well documented. In fact, research shows that people who live in close proximity to these wires are more likely to contract leukemia cancers. The BMC is aware of this, and may recommend relocation to such patients.

Television sets have been known for many decades to emit electromagnetic radiation that is hazardous if we sit too close to it. As a result, the BMC advises sitting at least 10 feet away from televisions and computer screens to avoid exposure to radiation. The BMC also suggests that its patients obtain a protective screen that can be placed in front of a computer monitor. All larger computer supply houses sell these screens. Although I spend many hours each day in front of a computer screen, I have chosen to use piezo electric crystals to deflect the electromagnetics.

These crystals come in a pouch and their affects on us can be tested through kinesiology. Kinesiology, is a holistic diagnostic testing procedure that measures a person's strength when they come into contact with unhealthy substances. When touching devises that emanate EMR, or touching substances we are allergic to, our muscular strength drops dramatically, and when holding or ingesting crystalline substances, our strength dramatically increases. When these energetic responses are measured, accurate determinations are able to be made about specific things that are good or bad for an individual's health.

I was first introduced to kinesiology at a holistic health convention in Santa Ana, California, where I met Wayne Topping. Wayne W. Topping, PhD, LMT, has a doctorate degree from Victoria University in New Zealand, wrote 10 books on the subject, and has taught the art in 22 countries. He did a kinesiology demonstration with a girl from the audience who was tested for several allergies, and when her muscular strength in her arm dramatically weakened, she confirmed she was allergic to the substance she was holding in her hand. Next, Dr. Topping tested her arm strength while stating ages aloud to determine when a trauma related to the allergy may have occurred. When he stated age five, her arm weakened again. At that moment, she confirmed the psychosomatic link to her allergy, and Dr. Topping claimed he could not go any further because of her need for confidentiality. Needless to say, I was impressed. Within the past couple of years, when I tested several people who wore piezo electric crystals, and after ingesting natural crystals, such as sea salt and natural sugar, a dramatic strengthening effect resulted, even while touching electromagnetic devices that would normally weaken them. It was then I realized that EMR could be deflected with crystals, and in particular piezo electric crystals were most effective.

X-rays, Vaccines, Dental Compounds, and Cancer Treatments
The BMC, and other credible scientific sources, cite radiation from X-rays as a primary cause of cancer. Diagnostic X-rays in clinics and hospitals contribute to a cumulative build up of radiation in the body, which increases the risk of contracting cancer. In addition, some medical research suggests that radiation from just a single exposure can alter a person's DNA and cause a variety of illnesses, including cancer. Research also shows that women who get regular mammograms have a higher incidence of breast cancer.

Of all the forms of X-rays that we cancer patients undergo in an attempt to track our cancer's progress, CT scans have the most radiation, because it requires several X-rays from various angles to create a 3-D computerized image of the inside of the body. Some radiation tests have reported CT scans to have as much as 500 times the levels of radiation as one chest X-ray. Radiation levels of PET scans fall somewhere between CT scans and a chest, neck, or abdomen X-ray. Many cancers can be staged with simple low-level X-rays. In addition, there are many books available describing the safer, older method of using blood markers for tracking a person's cancer, and many physicians are still willing to use this approach if asked.

Traditional Medical Practices and Therapies
Dental fillings made of mercury have been a controversial area of immunotoxicology since the mid 1980s, when evidence suggested that silver fillings cause or worsen various health problems. Silver fillings are made of 52% mercury, as well as copper, tin, silver, and zinc. Research conducted by the University of Calgary in Canada documented that the act of chewing increased mercury levels in the mouth six fold in test subjects with silver fillings. Chewing and eating hot or acidic foods also caused the release of mercury vapor, from which residues could be found in the jaw tissue, lungs, and gastrointestinal tract. Other sites found to contain mercury included the brain, heart, and several endocrine glands.

Directly related to cancer is the effect of mercury fillings on the immune system. American dentist Dr. Eggleston did research on silver/mercury fillings, which was published in the 1984 *Journal of Prosthetic Dentistry*. He measured the T-lymphocytes on three patients before and after removing silver/mercury fillings. After removal, the percentage of T-lymphocytes (which serve as valuable cancer-killing cells) went up substantially. One patient showed an increase of 55 percent. After reinserting silver/mercury fillings in two of the patients, the percentage of T-lymphocytes decreased again. Dr. Eggleston conducted 30 more identical immune system tests, which showed an average improvement in T-cells of 30 percent.

Dr. Hal Higgins, a dentist with a master's degree in Immunology, conducted similar research and stated, "At the University of Colorado, I've measured T-cell rises of 100–300 percent after fillings were removed. These findings could mean that amalgams have some role in causing allergies and autoimmune diseases." Dr. Higgins reported that 90 percent of 2000 patients he studied with symptoms of fatigue improved after mercury-based fillings were removed. He claims that mercury interferes with the oxygen-carrying capacity of red blood cells, which leads to fatigue. In the 1975 *Critical Reviews in Toxicology*, even low levels of mercury in the body were found to slow the uptake of glucose into the brain, which is significant since glucose is the energy that fuels our brains.

If the American Dental Association were to admit that mercury-based fillings are harmful, they would also be acknowledging guilt. Such liability, in light of the fact that most people in the United States over the age of 15 have some silver/mercury fillings, would be very costly. American dentists would then be putting themselves into the position of providing free filling replacements and would be subject to an onslaught of legal action from people experiencing health problems related to mercury poisoning. For those with cancer, and others who comprehend the repercussions of carrying a poisonous compound around in their mouths, wise replacements may include porcelain, plastic and glass composite, and gold fillings. Dentists who specialize in such replacements have specialized equipment that eliminates further poisoning, which can occur from more dangerous exposure during the process.

Radiation therapy is statistically proven to cause the disease it temporarily eradicates. Although concentrated megadoses of radiation does actually kill cancer cells by frying them, this particular medical procedure also causes the build-up of radiation in the body, which statistically contributes to the recurrence of cancer in the future. Research suggests that those patients who do radiation therapy have a greater chance of contracting cancer for a second time, and the risks increase with age. The older a person who's had radiation therapy gets, the more likely he or she will contract cancer again. It appears that radiation therapy should be a last resort, because of these facts. However, if it means saving a life, and if there are no other options, perhaps it may be the best choice for some cancer patients.

Chemotherapy is the process of killing all newly-dividing cells in the body, cancer cells being the most rapidly dividing cells. But it also causes the same condition it attempts to cure. In fact, the oncologist from whom I got a second opinion showed me studies indicating that chemo treatments for Hodgkin's lymphoma show the highest incidence of return between five and thirteen years. Sometimes people get a worse strain of cancer, such as non-Hodgkin's lymphoma. In addition, there are a number of side effects that can lead to death or other diseases. When we take large megadoses of toxins in our veins, after all, it makes sense. Therefore, traditional medicine's prescription for remission that involves megadoses of chemotherapy drugs is not likely to be the best choice to extend our lives.

Nutritional Degradation

The American Cancer Society, in the November/December, 1999, *Clinician's Issue, Nutrition for the Person with Cancer, p. 347*, reports that a third of all cancers could be prevented by a change in diet and lifestyle—by increasing the intake of fruits and vegetables, reducing the consumption of red meat and animal fat, and increasing exercise. The Harvard School of Public Health claims that up to 65% of all cancers can be prevented by a change in diet and lifestyle.

In order to fully understand the correlation between cancer and nutrition, we need to look at some statistics related to certain cancers, and at the history of food production. Since the early 1900s the incidence of breast cancer has risen dramatically.

For example, approximately 100 years ago women in Japan rarely developed breast cancer. They had a diet of fresh rice, vegetables, and a small amount of fish. But studies show that if they eat the standard Western diet, consisting primarily of meat, dairy products, eggs, and foods that are processed, canned, preserved, and fried, the incidence of breast cancer will be higher.

As we examine the history of food production in the United States, we look back to the middle of the last century. That is when the introduction of mass food production, combined with the reduction in family farms, began the decrease in the nutritional value of food. This problem is spreading to other parts of the world. Mass production farming is becoming accepted as the way to greater profits. But at the same time, nutritional depletion results from over farming the land.

In addition, in order to increase profits, farming corporations have genetically modified seeds to make crops more resistant to bugs and frost and more likely to increase in size. These foods often have less nutritional value than home-grown, family farmed, or organically farmed foods.

Genetics

Genetic predisposition, or hereditary factors, is one of the most scientific explanations for why people contract various forms of cancer. In my case, contracting the exact same type of cancer as my mother had, at almost exactly the same age, showed there was some type of blueprint in my body. When the other factors of diet and environment were present, the illness was like a dormant seed planted in fertile soil.

I believe that if my stress level weren't at an all-time high with bringing up my teenagers, and if my diet hadn't been poor, I wouldn't have triggered the genetic code that caused my illness. Perhaps if science included all variables when researching genetics—such as diet, lifestyle, and environment—it would give us a better perspective on the role genetics play in contracting cancer.

Lifestyle

Scientific research shows that lifestyle plays an important role in contracting cancer. Everybody is aware that smoking increases a person's chance of contracting cancer. Approximately one-third of all cancer deaths in the United States are a result of smoking. Tobacco is highly carcinogenic. It has been linked to lung, mouth, throat, esophagus, bladder, pancreas, uterine, cervical, and kidney cancers.

In addition, specific eating habits have been linked to certain cancers. For example, a high-fat low-fiber diet has been linked to cancers of the breast, colon, endometrium, and gallbladder. Obesity has been linked to a variety of cancers. Cancers of the esophagus, throat, and liver have been linked to the heavy consumption of alcohol. Some research suggests that people who have been sexually promiscuous are more prone to cervical cancer. Also, it is common knowledge that excess exposure to the sun increases the risk of skin cancer. Finally, research is increasingly linking use of hormones by women to hormone-based cancers.

The immune system is a crucial component in causing cancer. For example, HIV patients, who have reduced immunity to many diseases, have been known to contract a wide array of cancers.

In addition, stress has been linked to degradation of the immune system. For example, a teen's stress over attending the prom often leads to a break-out of pimples or a rash. The immune system therefore has a direct mental component, which is discussed further in the chapter on mind-body interventions.

Consider modern stress factors alone (overworked families, hectic lifestyles from an unnaturally fast pace in our society, etc.) and we can hypothesize that cancer is an immune disorder largely connected to stress, because excess stress absolutely reduces our immunity to cancer cells, which normally exist in our bodies. An unhealthy amount of stress can lead to our immune system not recognizing these foreign cells, and they are then allowed to grow. We must learn tools to reduce stress, such as counseling, self-hypnosis, meditation, or imagery. These are further discussed in the final chapter of this book.

Exercise

Some research indicates that exercise is beneficial for recovering from cancer, partly due to its stress reduction capabilities. In addition, during and immediately after exercise, hypermetabolic cancer cells take up less glucose, while the muscles take up more. Therefore, the cancer cells are somewhat starved.

Exercise increases a person's ability to fight cancer by strengthening the body and increasing circulation. Laboratory studies have shown that cancer cells cannot grow in a highly oxygenated environment. As exercise increases blood oxygen levels, the double dividing cells that characterize cancer simply do not divide. Oxygen therapy grew out of this research, and is still used successfully to fight cancer by both traditional and alternative medicine doctors today. One theory is that those who contract cancer do not get enough oxygen. If this is true, then a person with cancer may benefit from increased exercise.

Another benefit of exercise is that it causes the nervous system to naturally release endorphins (a natural morphine), which provide a powerful stress relief. Exercise also allows for better sleep, a time when the body can repair and rebuild itself. Exercise allows people to enter into a deeper level of sleep and stay there for longer periods of time without waking. Sleep research shows that if we reach delta brain waves once or twice during our normal sleep cycle, we are much more rested upon awakening. Exercise increases the chance for delta sleep, which has cancer recovery benefits.

Sleeping Habits

Sleep deprivation not only leads to decreased antioxidant production, according to some recent research released in 2004, but also increases stress, counteracting a person's ability to fight cancer. Adequately sleeping between the hours of 10:00 pm and 2:00 am increases the body's natural production of antioxidants. Antioxidants reduce free radicals and therefore increase our immune system's ability to fight cancer and other intruding biomatter. For this reason, it is best for a cancer patient to go to bed by 10:00 pm and to get a full night's sleep.

The Sad Truth about the Limitations of Traditional Medicine

There are only three ways medical doctors in the United States are trained and licensed to treat cancer: surgery, chemotherapy, and radiation. They know nothing about alternative medicine (I will tell you why later in this chapter).

In the vast majority of states, if they were to practice anything other than traditional medicine they would either lose their license to practice medicine, get arrested for breaking the law, or risk lawsuits from patients or patients' family members. It is, however, ethical and legal for most physicians in the United States to advise their patients against using alternative methods. Most physicians generally do not know which ones are most effective, nor would they tell you if they did know, since it is generally too risky for them professionally.

If the patient asks, most doctors will often say that alternative medicine clinics are all ineffective and they will then avoid getting into trouble if the patient tries alternative medicine and dies. Therefore, most physicians' advice on alternative medicines and the clinics that use them is completely useless.

While we Americans cannot get good advice from our physicians, medical doctors in England, Germany, France, China, and Japan are prescribing herbal medicines for disease, and they are often incorporated into conventional medical therapies. We have an underground network of naturopaths practicing in most states, many of whom must find loopholes in the law in order to practice. This puts the advancement of our lopsided medical system significantly behind those of other developed countries.

If it weren't for the courageous natural medicine and supplement companies, and the natural health practitioners—and both are consistently threatened by the FDA—we Americans would have no other choice but to use pharmaceuticals, which often can result in other illnesses and even death. The sad truth is that it will be slow to change, because our current government structure allows the funding of government officials' campaigns through private interest groups.

In most cases, traditional medicine offers far less than an 80 percent success rate (which is what the BMC claims) in putting most cancers "in remission" for five years. Yet most Americans put their faith in those therapies because they are the only ones cancer clinics and doctors know or are allowed to use.

Now, with so many intelligent people in many pharmaceutical companies' research and development departments, we must ask ourselves why these companies ignore the natural medicines offering the highest cure rate, such as herbal medicines for cancer. Also, why aren't medical students taught about natural cures?

To answer these questions, we must look at the entire American medical system: its teaching institutions and its financial and political structure.

Traditional Medical Education and Treatment Programs

Medical science bases most of its findings on studies funded by the pharmaceutical industry. The only way a pharmaceutical company will fund such studies is if they can patent the synthetic chemicals they produce and thus recoup their research and development costs and make a substantial profit. Therefore, medical research produces statistics showing the effectiveness of pharmaceutical medicine, not alternative or natural medicine, because these cannot be patented.

The NIH generally does not commonly fund studies of alternative medicine programs, either. In their cancer research, which is highly limited, alternative medicine substances are measured for their ability to be cytotoxic (substances that kill cancer in a petri dish). The problem with this approach is that natural cures are not cytotoxic; instead, they mend bodily systems so the body fights illness through normalization.

Only when the NIH begins to fund studies on human subjects, and increases the data that support the efficacy of natural cures, will natural cures gain public credibility and have equal weight with traditional medical approaches. Until then, a high number of the studies cited on the NCCAM web site are derived from studies done overseas. In addition, there are many loosely funded valuable studies that have not entered public awareness.

So how is our government set up in a way that works to the advantage of corporate America, and not the consumer of medicine? We must ask ourselves how pharmaceutical medicines are regulated and sold in the United States. Why is it that we Americans are told that we must buy name-brand pharmaceutical products here in the United States, made by U.S. companies, when these same medicines are sold at a much lower cost in other countries as generic medicines? No wonder many Americans are trying to circumvent this structure. Why can't we buy these American pharmaceutical generics in America at lower prices? Perhaps these questions can be answered by looking at our political system—specifically at private interest groups and the political climate of the FDA.

On December 16, 2004, I saw Aaron Brown with CNN News discussing a revealing survey with 20-year FDA employee Dr. David Graham. The survey revealed the monetary motivations behind the pharmaceutical approval process. The survey showed that approximately 20 percent of the FDA researchers polled felt pressured by their superiors to approve drugs they thought were potentially unsafe for public consumption. Two-thirds are less than fully confident in the safety of drugs on the market.

On August 12, 2005, Lou Dobbs, also on CNN, reported that special interest groups spent a record $2.15 billion on lobbying members of Congress and 220 other federal agencies in 2004, according to *Political Money Line*, a nonpartisan research service that tracks campaign contributions. That figure represents an increase of 34 percent in lobbying spending in 2001. Dobbs discussed what he referred to as a "revolving door" between Capitol Hill and K Street, stating that 43 percent of the eligible congressional members who left the government have become lobbyists. Nearly 250 former members of Congress and federal agency chiefs have become lobbyists since 1998. Although lobbyists are required to report who pays them and how much money they are paid, nearly 85 percent of the top 250 lobbying firms have failed to file one or more required forms, according to the Center for Public Integrity.

Members of Congress have received $18 million to travel the world at the expense of private organizations, according to *Political Money Line*. More than 6,200 trips were funded for 628 lawmakers, both Democrats and Republicans.

Alex Knott, Lobby Watch project manager at the Center for Public Integrity, in an interview with Lou Dobbs indicated that a significant problem with our government exists when special interest groups "have a greater ability to influence members of Congress and agencies than average American citizens do."

Why would pharmaceutical companies want to fund research in alternative medicine if it isn't profitable? Now we know why people complain about limited research into natural cures. Again, you cannot patent herbs and diets, so it is unprofitable and therefore a waste of corporate America's time. In fact, it is potentially more profitable for them to spend money to block research into natural cures! One look at the documentary that exposes the danger to health freedoms, "We Become Silent" (on the web site of the Alliance for Natural Health, at www.alliance-natural-health.org), and we conclude that this form of oppression is occurring on an international basis.

Furthermore, oncologists in the United States do not need to be as concerned with their success rate as those at the BMC, because it doesn't affect their reputation and therefore their profit margin. If they lose a patient, they often tell the family something to the effect that the patient lived in an era before any (traditional medical) cure for his or her condition was known, expressing their condolences. The family usually claims, "Well, Dr.____ was a good doctor and did all that he or she could do. Someday there'll be a cure."

Conversely, if a patient dies after going to an alternative cancer clinic, even though these clinics often get the patients that allopathic medicine has given up on and sent home to die, the family may claim, "It was that quackery they practiced at that alternative clinic in Mexico that killed them." In these cases, we are obviously swayed to believe that Western medicine has all the answers here in this country—even though other developed countries are commonly implementing complementary, natural medicine therapies for a variety of illnesses with notable success! I could give numerous examples of natural cures used successfully overseas that the vast majority of Americans simply know nothing about.

To be fair, at the other end of the spectrum, the likelihood that some cancer treatment centers in Tijuana with useless therapies probably wind up killing some people, who might have lived if they'd followed a traditional medical approach, is real. A friend of mine had four children and a wonderful husband, whom she referred to as her "soul-mate." These people were both artists, love birds, two peas in a pod, and a joy to be around.

Her husband found a lump under his arm and let it grow to the point that it was uncomfortable. He finally got it checked by a traditional medical doctor and found that it was cancer, well advanced. He opted to go to a clinic somewhere in Mexico (not Tijuana). I remember that she and her husband checked into the clinic for several weeks and used all their money in an effort to cure him, to no avail. He came back with barely enough energy to die in his home with his family around him. It was a sad ending for all of us who knew them. My friend kept all of us apprised by e-mailing us her journaling of their daily and weekly trials and tribulations.

Oddly, I didn't even think about this when I chose the Hoxsey clinic, because I had done my research. I found the supportive documentation. I talked to many people who'd had Hoxsey therapy. I knew it would work before I went there, because I'd already started making progress on my own with similar herbal medicines. Essentially, it was a safe bet.

It is wise to stay abreast of new traditional and alternative cancer therapies. And even though I don't trust the political aspects of our medical bureaucracy, and our seemingly bribed government officials, I still want to make it clear that I believe in the humanitarian efforts of the majority of allopathic health practitioners. Although some physicians enter the field because of the money, most do so in order to help people. They are simply ignorant of natural cures, due to the political environment in America.

The Insights of Lorraine Day, MD

A good source of information on natural recovery methods that had insights into the political environment of the medical profession is a video called *Cancer Doesn't Scare Me Anymore*, by Dr. Lorraine Day, MD, a former teaching physician.

Dr. Day's story starts with her 15 years on the faculty at the University of California in San Francisco. During this time, she discovered she contracted breast cancer. After doing a thorough investigation into the clinical efficacy of traditional medicine's cancer therapies, she decided that the two most popular ones, radiation and chemotherapy, don't cure cancer, they actually cause it. She decided to treat herself through nutrition, lifestyle changes, and spirituality. She was close to death at one point, with the tumor the size of a grapefruit. But when she fully implemented her self-designed methods, she ended up curing her condition without any chemotherapy, radiation, or surgical removal.

Her methods include the following.

1. Diet—Consume a diet high in fruits, whole grains, and vegetables, and low in animal fats.

2. Exercise—Exercise regularly to increase circulation. Some research shows that four hours a week of exercise can result in a marked decrease in the chances of contracting breast cancer.

3. Hydration—Water is the best hydrating liquid. Caffeine and alcohol dehydrate the body; these diuretics take more water out of the body than they put into it. We lose 10 glasses of water each day just by living. Our body is 75 percent water; the brain is 85 percent water. Dehydration is a major cause of all diseases, including cancer.

4. Sunlight—Sunlight boosts the immune system and decreases the size of internal cancerous tumors.

5. Temperance—Eliminate all harmful substances, such as tobacco, caffeine, alcohol, sugar, aspartame, MSG, processed foods, food preservatives, food chemicals and dyes, and drugs—prescription and illegal. Rebuilding the body with natural food may allow one to eventually get off prescription medicines. Her theory is that the side effects of many of these medicines can contribute to the growth of cancerous tumors.

6. Fresh air—Outside air is essential for good health. Dr. Day's research shows that cancerous tumors grow twice as fast in patients who breathe mostly indoor air as compared to those who breathe mostly outdoor air.

7. Proper Rest—Healing hormones are produced after 9:30 pm, when all cancer patients should be in bed.

8. Stress—Stress should be combated with God. God has the ability to heal all illnesses.

9. Attitude of gratitude—Blaming others or God for an illness, or whining and complaining, will prevent one from getting well. Be thankful for your life and for what you have.

10. A spirit of benevolence—Pray for others. Don't watch television; the majority of news is bad news and therefore unhealthy. Read the Bible and high-quality Christian books; listen to Christian music. Eliminate every negative thought from your mind, so you have mostly positive thoughts.

Although I don't agree with every aspect of Dr. Day's methods, most are noteworthy. For example, people who aren't Christian could read books and listen to music from their own faith tradition and get the benefits of connecting to their higher power.

Her statistics about the benefits of increased circulation may be further documented by a study I ran across, involving 4,700 women, about wearing bras. Women who never wore a bra had the same incidence of breast cancer as men, in whom breast cancer is extremely rare. It is postulated by medical anthropologist Sydney Ross Singer that the lymphatic vessels are blocked by the bra, thus preventing lymphocytes (white blood cells) from destroying abnormal cells, such as cancer cells. From Professor Singer's results, it appears that it would be prudent for women to wear bras fewer than 12 hours at a time, to discard bras that leave red lines on the skin, which shows reduced circulation (underwires, push-up types), and never wearing them at night. Women who wear a bra 24 hours a day are 125 times more likely to develop breast cancer than women who don't wear a bra at all.

With the above methods, Dr. Lorraine Day's grapefruit-sized tumor (documented with pictures) disappeared, her cancer was put into a solid remission, and she rose from her deathbed to share her story and her methods. It is a phenomenal story of bravery, discovering the truth, and a combination of spiritual and physical healing.

A Teaching MD's Discoveries about Medical Politics

Dr. Lorraine Day saw what traditional medicine does to cancer patients and bravely walked away from it, committing to a path that would not inflict more misery and suffering or shorten her life. She confirms many of my opinions. She points out that pharmaceutical companies provide huge sums of money to fund medical research in an effort to discover more drugs that can be patented to treat disease. They are not going to provide funding for research into natural recovery methods, because they can't patent and market therapies such as proper sleep, a healthy diet, sunlight, exercise, water consumption, and other natural cures, because they need a return on their research dollar.

She makes it very clear that when pharmaceutical companies provide large research grants and hundreds of millions of dollars to medical schools, they have an enormous amount of clout, and they directly and indirectly control much of what is being taught to medical doctors in training. She emphasizes that doctors are not taught about the causes of cancer. She points out that a deficiency of radiation and chemotherapy does not cause cancer, so taking them does not prevent or cure it in the long run. It is a well-known fact that both these methods cause cancer. If the real causes of cancer were to be seriously considered in treating it, then the effective treatment would involve restoring deficiencies, changing the environment, and more.

If traditional medicine therapies don't kill cancer patients, they often maim them for life or result in cancers later in life. Unfortunately, children suffer the most, because their bodies are often scorched for up to three years with therapies so toxic that many of them who survive the treatment are left permanently disabled. Yet from the beginning of medical school these are the only methods physicians are taught for treating cancer; and, therefore, the only methods a medical doctor in the United States can legally recommend or administer. Sadly, in many states, if parents refuse to put their children through such tortures they could be breaking the law.

In fact, if physicians don't prescribe the three traditional medical treatments, they are likely to be severely disciplined by their hospital or other medical governing bodies. In addition, they may lose their license to practice medicine if alleged to be using non-FDA approved medicines, or unauthorized experimental research. In the vast majority of states, it is against the law for medical doctors to treat cancer with anything other than surgery, radiation, or chemotherapy. And in many states, such as California, a doctor can refuse to provide care for a cancer patient if he or she refuses traditional therapy.

How the Hoxsey Therapy Works

Hoxsey therapy works with the causes of cancer. I will explain the system as I know it through the naturopathic research I discovered, which included several interviews with Dr. Gutierrez, a physician at the BMC.

Our immune system has multiple defense categories, but once cancer immunity is compromised, the intruding cancer cells that regularly form within a normal human body proliferate, increasing in size and territory. Eventually cancer cells take over vital organs and lead to death, if every last cancer cell is not completely destroyed by either the immune system or traditional medicine's toxic treatment programs.

White blood cells, called T lymphocytes, identify and then destroy cancerous cells, viruses, and microorganisms like bacteria and fungi. The thymus is the most important gland of our immune system, and from it T-cells mature, thus the "T" in the name. This is where the T-cells learn to differentiate between "self" and "non-self" cells, and either tolerate ("self") or destroy ("non-self") them.

Unfortunately the thymus is susceptible to stress overload, and therefore to a breakdown in efficiency. This may lead to the immune system not recognizing a cancerous cell or foreign invader, and therefore adopting the cell as part of "self." This chain reaction has been linked to a variety of conditions, including cancer.

The goal of the Hoxsey therapy is to rebuild the immune system so that it learns to recognize the "non-self" cells again—those that are cancerous— and to destroy them by eating up tumors from the inside out. The system entails the following:

1) Supplements rebuild deficiencies and inhibit or eliminate cancer cell growth.

2) Herbal blood purifiers cleanse the organs of toxins. Many organs contribute to normal immune function and stimulate the growth of bone marrow immune cells that are toxic to cancer cells. Some of the external herbal therapies form a barrier of white blood cells that kill all the cancerous tissue around tumors, allowing for escharotics, or the extraction of tumors near the surface. In addition, the internal herbal compounds kill viruses, bacteria, intestinal microorganisms, candida, and other precancerous microorganisms, while the potassium iodide base helps break down the fibrotic (tumor) tissues and provide improved body fluid alkalinity.

3) An all-natural, alkaline-forming diet inhibits cancer cell growth and increases vitamin and mineral nutrients in the body, contributing to increased immune response and carcinogen and toxin elimination

4) Lifestyle counseling helps discover environmental factors, such as toxins in one's community, home, or place of work; and stress reduction, including an analysis of stress triggers.

5) Other natural therapies may be added that have been proven to be helpful in addition to the traditional Hoxsey therapy above, which may include Chinese medicines, special plants such as cactuses, or vaccines that have proven to be especially effective with specific cancers.

What is It Like to Encounter Obstinate Allopathic Physicians?

Sometimes people with various health challenges, particularly cancer, ask me what I think about obstinate or close-minded allopathic physicians. I tell them that in this day and age, when holistic health and alternative/complementary medicines are reaching an all-time high in public interest, wider use, and effectiveness, they have a right to choose their physicians. If a doctor's advice is to stay away from alternative/complementary medicine, I tell the patient that he or she may want to find another physician who is better educated or more open-minded.

However, if the doctor claims that the alternative/complementary methods do not have as much research to support their claims, this may not necessarily be untrue. Many of these therapies do not have the financial backing behind them, such as pharmacological medicines, because natural health nutrients or compounds cannot be patented.

However, as time goes on, there is more valuable and convincing research being conducted by natural health manufacturers that demonstrates that natural health products are at least as effective as pharmaceuticals, and often are proving superior, as they often lack dangerous side effects. For example, one natural health manufacturing company—NutriCology/Allergy Research Group, has an advisory board with several NDs and MDs on it who obviously believe in exercising their right to treat patients with natural therapies. In my opinion these physicians believe in practicing with a patient-first philosophy.

I've talked to many nurses and doctors about the research I've discovered into herbal cancer cures. Many of them *actually tell me* that the reason the United States doesn't offer these therapies is because it's about money. In the majority of these conversations, which occurred before the release of this book, I hadn't alluded to this concept; they were the ones saying it first. So I know that some medical professionals are aware of the problems with the medical system in this country and would like to see it changed.

I've also met numerous physicians and nurses, many in oncology, who have anonymously told me that they've seen what chemo and disfiguring surgeries have done to patients and would choose the alternative cancer route if they contract cancer themselves.

I was told by one physician, who attended a seminar I put on at a health symposium, "We allopathic physicians are apprehensive about discussing natural health with our patients, such as herbs and supplements, since we simply didn't receive any training in this area in medical school." Others have made similar statements, and I always smile and proceed with my discussions, to take the focus off this deficiency and make them feel more comfortable when talking to me. One of my goals is to communicate openly with traditional health practitioners.

Sometimes I have been told by allopaths (particularly allopathic pharmacists) that I am dabbling in unproven and unsafe therapies. I'll never forget my daughter's physician, who said, "Tell your father to stay away from those clinics, because if he doesn't they will kill him."

Granted, there are many clinics, particularly cancer clinics, operating in Mexico—five or more just over the border in Tijuana—and not all of them have the high cure rate that the Biomedical Center has. Therefore, it is a good idea to talk to at least a few people who have survived cancer through treatment at such a clinic before committing to one. I did my research and found the Hoxsey therapy and the Biomedical Center to be the oldest, most reputable, least expensive, and most well-documented alternative, natural cancer therapy clinic in the world.

So, yes, we need to be selective, not only in the therapy we choose, but also in the physicians we choose to treat us and the opinions we decide to believe in and follow.

Summary

I must reiterate that I was fortunate to have an oncologist who was spiritually evolved enough to give me the freedom to choose my cure. At the same time he assisted me with the best tests Western medicine could provide, so I could more effectively track my progress. He stayed with me out of a sincere desire to see me get well. But my life choices were my own, unique and independent.

It is important to understand that the longevity of the Biomedical Center is based on its success rate. It's lasted more than 80 years, surviving a slew of lawsuits and harassment by the American and Mexican governments before, during, and after the time it fled the United States in 1962. It has sustained itself through an international circle of tens of thousands of cancer patients who've cured themselves with a small financial and personal investment. These people have passed the information along to others who will listen and accept that *God has left a natural cure for cancer to us on planet earth. It grows naturally, and it can be found in its most pure form at the BMC in Tijuana, Mexico!*

As Dr. Gutierrez once said in an interview I had with him about the Hoxsey system of recovery, "It won't make you more sick." The beauty of the system is that people may truly *kill their cancer without killing themselves.*

Cancer is a huge multi-billion dollar industry. Therefore, when a large amount of money is involved, in my opinion, those in control of the purse strings, figuratively speaking, should not be trusted. Money supports medical research, which results in a big business. Big business funds politicians, and politicians make laws to pay back big business's donations. The direct result is what the consumer, or cancer patient, is offered in the United States.

Anybody can understand the political system in America, in terms of what consumers are offered to cure their illnesses, except those prone to "blind acceptance," in the form of what they call patriotism. While I am extremely patriotic, my version of patriotism involves questioning the system so that the U.S. government is "for the people and by the people," as it was intended by our forefathers.

Some don't question, while some do. Some, like me, are survivors and find a way, regardless of peer pressure. They take a risk, they dare to venture out, to gamble a little bit, and they often win. These, truly, are the "exceptional patients." These are the real survivors.

I hope that some day people will band together to help change the laws in the United States and help Hoxsey therapy save more lives. People are dying needlessly, especially children with cancer. Children's cancers are under funded in pharmaceutical research, because the vast majority of people who contract cancer are adults. Of the 1.4 million Americans stricken with cancer in 2005, 12,400 are people younger than the age of 20. Pharmaceutical companies typically invest 10 years and $800 million dollars to bring new drugs to the market, according to the statistics of the Tufts Center for the Study of Drug Development. Because pediatric drugs for cancer are low-profit, even if they're discovered they're often not developed and made available. As a result, there have been several cases where children don't have access to life-saving cancer treatments.

A cover story by Liz Szabo in a July, 2005, issue of USA Today, titled, *Who's Fighting Cancer In Kids?* was a real eye-opener regarding how lethal medical politics can be to our children. It described how not one pharmaceutical company was willing to produce the drug called 131 I-MIBG, which university research pharmacists recently discovered would successfully treat a rare cancer called neuroblastoma. This reluctance is because only 650 children are afflicted with this disease each year; therefore, there simply is not enough profit in saving these kids' lives. Now tell me there isn't something wrong here! God help us...and this is the same country that our founders committed to being a "nation, under God." We're missing the big picture here as we suffer from the inadequacies of a system that relies on self-serving medical politics to cure life-threatening illnesses.

Don't get me wrong; I am very patriotic. I believe the United States is a great country, obviously the number-one world power, which offers unmatched opportunities to become a success doing whatever you desire. I certainly appreciate our freedom of speech laws that prevent people like me from getting killed or locked up for our opinions.

I simply believe that with the right political powers at the helm, we could become a leader in alternative medicine, rather than being considered behind the times by other developed countries. Most other developed countries are more educated and proficient in utilizing natural medicines in place of or in conjunction with traditional medicine.

Cancer is a multi-billion dollar industry. We need to put healing first, and making a profit from illness and disease secondary.

"The love of money is the root of all evil." 1 Timothy 6:10

For more facts about the relationship between environmental factors and health, explore the research listed on the web site of the World Health Organization, at www.WHO.org. For more information on world health politics and our freedoms, go to www. alliance-natural-health.org.

Chapter 8

The Anti-Cancer Herbs

In this chapter we will examine and compare the cancer-curing herbal formulas from three primary sources: the mystic and naturopath Edgar Cayce; the naturopath Harry Hoxsey, founder of the Biomedical Center, and the research and development labs at Parke-Davis and Company at the turn of the twentieth century, when herbal medicines were prominent in the treatment of disease.

Edgar Cayce's Anti-cancer Herbs

Cayce's herbal formulas surfaced while he was in a state of hypnosis and, therefore, many people believe they were divinely inspired. Regardless of this, they have been proven to be effective in curing various illnesses, and for our purposes, particularly cancer. In order to examine Cayce's cancer-curing formulas, we must, therefore, explore Cayce's readings. As we do so, readers should keep in mind that Edgar Cayce, when he spoke from the meditative state from which he gave his readings, used a syntax that is somewhat difficult to follow.

Now we will proceed to look at one specific case, where Cayce received information from the collective unconscious, or the spirit realm, for the purpose of helping a person with throat cancer:

Case #4695-1
"In the blood supply, we find this deficient in the rebuilding properties and an excess of the white blood supply, with a deficiency in the red blood, and that bacilli carried in the blood stream showing the cause, the character, or conditions as exist in the system, for the system attempts to create that necessary to war against the ravages of the sarcoma germs in the blood supply...this produces the condition in blood supply, the condition over the whole system, and especially that as causes the condition in the circulation through the capillary... the specific condition as found in the cuticle, for with the system attempting to eliminate, and so much of the leukocyte forces used in the destruction of the bacilli in blood supply, the capillary circulation becomes clogged and choked, and dross left without the elimination being properly cared for.

In the nerve system, we find in this much of the condition of taxation, for with the vital forces in body being attacked by these bacilli, the nerve centers become depleted in their ability to function in the normal manner. Hence, the tired debilitation at times that appears in the body, the feelings as if there is no use to fight against existing condition, lack of vital forces in nerve supply to meet the needs of the physical forces in the body.

In the organs of the body, in the throat, lungs and larynx: In the portion of the throat at the base, or root, or tongue, we find this condition where cellular forces show the surrounding of those conditions producing the ravages in the system, first produced by too much of certain elements in the system as taken for cathartics, and with other stimulation produced the irritation that brought about the condition which separates itself, and because the germ forces as created in the system itself... In the functioning of other organs, we find those of the system that produce the change in circulation by the action of that organ's secretions, as we find in spleen, pancreas, liver, and kidneys. All engorged to meet the needs of the system, a normal condition for existing conditions in the body. These conditions may be assisted and the condition brought to that of little effect in the system if cared for in proper manner. Then do this: We would take first in the system these properties:

Tincture Wild Cherry Bark	1/2 ounce
Tincture Stillingia	1/2 ounce
Tincture Yellow Dock Root	1/2 ounce
Tincture of Poke Root	1/2 ounce
Tincture of Burdock Root	1/2 ounce
Iodide Potassium	3/4 ounce
Sufficient Simple syrup to make 6 ounces	

Shake solution well together until all is dissolved. The dose would be half a teaspoonful four times each day—letting one dose be just before retiring. And apply to the body through the solar plexus center, and at the second cervical, the plates or vibrations that will be found in the Abram's Oscillator for the sarcoma germ. This will, within three to five weeks, reduce the condition to that of almost nil. Then the general health afterwards must be kept. We will find through these forces we will bring the better conditions for this body."

According to documented correspondence, the man referenced above went into remission in three to five weeks. In another case, where there was a skin tumor, lack of blood supply, and other precancerous conditions, the following herbal regimen, with colonics, was recommended:

Case #1012-1:

"Then, in meeting the needs of the conditions of this body, as we find in the present, it would be in making the condition within the organs themselves so that there would be a purification, as it were, of the blood stream. Then the more perfect coordination in the eliminating forces of the system itself. And then the correction or absorption of the conditions that have already taken on the form of segregation in a manner.

Do not operate, then, in the present; else the body would not, under the present conditions, ever be as well again—if it were operated on in the PRESENT, see? For the body necessitates being built up. Then if built up, there may be produced that in the condition of the body where absorption, eliminations, coordinations of a more perfect blood supply, nerve energies, would make for revivifying. For the conditions are not in that state where they have separated themselves entirely, but there IS that combativeness yet in the vital forces of the body. But it is losing ground rather than gaining, in the present. We would begin, then, with first preparing a compound to be taken internally, in this manner:

To 1 gallon of Distilled Water, add:

Wild Cherry Bark	1/2 ounce
Sarsaparilla Root	1/2 ounce
Yellow Dock Root	1/2 ounce
Burdock Root	1/2 ounce
Prickly ash Bark	1/4 ounce
Elder Flower	2 ounces

...We would begin almost immediately with high enemas. And this doesn't mean just an ordinary enema. Use the colon tube, to eliminate or evacuate the whole of the colon tract. Take one such colonic irrigation every week for three weeks. THEN take one every THREE weeks, see?"

Colonics were often recommended in addition to herbal and other treatments, in order to reduce toxicity in the organs. A common denominator in the cancer readings is descriptions of the organs that are responsible for proper immune function and the forces at work in a body that is challenged with cancer. Edgar Cayce consistently used the words "segregation," "separation," or "creative in itself" in order to describe hypermetabolic cellular activity, or cancer cells and tumors. He also used "purification" of the "blood" relative to organ cleansing and detoxification.

It is important to consider that each reading had different combinations of herbs that were suggested for the specific, causative health conditions that preceded the onset of cancer. Therefore, as with all herbal cancer therapies, not only was the cancer being eradicated, but the causative conditions within the body that preceded the illness were being rectified as well, allowing for a more effective, long-lasting cure. This causative diagnostic characteristic may also be noted in the following reading:

Case #409-7, Cancer Warning?:
"The throwing off of refuse and its being able to be centralized, or sufficient of the properties in body—or the lymph and blood—to

segregate same, should be taken as a good omen, of the ability to create in system those of the proper coagulating elements in system. This is a very good study here, taken properly. Where these have been segregated, and where it has been taken up by the lower portion of the epidermis formation, these should be brought to the surface by the applications of properties that will cause same to SEPARATE itself from the system, or in an ASTRINGENT in the nature of an antiseptic in its reaction, that there may not be in the destroyed tissue that which will cause any condition to become in the form of the creative in itself."

The consensus among naturopaths is that cancer is an immune disorder caused by an immune deficiency. A compromised immune system results from the organs, such as the liver, essentially getting clogged with contaminants (metals, toxins, etc.). So the goals of herbal medicines include "the throwing off of refuse," as Cayce states above, by using herbs known as blood purifiers, or blood cleaners, which were recommended by Cayce and, as we will see later, by other great naturopaths at that time in medical history.

There were several readings recommending that the patient find the herbs growing in their home town area, pick them, and prepare infusions— that is, simmer the medicinal parts of the plants (roots, berries, leaves, flowers) in water to create an extract. In some cases, Cayce suggested that his clients find the plants dried and packaged for sale. Sometimes tinctures were recommended that had already been prepared with alcohol or glycerin, a process that allows the herbs to be suspended in a solution that does not require refrigeration. Sometimes combining the herbs with potassium iodide was recommended.

Today, as far as I am aware, all herbal manufacturers in the United States use alcohol suspension, which is not ideal for the medicinal treatment of cancer. The process of suspending herbal medicines in alcohol has the effect of reducing its potency.

The herbs that Cayce most consistently recommended for cancer are those I refer to as Cayce anti-cancer herbs; they are listed below.

Potassium Iodine
Licorice
Red Clover
Burdock Root
Stillingia Root
Berberis Root
Poke Root
Cascara Sagrada
Prickly Ash Bark
Buckthorn Bark
Wild Cherry Bark
Yellow Dock Root
Elder Berry/Flower
Sarsaparilla Root

In addition to the herbs recommended above, the herb *plantain* was often recommended, most often for the treatment of external cancers. Cayce patients were told to create a plantain salve to be applied to the skin, forming a white blood cell barrier around the tumor. This causes the tumor to die and come to the surface, where it is able to be extracted.

Of the Cayce anti-cancer herbs, two were also commonly used by Native Americans and naturopaths (they were called eclectic physicians around the turn of the twentieth century): red clover and burdock. Cayce most often combined these powerful blood cleansers with prickly ash, yellow dock, and other blood purifiers.

Burdock was recommended approximately 160 times by Cayce for various health conditions, including 40 cases where he recommended it for cancer. In one case, Cayce also recommended poke weed for cancer as follows:

> Case #3515-1:
> "Eat very young poke—the tender shoots of the pokeweed to act as a purifier for the body. Prepare it in this manner: When cutting sufficient to make a small dish or salad, put in cold water and let come to a boil. Strain or drain off, as in a colander—or put in a colander and let all the juice drain off. Then prepare or cook the remaining leaves with other greens, especially such as lamb's tongue and wild mustard—about an equal quantity. This eaten once a week will purify the whole body."

Cayce specified the use of poke in approximately 50 cases, often with the use of the herbs stillingia and burdock (also used by Hoxsey), and the alkalizer compound Hoxsey recommended, potassium iodide. In another case involving cancer (#5521-1), most likely a type of lymphoma, Cayce recommended poke with another blood cleanser, wild cherry, and the well-known lymphatic restoring herb elder berry/flower—which maintains a cleansing action for the lymphatic system.

The action behind prickly ash, also a Hoxsey herb, was summarized in the following case, #1012-1, involving cancer:

> "The prickly ash bark acts directly with the activative forces in the liver itself, in the gall duct, and as a stimulant to the pancreas and spleen's activity."

Prickly ash was recommended in more than 100 cases, 50 of them combining it with burdock.

Cayce also recommended the use of stillingia more than 200 times, most often for liver function and eliminations. In 59 cases it was combined with potassium iodide.

> Case #5509-1:
> "Stillingia—an active force in the functioning of the liver, as related to the pancreas..."

Case #404-4:
"Other properties; as in stillingia, make for that activity with the pulsations between the liver, the heart, the kidneys, in such a manner as to still the circulatory forces there."

Licorice and cascara sagrada were often recommended together in the same compound. Licorice was suggested more than 60 times, and in 40 of these cases it was combined with cascara sagrada.

Potassium iodide, a compound of iodine and potassium, was suggested by Cayce on more than 200 occasions, and often in combination with herbal blood purifiers. For rectifying conditions involving blood toxicity, such as in case numbers 3996-1 and 4697-1, he recommended using potassium iodide with yellow dock, burdock, stillingia, and poke.

In the following case involving cancer, he listed several herbs and their actions:

Case #1012-1,
"...The first ingredient, the Wild Cherry Bark, is a direct activative force upon the pneumogastrics and the pulmonary system.

The Sarsaparilla works with the gastric juices of the stomach, and the eliminations in the peristaltic movement through the intestinal tract.

The Yellow Dock acts with the DIGESTIVE fluids themselves. The Burdock is an activative force with or in the juices through the hydrochloric area, or in the pylorus.

The Prickly Ash Bark acts directly with the activative forces in the liver itself, in the gall duct, and as a stimulant to the pancreas and spleen's activity.

The Elder Flower acts with the increasing flow for the NATURAL eliminations through the system to the organic activities of the system in its relation to the sex activities of the body.

Then the preservative, with the activative forces in the gum, makes for an effectual activity without producing a disagreeable effect in the activity of the others."

Summary of Cayce's Anti-Cancer Herbs

Of the dozens of prescriptions given specifically for the treatment of cancer, some people did not report back their results, and many results were not documented because they were not in the form of written correspondence. As a result, the half dozen cures that were recorded include:

#570	male- cancer of the abdomen
#757	female- cancer of the skin
#1500	female- sarcoma of the breast and legs
#1967	male- cancer of the ear
#2457	female- cancer of the breast
#4901	male- cancer of the lip

Most people would agree that the way this great naturopath accessed his information was nothing short of miraculous. Treating the causative conditions in the body proved he was ahead of his time. Today, medicine treats cancer by directly targeting cancer cells, ignoring the disease's causative factors. This was not Cayce's way of treating cancer. Therefore, under this premise, his patients probably received a more permanent cure than patients using traditional medicine.

Harry Hoxsey's Anti-cancer Herbs

Some writings I've encountered in my research indicate that the formula in the most commonly used tonic, the "black tonic," has been altered over the years, for the purpose of treating various modern cancers more effectively. Listed below are the original ingredients, which were published in the June 12, 1964 issue of the *Journal of the American Medical Association* (JAMA) after an "investigation" into the Hoxsey Cancer Clinic of Dallas, Texas. Naturopathic physician Harry Hoxsey had been given orders to properly label the tonic for the purpose of shipping and commerce. As a result, the Hoxsey Tonic was able to be analyzed by the AMA laboratories. They found that in a 16-ounce bottle, each 5 cc. contained the following:

Potassium Iodine	150 mg.
Licorice	20 mg.
Red Clover	20 mg.
Burdock Root	10 mg.
Stillingia Root	10 mg.
Berberis Root	10 mg.
Poke Root	10 mg.
Cascara Sagrada	5 mg.
Prickly Ash Bark	5 mg.
Buckthorn Bark	20 mg.

Three other herbal compounds are used at the Biomedical Center: the "red tonic" (another internal compound), and then two external compounds, referred to as the "red salve" and the "yellow powder." Like the black tonic, the red tonic is used for internal cancers. Its formula is a slight variation of the black tonic and is used for people who have difficulty tolerating the black tonic's occasional side effects in the digestive tract, such as nausea, bloating, stomach ache, and diarrhea. In Roger Bloom's 2002 book, *Cancer Medicine From Nature,* he states that when he interviewed the Hoxsey clinic about the ingredients of the red tonic, they claimed they add lactate of pepsin, and remove cascara sagrada, burdock, and prickly ash, from the black tonic formula.

The two other herbal compounds, which are used specifically for external cancers (tumors near the surface of the skin), are the yellow powder and the red salve. According to Harry Hoxsey's autobiography, "The yellow powder contains arsenic sulphide, yellow precipitate, sulphur and talc; the red paste has antimony trisulphide, zinc chloride, and blood root; the liquid is trichloro-acetic acid." These escharotics use a mild caustic with cancerolytic phytochemicals to first kill the cancer, then stimulate the body's own immune system to form a white blood cell barrier around the tumor. From there, it's extracted through the skin, and the body naturally repairs the underlying tissue (see story reprinted from Harry Hoxsey's autobiography in Appendix B).

The black tonic is the most common of the four primary herbal compounds used to treat cancer at the Biomedical Center. I went to several naturopathic medicine texts in order to document the purpose, action, and potential side effects of each herb in the black tonic. My findings were as follows:

Potassium Iodine (KI)—Also known as "potash," potassium iodine is derived from wood ashes and is therefore a strong alkali. It serves several functions, one of which is suspending the herbs in a concentrated form, thereby providing a base for the herbal tonics. It also has alkaline-forming properties for the arterial blood and body fluids. Its history dates back to the turn of the twentieth century, when eclectic doctors used it to treat a wide variety of diseases. It had a reputation for curing skin conditions, ulcerations, and thyroid problems, and was used as a powerful expectorant. It influences the glandular system and the serous and mucus membranes. It was also historically used as a base for a variety of medications.

In 1926 and 1930 Arthur Bryan, a Baltimore veterinarian published the AMA's findings of potassium iodine's anticancer action in *The North American Veterinarian* and in *Veterinary Medicine*. In the 1950s, he experimented with injecting solutions, or placing crystals, of potassium or sodium iodide within the cancerous tumors of domestic animals. This frequently resulted in the breakdown and disappearance of tumors of a wide variety of neoplasms (cancers) within a few weeks or less. In some cases, tumors larger than a pumpkin in horses and cattle dramatically disappeared.

The first record of using potassium iodine on humans with cancer can be found in the 1940s and 1950s, when Dr. Kleiner, professor of biochemistry at New York Medical College, and Dr. M. M. Black of the Brooklyn Cancer Institute, treated patients with advanced cancer and noted significant results.

Years later, U.S. public health officials were documented dispensing potassium iodine pills to people who lived near Three Mile Island, a few days after the near-nuclear accident there. It is believed that it blocks ionizing radiation from damaging the thyroid gland. The Russian government also dispensed potassium iodine pills to people in close proximity of the Chernobyl nuclear disaster; it later measured significantly low levels of radiation in the thyroids of those residents. This is significant because the thyroid is an integral component of the immune system, and when the thyroid absorbs high levels of radiation, various cancers are likely to result. On the occasion of both these accidents, the treatments involved the use of high dosages of potassium iodine, and no serious side effects from those higher doses have ever been reported.

Licorice Root (Glycyrrhiza Glabra)—Licorice is indigenous to southern/ southeastern Europe, southwest/western Asia, and Iraq. This extract not only covers up the bitter taste of the roots in the black tonic, it also serves as a gentle laxative, stimulating the entire digestive mucous membranes. It has estrogen-like properties, enhances immune function, and has antiviral capabilities. In has long been used as a blood purifier, anti-inflammatory, and an antibacterial agent. In animal laboratories, it has demonstrated anti-tumor activity.

Licorice is used extensively in Chinese medicine for its synergistic effects in combining herbal medications. In high dosages (above 50 gm/day), used for extended periods of time, it has been known to be toxic, sometimes leading to hypkalemia, hypernatremia, edemas, hypertension, and cardiac complaints, and in rare cases myoglobinemia. The *PDR (Physicians Desk Reference) for Herbal Medicines* recommends against taking high dosages of licorice extract for more than six weeks, which is not a concern for Hoxsey patients, who generally take a moderate dose.

Red Clover (Trifolium Pratense)—This herb is gathered when in bloom, because the flower heads hold the medicinal properties. The plant is indigenous to Europe, central Asia, and northern Africa, and is naturalized in many other parts of the world. It's been known to assist in capillary circulation, a variety of skin conditions (psoriasis and eczema), indolent ulcers, and as an antispasmodic or expectorant for respiratory conditions, such as whooping cough.

It is the primary ingredient in Winter's Tea, which was developed by the Hollywood stunt man Jason Winters. After he was told by his doctors that his cancer was terminal, he traveled the world in search of alternative cures. After combining various herbal tea mixtures, he discovered one that reversed his disease: it contained a significant amount of red clover.

Jethro Kloss (1863-1946), who was famous for researching and popularizing herbal medicines around the turn of the twentieth century, is worth quoting for his reference to red clover in his book *Back to Eden.* "...one of God's greatest blessings to man; very pleasant to take and a wonderful blood purifier...an exceedingly good remedy for cancer on any part of the body." After studying many cases of cancer, he claimed significant success in using a tea made up primarily of red clover, with the addition of burdock, poke, and yellow dock.

Popular herbal medicine researcher Jonathan Hartwell, who wrote *Plants Used Against Cancers*, noted that thirty-three cultures around the world use red clover to treat cancer. Research indicates that red clover is antiangiogenic, meaning that it prevents the formation of new blood vessels, thereby reducing or eliminating the blood supply to tumors. It is also known to contain genistein. This is the same estrogenic isoflavone found in soybeans, a food consumed regularly in Asia, where the incidence of breast and other female reproductive cancers is significantly lower than in the United States.

In addition, red clover contains many biologically active compounds, including phytoestrogens, which are also found in soy. Recent research suggests that soy, a dietary source of these phytoestrogens, lowers risks of leukemia and breast, lung, and prostate cancers. Red clover may also be effective in reducing the side effects of menopause and premenstrual syndrome. No adverse side effects for using high dosages of red clover are reported in the *PDR for Herbal Medicines*.

Burdock Root (Arctium Lappa)—Burdock is indigenous to Europe, northern Asia, and North America. It contains compounds with potent immune-enhancing qualities. Back in the early 1900s, famous herbalist Eli Jones cited burdock's use in treating cancer. Various Native American tribes have used burdock for hundreds of years in the successful treatment of cancer.

Burdock is also the primary ingredient in Essiac Tea, a tea discovered in 1922 by a Canadian nurse named Renee Caisse. Ms. Caisse's search for a cancer cure was stimulated by her aunt's contracting an inoperable, terminal cancer. She found a woman who had cured herself with an Ojibway Indian tea that consisted of burdock, sheep's sorrel, slippery elm, and Indian rhubarb root. All are blood purifiers. After her aunt was cured, she named the tea after her last name, Caisse, spelled backwards; thus, the name "Essiac."

Burdock has historically been used in folk medicine to relieve lymphatic congestion, inflammations of the skin, rheumatic conditions in their inflammatory stages, and for ulcerations and new growths. It has also been used as a folk cancer remedy in Chile, India, China, Canada, Russia, and the United States. Herbalists commonly use it as a blood purifier. Cancer studies in Hungary and Japan showed it has significant anti-tumor activity. It has been well documented to be useful in the treatment of leukemia and lymphoma. It has no known side effects.

Stillingia Root (Stillingia Sylvatica)—Indigenous to the southern United States, it is also known as Queen's root. It is a blood purifier, which was commonly used at the turn of the twentieth century for digestive disorders and to treat liver, gall, and skin diseases. Eli Jones, in his book *Cancer: Its Causes, Symptoms and Treatment* (1911), listed stillingia as an effective remedy for internal cancer.

In 1980, German scientists documented two anti-tumor properties in the root. In addition, an alcohol extract of stillingia was shown to significantly reduce breast cancer tumors implanted in mice in a report put out by Taylor A. McKenna (1962) called *Screening Plant Extracts for Anti-cancer Activity*. The *PDR for Herbal Medicines* cautions that this extract is a skin and mucous membrane irritant; it has been known to cause nausea and vomiting when used as an emetic, and diarrhea when used as a laxative.

Barberry (Berberis Root)—Barberry's natural habitat is Europe, northern Africa, parts of America, and central Asia. In folk medicine, the barberry plant was used as a valuable anti-diarrheal and anti-infective agent. It demonstrates powerful antibiotic and antimicrobial activity against a wide range of microorganisms. In some studies, it has been shown to be a potent activator of macrophages—cells responsible for destroying bacteria—and to be highly effective against viruses, yeast, and tumor cells. There's some significant research showing how berberis root blocks oxygen uptake to cancer cells.

Its action against *candida albicans*, a common precancerous condition referred to as candidiasis, is well documented. Candidiasis, a chronic overgrowth of yeast in the intestinal tract, is perhaps the leading cause of immune system degradation and its inability to recognize and destroy cancer cells under normal conditions. Early BMC Director Mildred Nelson theorized that the Candida yeast condition generally preceded the onset of cancer.

Naturopathic scientific research links the overgrowth of Candida to the prolonged use of certain drugs, such as antibiotics. Essentially, bacteria in the intestinal tract that prevent yeast overgrowth are often destroyed by antibiotics, and Candida overgrowth is the result. Candidiasis makes us more prone to viruses and viral infections lead to bacterial infections. Then we take antibiotics again for the bacterial infections, which kills the bacteria that controls the growth of Candida, and the cycle continues.

Other drugs that cause Candida overgrowth are steroids. These are often used for asthma, arthritis, and commonly prescribed oral contraceptives, anti-ulcer medications, and more. (In my case, I pinpointed my own condition of candidiasis from using steroid inhalers to combat dust allergy-induced asthma during the winter.)

People with Candida often experience a cleansing effect when they take barberry, known as the herxheimer reaction, in which the yeast dies off and the symptoms of diarrhea, psoriasis, PMS, and chemical and allergen sensitivities worsen for a short period of time. These are indicators that chronic Candida has been the result of the liver not purifying the blood properly. When the liver is clogged, immune suppression results, with the potential of cancers.

Because of the herxheimer reaction, some naturopathic researchers recommend undergoing a liver cleansing before and/or in conjunction with taking a yeast-killing herb such as barberry, because the yeast releases toxins into the blood during necrosis. Those who desire to rid themselves of candidiasis may consider the liver-cleansing systems of various natural health manufacturers. For Hoxsey patients, the daily prescribed dose of grape juice—one quart per day, diluted with water—may suffice as an effective liver cleanser.

Research botanist James Duke, during his career with the USDA, found berberis root to be high in alkaloids (bitter organic bases found in plants). As a result, it has a wealth of anticancer, antitumor, and antioxidant properties, including valuable cellular mutation preventative actions.

The *PDR for Herbal Medicines* suggests that no health hazards or side effects are known with the proper administration of designated therapeutic dosages. Overdoses of over 4 mg. have been known to bring about a light stupor, nose bleeds, vomiting, diarrhea, and kidney irritation. In order to create a tea infusion, it is recommended to add 150 ml. of hot water to 1 to 2 teaspoons of whole or squashed barberries and strain after 10 to 15 minutes. The common tincture dosage is 20-40 drops. The Hoxsey tonic demonstrates a safe dosage.

Poke Root (Phytolacca Americana)—Poke grows in North America and also in Mediterranean countries. Its medicinal value comes from the root and berries. Its active compounds have demonstrated anti-inflammatory and anti-rheumatic properties. In folk medicine, it has been used to aid digestion.

Hundreds of years ago, Native Americans used the powdered poke root for cancer recovery, and early settlers successfully used the berry juice on skin cancer. In eclectic medicine, around the turn of the twentieth century, the berries, leaves, and roots were often used in a salve or ointment. Famous eclectic physician Eli Jones, described by science writer Ralph Moss as "one of the founders of modern oncology," considered poke the most valuable general remedy in treating cancer.

In 1998, in *Antimicrobial Agents and Chemotherapy*, the official journal of the American Society for Microbiology, a study was published indicating that a promising new drug eradicated HIV infection (AIDS) in mice. This new agent contained a powerful anti-viral protein from the poke weed plant. All the mice in the study were cured of human AIDS without side effects. Thereafter, more study was approved by the FDA, but I am unaware of any current research.

There are multiple studies that indicate poke's ability to activate a stronger immune response, which is an integral part of killing cancer in the Hoxsey method of therapy.

However, poke can be highly toxic, and should not be self-administered. According to the *PDR for Herbal Medicines*, an overdose may lead to bloody diarrhea, dizziness, hypotension, severe thirst, somnolence, tachycardia, vomiting, and in rare cases respiratory failure and death. It goes on to warn that "up to 10 berries are considered harmless for an adult, but could be dangerous for small children. Adults who consume more than 10 berries, and small children who consume any berries, should be treated for poisoning." The *PDR for Herbal Medicines* suggests that cooking poke destroys the lectins, thereby reducing its toxicity. Yet the dosages used in the Hoxsey tonic are minimal. Certainly in comparison to the mortality rates of modern chemotherapy, it may be considered relatively safe.

Cascara Sagrada (Rhamnus Purshianus)—This herb is indigenous to the western part of North America, on the Pacific coast of the United States and Canada, and to eastern Africa. Its medicinal properties are in the bark. It is well known for its laxative effects. It is contraindicated in intestinal obduration, acute inflammatory intestinal disease, and appendicitis. Research showed that in extract form, it successfully inhibited tumor growth when breast cancer tumors were implanted in mice.

The shortening of time for solid digestion in the intestinal passage reduces liquid absorption, so without proper hydration, drinking hydration-fostering liquids, cascara could lead to loss of electrolytes. According to the *PDR for Herbal Medicines*, in very rare cases, heart arrhythmia, edemas, and bone deterioration can result. However, an overdose of most laxatives would probably cause similar adverse effects. It appears that cascara in moderate doses is relatively safe, provided there is conscientious hydration, such as in Hoxsey therapy.

Prickly Ash Bark (Zanthoxylum Americanum)—Native to North America, the medicinal parts of this plant are the root, bark and berries. It contains a COX-2 inhibitor known as Berberine, which may alleviate symptoms of Alzheimer's, arthritis, and colon cancer. It also contains cherlerythine, which has proven to be cytotoxic (cancer cell-killing) in tumor cell tests. Another inherent compound, referred to as nitidine, was found to be highly cytotoxic in leukemia cell tests.

Several Edgar Cayce readings referred to this herb's ability to cleanse the liver, in addition to the gall duct, and to stimulate the pancreas and spleen, key organs in immune response. It has been used in eclectic medicine for low blood pressure, rheumatic disorders, fever, and inflammation. There are no contraindications, overdoses, or adverse reactions to be found.

Buckthorn Bark (Rhamnus Frangula)—This plant is indigenous to all of Europe, western Asia, and Asia Minor, and has spread to the wild in North America. It has long been used for blood cleansing, liver disorders, and for constipation. It has proven to be effective against several types of tumors, including those of leukemia cells. It is contraindicated for use with intestinal obduration, acute intestinal diseases, and appendicitis.

The *PDR for Herbal Medicines* states that vomiting and spasmodic gastrointestinal complaints may occur as side effects, particularly with overdoses. It cautions against long-term use at high doses, which may lead to loss of electrolytes, in particular K+ions. Therefore, consistent hydration is important with its use.

Summary of the Hoxsey Herbs

Generally, these herbs are commonly referred to as blood purifiers or blood cleansers; they cleanse the organs and reactivate immune response. They not only reduce blood supply to tumors, reducing or eliminating tumor growth, but they also change the arterial blood and body fluids to an alkaline state, which further inhibits cancer cell proliferation.

Most importantly, the herbs help to rectify the original cause of the cancer in the body, the malfunction that created the fertile environment for cancer to exist in the first place. Unlike cytotoxic synthetics (chemotherapy drugs) or radiation (radiotherapy), which are tested for their kill-rate in petri dishes, taking herbal medicine tinctures or tonics tends to adjust the inner environment of the body. This allows the body to repair certain altered or damaged cells and tissues and restore the efficiency of the organs and glands involved in our immune system response. Healing is often accomplished naturally, without adverse side effects in the majority of cases. Therefore, the causative, precancerous conditions are transformed, and cancer cells and tumors are eradicated by the body, almost as if building an immunity to the cancer cells.

In addition, many of the herbs are anti-viral, anti-bacterial, and anti-parasitic, and modern science has linked all these things to the development of cancer. Viruses in particular have been proven to be linked to cancer by conventional medicine, which Harry Hoxsey asserted in the late 1950s in his autobiography.

Next, we will do a comparative analysis of the herbs recommended by the two fathers of natural cancer cures.

Comparative Analysis
A. Hoxsey Black Herbal Tonic
B. Cayce's Anti-Cancer Herbs

Potassium Iodine	Hoxsey and Cayce
Licorice	Hoxsey and Cayce
Red Clover	Hoxsey and Cayce
Burdock Root	Hoxsey and Cayce
Stillingia Root	Hoxsey and Cayce
Berberis Root	Hoxsey and Cayce
Poke Root	Hoxsey and Cayce
Cascara Sagrada	Hoxsey
Prickly Ash Bark	Hoxsey
Buckthorn Bark	Hoxsey
Wild Cherry Bark	Cayce
Yellow Dock Root	Cayce
Elder Berry/Flower	Cayce
Sarsaparilla Root	Cayce

In my research, I discovered that wild cherry and yellow dock are also blood cleansers, and are often recommended for cleansing and toning the digestive tract. In other texts, I found documentation supporting elder berry's benefits to the lymph system, drawing the conclusion that it may be particularly beneficial for cases of lymphoma, in conjunction with other herbs. Although the *PDR for Herbal Medicines* lists many of the herbs as not indigenous to North America, Harry Hoxsey and Edgar Cayce both indicated that all of the herbs above could be found growing in the United States.

Investigation of the Hoxsey Herbs

There have been several studies and anecdotal research projects involving Hoxsey therapy over the last seventy years that clearly prove its efficacy in curing cancer. It is important to note that these studies were conducted on various populations; some had been newly diagnosed and the cancers were in their early stages, and some were well advanced. Just as in traditional medicine, the earlier a cancer is detected and treated, the more likely Hoxsey therapy will lead to a cure.

Some studies were conducted in the 1940s, when eclectic physicians were getting heat from conventional physicians (who were using synthetics) and their governing boards. One study was launched by Sam L. Scothorn, who took his wife to Hoxsey to treat her ovarian cancer after radiation had failed. His wife was cured. Scothorn then enlisted several physicians to review twenty-seven cases, using the biopsies they'd performed themselves to document the certainty of all twenty-seven cancer patients in the study. Twenty-four of the twenty-seven in the study went into complete remission.

In Harry Hoxsey's 1956 autobiography, *You Don't Have To Die*, he cited the following statement by a group of ten physicians from around the country who spent several days, just before the release of his book, examining the treatment program, the clinic records, and the patients:

"We find as a fact that our investigation has demonstrated to our satisfaction that the Hoxsey Cancer Clinic at Dallas, Texas, is successfully treating pathologically proven cases of cancer, both internal and external, without the use of surgery, radium or x-ray.

Accepting the standard yardstick of cases that have remained symptom-free in excess of five to six years after treatment, established by medical authorities, we have seen sufficient cases to warrant such a conclusion. Some of those presented before us have been free of symptoms for as long as twenty-four years, and the physical evidence indicates that they are all enjoying exceptional health at this time.

We, as a Committee, feel that the Hoxsey treatment is superior to such conventional methods of treatment as x-ray, radium, and surgery. We are willing to assist this Clinic in any way possible in bringing this treatment to the American public. We are willing to use it in our office, in our practice on our own patients when, at our discretion, it is deemed necessary.

The above statement represents the unanimous finding of this Committee. In testimony thereof, we hereby attach our signatures."

S. Edgar Bond, M.D. (Richmond, IN)
Willard G. Palmer, M.D. (Seattle, WA)
Hans Kalm, M.D. (Aiken, SC)
A.C. Timbs, M.D. (Knoxville, TN)
Frederick H. Thurston, M.D., D.O. (Boise, ID)
E.E. Loffler, M.D. (Spokane, WA)
H.B. Mueller, M.D. (Cleveland, OH)
R.C. Bowie, M.D. (Fort Morgan, CO)
Benjamin F. Bowers, M.D. (Ebensburg, PA)
Roy O. Yeats, M.D. (Hardin, MT)

In 1984, a well-respected naturopathic doctor from Oregon, Steve Austin, ND, conducted a preliminary review of Hoxsey patients. The study followed a group of people from the Pacific Northwest with advanced cancers. They went to three of the most popular Tijuana alternative cancer clinics, which offered, respectively: Hoxsey therapy, Gerson therapy (a dietary approach), and laetrile (an extract of apricot pits).

The review was published in the *Journal of Naturopathic Medicine*. It found that six of sixteen Hoxsey patients survived for five years, disease-free. These included two cases of melanoma and two of lung cancer, which are often fatal. Dr. Austin said, "We noted that several long term survivors had very poor initial prognosis." This was obviously due to the fact that many people who try alternative cancer therapies in Tijuana have well-advanced, often metastasized cancer deemed terminal, and come to Tijuana as a court of last resort, figuratively speaking. Patients who start Hoxsey therapy earlier, without ravaging their systems with traditional therapies, would probably have had better results. He went on to conclude: "...any apparently successful treatment of late-stage lung cancer and melanoma should prove of interest." There were no survivors from the other two therapies under his study.

Dr. James Duke is a botanist who, while working under the United States Department of Agriculture, founded a world-class data base on plant medicine, and collaborated for many years with the National Cancer Institute to discover anti-cancer remedies found in plants. For example, he was part of a team of botanical researchers who discovered the cancer-curing properties of the pacific yew tree, which resulted in taxol, a popular chemotherapy drug. According to Duke, at least three of the herbs in the Hoxsey tonic—barberry, cascara sagrada, and buckthorn—contain compounds that have been studied by the NCI and found to be effective in some tumor systems.

In 1988, Duke's article about his research appeared in *Herbal Gram,* a peer review journal of the American Botanical Council. It revealed that eight of the nine herbs in the internal tonic showed anti-tumor activity in controlled animal laboratory tests. Five of the herbs showed antioxidant properties, which protect against cancer. All nine herbs showed antimicrobial properties, which involved activity against viral or bacterial infections that likely precede, or commonly coexist with, contracting cancer.

Around the same time, medical historian Patricia Spain Ward, Ph.D. contracted with the federal Office of Technology Assessment to get to the bottom of whether or not alternative cancer treatments were effective. After she examined patient records from the Hoxsey clinic, her findings were similar to James Duke's in that the treatment was found to be very effective. However, according to Kenneth Ausebel's book *When Healing Becomes a Crime*, interviews conducted with Ms. Ward revealed that the board governing the report suppressed much of her pro-Hoxsey findings. Apparently, they believed she was biased when she reported an overwhelming percentage of long-term remissions at the clinic.

One segment of Ausebel's book described how investigators from the Office of Alternative Medicine (OAM), under the NIH, started a preliminary investigation of the Biomedical Clinic in 1998. They discovered that this clinic was the preeminent herbal treatment facility for people in the United States, Western Europe, and Australia, with about 1,200 people visiting each year at that time (it is now almost double), making it the largest alternative medicine cancer clinic in the world. They pulled the records of 150 patients from 1992 to 1997 who used exclusively escharotics and/or the herbal tonics, to examine the results of the Hoxsey method. They found that though many patients could not be located, of those who could, the results were "noteworthy." Mary Ann Richardson and her team reported the following preliminary government review of these patient records in 1999:

> "A best-case series of more systematic prospective monitoring of patients is justified not only because of the public health issue to justify the large number of patients who seek treatment at this clinic, but also because of the several noteworthy cases of survival."

The NCI performed laboratory testing on all the Hoxsey herbs to discover their cytotoxicity. In other words, the herbs were incorrectly tested; the tests measured their kill rate by using cancer cell lines in petri dishes, just as toxic synthetic medicines are tested before being approved as chemotherapy drugs.

In a report called *Unconventional Cancer Treatments*, by Congress's Office of Technology Assessment, the results of these tests were posted as negative, because although they showed some degree of cytotoxicity, they did not kill all the cancer cells in the petri dish. In contrast, naturopaths using herbal medicines treat the systems of the body that are at the cause of various cancers. They essentially increase vitality and restore capabilities for obtaining homeostatic conditions in the body. Once homeostasis is achieved, the body kills its own cancer cells. Apparently, the major problem with the NCI protocols used for screening herbal medicines was that they did not test the herbs the way naturopathic physicians tend to use them. Therefore, cytotoxicity testing is virtually useless.

This may be better understood as we examine Harry Hoxsey's own words. In his autobiography, he documents exactly how the Hoxsey system of therapy effectively kills cancer in the human body:

> "We are convinced that cancer cannot be cured successfully as an isolated phenomenon, unrelated to basic body processes. We attempt to get at the roots of the disorder, rather than deal merely with its end result. Our primary effort is to restore the body to physiological normalcy. We have a basic medicine which, taken orally, accomplishes this purpose. It stimulates the elimination of toxins which are poisoning the system, and thereby corrects the abnormal blood chemistry and normalizes cell metabolism. Its ingredients are not secret. [He goes on to list the formulas and uses for external and internal cancers and states,] ...the exact ingredients and dosage vary, depending on the individual patient's general condition, the location of the cancer, and the extent of previous treatment."

Pharmaceutical Companies and Herbal Medicine

According to Ausebel, in the late 1800s pharmaceutical companies were manufacturing remedies with the same herbs that Hoxsey later used for the treatment of cancer. Francis Brinker, a naturopathic scholar who investigated the Hoxsey formula, found evidence that in 1890, Parke-Davis and Company produced an herbal compound advertised as effective against cancer called Syrup Trifolium; the ingredients are listed below.

Potassium Iodine
Red Clover
Burdock Root
Stillingia Root
Berberis Root
Poke Root
Cascara Amarga
Prickly Ash Bark

This formula is identical to the Hoxsey formula, except for the lack of Buckthorn and Licorice.

Apparently, in the late 1800s and early 1900s, herbal cancer remedies were being used successfully by naturopathic physicians, also known as "eclectic" or "irregular" physicians. Eli Jones, a popular eclectic physician mentioned earlier, wrote three definitive books outlining the advancements in cancer therapy (before the AMA and synthetic medicines became popular): *Cancer: Tumors and Malignant Growths Both External and Internal Permanently Cured without a Surgical Operation* (1905); *Definite Medication* (1910); *and Cancer: Its Causes, Symptoms and Treatment* (1911). Regarding the success rate of natural medicines of that time, Dr. Jones stated:

> "The Eclectic school of medicine was the pioneer in the successful treatment of cancer by internal medication. By my method of treating cancer as a blood or constitutional disease (as I was taught in the Eclectic college over forty years ago), I have cured 80 percent of the cases of cancer which have come under my treatment. I honestly believe, from my own experience, that 95 percent of the cases of cancer in our country could be cured by medicine if treated before an operation or the use of X-ray (radiation therapy)."

I believe Dr. Jones was referring to Parke-Davis's Syrup Trifolium, a nontoxic chemotherapeutic herbal compound that physicians used at that time to cure cancer. Interestingly, he claimed the same success rate that the Biomedical Center claims today. If used as a first defense, before surgery or radiation, he claimed a 95 percent success rate!

This is due to the detrimental side effects of traditional medical treatments, which often cause the recurrence of cancer, in addition to depleting the body of its natural healing abilities. When the side effects of traditional medicine are circumvented, and a comprehensive herbal medicine regimen is applied, the immune system is kept intact and the success rate is even greater than 80 percent, with a very low rate of recurrence.

Now let's do a comparative analysis of all three highly successful, turn-of-the-century, pre-AMA, pre-synthetic era cancer remedies.

Comparative Analysis
A. Hoxsey's Black Herbal Tonic
B. Cayce's Anti-Cancer Herbs
C. Parke-Davis's Syrup Trifolium

Potassium Iodine	Hoxsey, Cayce, Parke-Davis
Red Clover	Hoxsey, Cayce, Parke-Davis
Burdock Root	Hoxsey, Cayce, Parke-Davis
Stillingia Root	Hoxsey, Cayce, Parke-Davis
Berberis Root	Hoxsey, Cayce, Parke-Davis
Poke Root	Hoxsey, Cayce, Parke-Davis
Cascara Sagrada	Hoxsey, Parke-Davis
Prickly Ash Bark	Hoxsey, Parke-Davis
Licorice	Hoxsey, Cayce
Buckthorn Bark	Hoxsey
Wild Cherry Bark	Cayce
Yellow Dock Root	Cayce
Elder Berry/Flower	Cayce
Sarsaparilla	Cayce

Looking at this comparison, we can conclude that the most effective herbs for curing cancer include red clover, burdock root, stillingia root, berberis root, poke root, and the alkaline-forming suspension potassium iodine, or potash.

Summary

It appears that we really did not need to reinvent the wheel by using chemotherapy, radiation, or surgery to kill cancer, when these herbal cures that were so widely used at the turn of the twentieth century proved to be so successful. Most cancers aren't like viruses, mutating over time and requiring the development of new treatments for their eradication. With the age-old philosophy of "Physician, do no harm," it seems a more ethical approach to ensure that medical doctors in the United States receive the proper education, and legal right, to prescribe methods that won't risk making people sicker or killing them. The more invasive procedures that allopathic medicine offers should be a last resort. It makes sense that people should be legally allowed to try herbal cures in more states than just the thirteen states which currently allow naturopathic doctors to practice (Alaska, Arizona, California, Connecticut,

Hawaii, Kansas, Maine, Montana, New Hampshire, Oregon, Utah, Vermont, and Washington).

Why should people have to go all the way to Tijuana, Mexico, to get natural cures that won't make them more sick, disfigure them, or give them more cancers? In other words, let us stand up for our right to choose, our right to use the natural therapies that commonly have fewer side effects.

I feel blessed to live in the state of North Carolina, where, at least in my home town, it is common for people see a naturopath before an allopathic doctor for common ailments, unless they have a problem that calls for traditional medical approaches. In those states where traditional medicine has a noose around the necks of both natural health practitioners and traditional medical doctors, natural health treatment programs are simply taking place underground, or people are traveling out of their home state or out of the country to access them. This will continue until we the people, in every state, stand up for our right to choose the therapies we believe will improve our health. We are in the information age, and a self-managed health care system, so why not? We're certainly educated enough.

If we're looking for a track record for success before trying herbal medicines for cancer, then what's wrong with the 100 to 200 years' worth of Hoxsey therapy? In my opinion, it's the correct choice for a first line of defense.

Chapter 9

The Anti-Cancer Diet

"Up until 200 years ago, 80 percent of our diet came from plant products. That has now decreased to less than 50 percent, and because our bodies are not genetically adapted to that change, we are experiencing an epidemic of cancer and heart disease that is potentially avoidable."

Oliver Alabaster, Institute for Disease Prevention,
George Washington University Medical Center

My primary goal for this chapter is to give readers a simple recipe for health without their having to be nutritionists. It is intended to serve as a good resource for both cancer patients and genetically cancer-prone individuals interested in prevention. It covers the detrimental aspects of large-scale farming, food processing, and the degradation of the environment, and how they negatively affect our nutrition, and various toxic or carcinogenic chemicals inherent in our food chain, food production, and our modern lifestyles.

We will look at what I consider to be a cancer prevention diet, the *Cayce alkaline diet*, and the one I used to stifle my cancer in June of the first year of my recovery. We will thoroughly examine what I consider to be a cancer recovery diet, the Hoxsey diet, which is the one I used in August of first year of my recovery. The Hoxsey diet is commonly recommended by the Biomedical Center as a complement to the herbal tonics; together they create a respectable success rate.

The primary objective of both diets is to create an alkaline environment in our bodies, or, in other words to turn our body fluids alkaline. I will explain later why this is important for health. In this effort, it is important to eliminate the foods that we commonly consume that help create an acidic environment. Stress also creates an acidic environment (hence the need for the chapter on mind-body approaches).

This chapter will also lay out traditional medical scientific research pertaining to diet, in addition to the discoveries of Edgar Cayce and Harry Hoxsey. Both of them understood the benefits of an alkaline diet a century before most people had even heard of the concept. We will focus primarily on the dietary recommendations of the Biomedical Center—the Hoxsey diet— which has cured hundreds of thousands of people of cancer by combining a simple, easy to follow, straightforward dietary approach, in conjunction with the anticancer herbs previously mentioned. Later in this chapter, I will also present to readers a way to test their pH level, or the pH levels of their loved ones. This is how to test the body's acidity or alkalinity levels.

Scientific Proof of the Importance of an Anticancer Diet

There is solid evidence that improved nutrition strengthens the immune system, slows or eliminates the growth of tumors, and protects against metastasis (the spread of cancer). A study done at the University of Victoria in British Columbia examined 200 cancer patients who had experienced spontaneous regression; i.e., an inexplicable cure or tumor reduction. Eighty-seven percent of these patients had made significant changes in their diets.

"Nutrition recommendations usually stress eating lots of fruits, vegetables, and whole grain breads and cereals; including a moderate amount of meat and dairy products; and cutting back on fat, sugar, alcohol, and salt."

Eating Hints for Cancer Patients, 1999 edition,
by the National Cancer Institute

Diets high in saturated fat have been shown to stimulate the growth of cancer. Some natural cancer recovery experts go so far as to recommend eliminating virtually all sources of saturated fat, which includes meat and dairy products, and all processed foods, because of their saturated fat and trans fatty acid content. This is often recommended when diet is the only form of cancer treatment. Both the Hoxsey diet and the macrobiotic diet allow only small quantities of these things, and report high success rates.

Most experts agree that the most important dietary change a person can make to prevent or eliminate cancer is to reduce fats while consuming more foods containing phytochemicals, such as fruits, fiber-rich vegetables, herbs, legumes, whole grains, and other plant foods. (*Phyto* is the Greek word for plant.)

It is important to be mindful that the nutrients our bodies need are found naturally in a good diet, one containing foods that are rich in things such as vitamins, macro minerals (i.e, zinc, magnesium, phosphorous), and micro minerals (i.e., vanadium). However, because of mass food production and soil depletion, many foods in America are losing their nutritional value. Therefore, as we will see in the next chapter, taking concentrated supplements is wise for cancer patients, particularly since they are likely to be low in specific nutrients that the body needs to support a healthy immune system.

This is why the BMC requires specific, nutrition-based blood tests to evaluate their patients' nutritional levels after being on the Hoxsey program.

The Immune System Relative to Cancer

In order to understand the importance of an anticancer diet, we must explore the concept of immune function, because the premise behind dietary cancer therapy is that boosting the immune system will help the body to kill its own cancer. Essentially, an anticancer diet and herbal medicines increase our body's immune activity.

According to several oncological health resources, cancer results from the degradation of a person's immune function, which in turn results from changes in his or her DNA. Scientific opinions vary as to the exact cause of this change, but we know that it is normal for cells to randomly double-divide in the human body. When the person is healthy, this signals the immune system that a foreign invader cell is present that could be hypermetabolic and potentially cancerous. In a healthy body, the immune system then attacks these foreign invaders, recognizing that they do not fit the code for good health, so to speak, and destroys them before they grow into tumors.

In a body with a compromised immune system, such as a cancer patient's, the immune system does not attack these double-dividing cells. They can develop into tumors. The tumors eventually spread and engulf vital organs, a process with mortal consequences unless it is stopped.

For the scientifically-minded person, the next two paragraphs will further examine the immune system's function and how this complex system works. By the way, medical science is still trying to understand it.

Antibodies, immunoglobulines, T-lymphocytes, B-lymphocytes, monocytes, and leukocytes: all are types of white blood cells that fight foreign invaders such as bacteria, viruses, and cancer cells. Of these white blood cells, the lymphocytes and monocytes are of utmost importance in the immune system's ability to fight disease. They are produced by the lymph system. The lymph system helps in the process of singling out bacteria and dead cells reaching the end of their life cycle, and other debris, and preventing them from entering the blood stream and thereby decreasing immune efficiency.

In naturopathic medicine, the liver and thymus gland play integral roles in proper immune function. The liver's primary role is to filter out various toxins or carcinogens, such as: tobacco, alcohol, food preservatives, chemicals in meat, environmental pollutants, pharmaceuticals, chemotherapy drugs, and other synthetic chemicals. It also filters out waste materials such as dead cells and tissues, and digestive waste secretions that are not being eliminated from the colon, but instead are being secreted back into the blood stream. Essentially, the liver, in conjunction with other organs and glands, acts as a screen for filtering the blood, similar to a filtration system in a swimming pool. When the liver is clogged from too many toxins, immune function drops and cancer cells are allowed to proliferate. Other illnesses may also develop.

Yet the liver does not act alone in the overall picture of immune function. In conjunction with the liver, the spleen manufactures different types of immune cells, which also assist in filtering out bacteria and dead or damaged red blood cells from the immune system. Another important gland tied into the immune system is the thymus gland. The thymus gland contributes to the regulation of cancer-fighting cells, often referred to as T-cells. When we are under high amounts of mental stress, we produce fewer T-cells. This highlights the vital need, in people with normal immune function, to reduce stress to maintain their health. For cancer patients, who have a compromised immune system, it's a necessity.

In addition, hereditary factors play a part in immune function. We each have genetic codes for health, longevity, and disease, which we can refer to as *genetic predispositions*. Our DNA, a code passed down to us from our ancestors, plays an important role in our cellular regulatory systems. What triggers our DNA is unknown to medical science, yet it is known that forms of radiation affect our DNA, particularly in people with a genetic predisposition to cancer. Even in people with no predisposition to cancer, excessive radiation exposure also has been shown to cause cancer, when the radiation enters the thymus gland. It is therefore logical to avoid such things as radiation therapy, particularly if cancer is in one's family.

Naturopathic medicine focuses on restoring organ and glandular functions relative to the immune system, as an integral component of the cancer recovery process. The Hoxsey therapy, the natural system of cancer recovery achieves this by:

> a) taking supplements, which assist in restoring deficiencies in the body;
> b) implementing an all-natural, alkaline diet, which helps the body restore deficiencies, normalize immune function, and stifle the growth of cancer cells and tumors; and
> c) taking specific herbal medicines that increase alkalinity, cleanse mucus membranes and bowels, cleanse the blood, and detoxify the organs and glands that are essential to proper immune function.

How Important Is Diet?

The most significant recommendations I found in my research were those of health mystic Edgar Cayce, naturopathic doctor Harry Hoxsey, (author of *You Don't Have To Die*), medical doctor Lorraine Day (teaching physician), medical doctor Bernie Siegel (author of *Love, Medicine and Miracles*), medical doctor James Balch (author of *Prescriptions for Nutritional Healing*), and pharmacologist Richard Harkness (author of *Reducing Cancer Risk*). They are relatively consistent with each other in recommending or not recommending specific foods, based on whether they facilitate or detract from proper immune function. Two other dietary cancer therapies worth noting are the Gerson diet, which is made up primarily of raw fruits and vegetables, and the macrobiotic diet, which is very similar to the Hoxsey diet and recommends low amounts of healthy meats and high amounts of fruits, vegetables, and whole grains.

Edgar Cayce was the first to discover the health benefits of an alkaline diet in conjunction with blood-cleansing herbal compounds, and the Hoxsey diet has been tested on humans and perfected over the past 80 years with similar compounds. For these reasons, the Cayce and Hoxsey therapies are probably the most effective nutritional cancer therapies available today. Therefore, we will focus primarily on the Cayce and Hoxsey diets as our cancer prevention diet and our anticancer diet, respectively. For the benefit of readers who are attempting to rid themselves of cancer, we will provide more emphasis on the Hoxsey diet.

The Importance of an Alkaline Diet

According to Cayce, Hoxsey, and a number of other nutritional and naturopathic medicine researchers, when our body fluids are acidic, it provides fertile soil, figuratively speaking, for cancer to grow. When our bodies are alkaline, cancer generally cannot grow, particularly when it's in an inactive state as opposed to an active state.

At this point, readers might ask what the difference is between cancer being in an active state and an inactive state. The only time I heard these terms used was at the Biomedical Center. According to the center, a patient's cancer is considered active when the cancerous tumors are aggressively growing and cancer cells are moving to other areas of the body. Cancer is inactive when cancer cells still exist in the body but are either stifled or dying, causing tumors to regress. The goal, of course, is to bring cancer into an inactive state.

Furthermore, a highly dangerous cellular process that takes place in every cancer patient with active cancer is the lactic acid cycle. This is what I call the "double whammy effect." In the natural process of cancer cells' hypermetabolic reproduction, lactic acid is produced, turning the body more acidic and thus enhancing the process. As a result, cancer patients experience a double whammy! Their body fluids were in an acidic state when they contracted cancer; the more their cancer progresses, the more lactic acid is produced, which accelerates the process. The more cancer, the more lactic acid; then more acidity, and more cancer, and so the repetitive cycle continues.

As a result, one primary goal of the Hoxsey system of therapy is to quickly move the patient toward an alkaline state by using high alkaline-forming natural components, such as: the potassium iodide in which the herbal tonics are suspended; lifestyle counseling and stress management techniques; and the high alkaline-forming foods in the Hoxsey diet.

The Alkaline-Forming Diet

To understand the importance of an alkaline-forming diet, which we will refer to as an *alkaline diet*, we must examine how both acidic and alkaline-based foods are either acid-forming or alkaline-forming, relative to our body fluids. The goal is to adjust our body fluids so they consistently stay in an alkaline state. We must also understand that foods that are acidic are not necessarily acid-forming. For example, citrus foods are acidic before entering the body, but they become alkaline-forming when digested.

There are numerous books available on the subject, which the cancer patient may be tempted to use to compose an intricate scheme of consuming the most correct combination of acid and alkaline-forming foods, in an effort to turn their body fluids alkaline. However, I must warn that most books published on the subject are not valuable to the cancer recovery patient, who must succeed in achieving a high alkalinity level, since their life depends on it. For this reason, I will critique the books that attempt to assist people in creating an alkaline environment.

For example, the book *Acid and Alkaline* does a wonderful job in breaking down the acid-forming and alkaline-forming values of foods and in emphasizing the macrobiotic diet, which is a good one to alkalize with, because it is a well-balanced, mostly vegetarian diet that has a reputation for helping cancer patients recover from their illnesses. The book also goes into detail as to how the elements found in foods, such as magnesium and other things, contribute to pH.

But the book doesn't target people with health issues, and therefore some acid-forming foods, such as garlic (which is very mildly acidic), are not recommended when they actually help in the prevention and recovery from cancer, according to Japanese medical studies and those compiled at the NIH. In addition, it doesn't discuss the importance of avoiding fermented or malted food products, the number one acid-forming agents.

Another book, *Alkalize or Die,* shows which fruits and vegetables are alkaline and acid-forming, and it also reveals which meats and starches are acid-producing. This is valuable information for the cancer patient. However, this book also says nothing about the dangers of malted or fermented products. It even offers recipes in the back that include salad dressings with vinegar—a big no-no.

One of the most accurate and informative books on the subject of alkalizing for health is *The pH Miracle*. This book offers an 80/20 alkaline to acid balance, similar to the Cayce alkaline diet, which is discussed later. It's the only book I found that lists acid-forming foods and emphasizes the importance of avoiding them, something that is key to a cancer patient's recovery. Most foods in the list are malted or fermented foods. The list in the book is almost identical to those the Hoxsey diet also recommends eliminating:

Vinegar
Mustard
Ketchup
Steak Sauce
Soy Sauce
Tamari
Mayonnaise
Salad Dressings
Chili Sauce
Horseradish
Miso
Monosodium Glutamate (MSG)
Any form of alcohol
Pickled Vegetables (relish, green olives, sauerkraut, pickles)
Malted Milk
Candy

The book emphasizes how many foods are manufactured with acetic acid/vinegar, and how sugars commonly transform into ethyl alcohol or vinegar after they enter the body. However, although *The pH Miracle* is an excellent resource, it fails to mention one specific food that the Hoxsey and Cayce diets both cite as acid-forming: tomatoes and tomato products. Otherwise, this book is the most accurate in giving a well-researched and plausible explanation of the dietary pH factor.

The book *Edgar Cayce on Diet and Health* was way ahead of its time; our society is just now beginning to recognize the medicinal value of diet. As a medical intuit, Edgar Cayce proved time and time again that he could read conditions in the body with the accuracy of X-ray vision and laboratory tests, even before X-rays and modern lab tests were invented. Regarding alkalinity, he states in reading 480-19:

"If an alkalinity is maintained in the system—especially with the lettuce, carrots, and celery, these in the blood supply will maintain such a condition as to immunize a person."

According to Cayce, colds and viruses are unable to exist in an alkaline environment. This is particularly important because traditional medical research has recently discovered links between specific viruses and various cancers, a theory Harry Hoxsey held almost a hundred years ago and documented in his autobiography in 1956.

In health reading 808-3, Cayce states:

"Colds cannot—does not exist in alkalines."

Because we may get confused by all the information available about alkalizing diets, it may be important to choose a formula proven over many decades to get results, such as the Cayce diet or the Hoxsey diet, both of which are explained below. The best way to see if your diet is effective in creating an alkaline environment is to do what Cayce suggested, which is to check your pH level, preferably on a daily basis. (There's a discussion of testing procedures in the following segment.)

The Cancer Prevention Diet

The Cayce Diet

Although Edgar Cayce recommended a wide variety of health diets for specific individuals, depending on their illnesses, the Cayce diet was routinely recommended for people to maintain optimum health. It was one that led to keeping the body fluids in a slightly alkaline state. Cayce recommended that an optimum balance for maintaining good health was "about 20 percent acid to 80 percent alkaline-producing" (Case 1523-3).

Edgar Cayce also regularly recommended lemon juice, which is a high alkaline-producing food, and he recommended against excessive amounts of sugar because it ferments in the digestive tract. He also recommended against pork and excessive starches or carbohydrates, which are also acid-forming. All of these recommendations are consistent with the Hoxsey diet. In addition, Cayce warned against a sedentary lifestyle, which tends to be acidic-forming. He emphasized the health benefits of regular exercise, particularly for the cancer patient.

Note the following Cayce suggestions:

Case 798-1:

The less activities there are in physical exercise or manual activity, the greater should be the alkaline reacting foods taken. Energies or activities may burn acids; but those who lead the sedentary life or the non-active life can't go on sweets or too much starches...these should be well balanced.

Case 593-1:

As to the matter of diet, be mindful that the food values are kept rather in an alkaline-reacting state; or that the test of litmus paper— both for the spittle and for the urine—show an alkaline reaction, see? This should be maintained more by the diet than by other efforts, you see...

Case 681-2:

Q-6: What diet should be taken?

A-6: There might be one diet given today and then next week you would have another! That which keeps the spittle or salivary reaction alkaline. That which keeps the blood reaction, by test, negative. That which keeps the urine eliminations as a balance at twenty-four without albumin, without sediment, and with an alkaline tendence; but not too great a tendence. That which makes for the proper eliminations and body-building without becoming superfluous flesh, or drainage to

A Brand of Litmus Paper

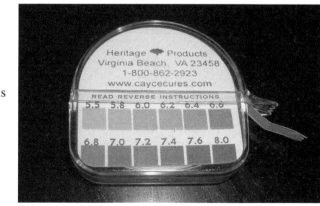

Basic Diet

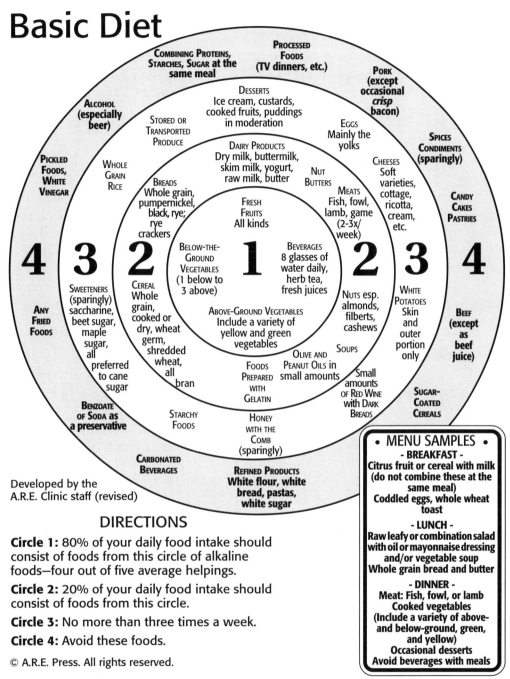

Developed by the
A.R.E. Clinic staff (revised)

DIRECTIONS

Circle 1: 80% of your daily food intake should consist of foods from this circle of alkaline foods—four out of five average helpings.

Circle 2: 20% of your daily food intake should consist of foods from this circle.

Circle 3: No more than three times a week.

Circle 4: Avoid these foods.

• MENU SAMPLES •
- BREAKFAST -
Citrus fruit or cereal with milk
(do not combine these at the same meal)
Coddled eggs, whole wheat toast
- LUNCH -
Raw leafy or combination salad with oil or mayonnaise dressing and/or vegetable soup
Whole grain bread and butter
- DINNER -
Meat: Fish, fowl, or lamb
Cooked vegetables
(Include a variety of above- and below-ground, green, and yellow)
Occasional desserts
Avoid beverages with meals

This summary of the principles of the Edgar Cayce readings is recommended for maintenance-level weight control.

For the purpose of *losing* weight, only a few minor changes need to be made.

same—see? Hence these are to be kept by constructive measures and forces, see?

Notice the suggested use of litmus paper to determine alkalinity within the body fluids. I purchased this pH test paper kit from Heritage Products (see reference list in the back) and began using it shortly after I started using the Hoxsey herbs. I didn't find validity in the test using urine; however, I found it to be accurate using saliva, provided I didn't eat anything for a six to eight hour period beforehand. Therefore, I often tested my saliva in the mornings.

To take a more in-depth look at what is referred to as the Cayce diet, I've included the following diagram, with permission of the Association for Research and Enlightenment in Virginia Beach, Virginia.

Perhaps the most frequent recommendation in the readings for the diet of people who had all types of cancer was the high consumption of raw vegetables. For those with advanced stages of cancer, he recommended that his client eat "that that a cow or rabbit would eat." This is consistent with Dr. Day's recommendations and the recommendations of the BMC.

Although Cayce did not recommend eliminating tomatoes from a person's diet, he did caution about their volatility and therefore their risks to a person's health, such as the advice given in the following case:

Case 584-5:
"Quite a dissertation might be given as to the effect of tomatoes upon the human system. Of all the vegetables, tomatoes carry most of the vitamins in a well-balanced assimilative manner for the activities in the system. Yet, if these are not cared for properly, they may become very destructive to a physical organism, that is, if they ripen after being pulled, or if there is the contamination that in most instances, because of the greater uniform activity, is preferable to be eaten after being canned, for it is then much more uniform."

Back in Cayce's day (the early 1900s), canning involved putting tomatoes in jars. Nobody had canning manufacturing facilities at home; therefore the word "canning" meant "jarring" to the farm families of the time. In addition, canning then did not involve high amounts of salt and preservatives, as it does today.

Being "much more uniform" appears to point to the stage of ripeness relative to acidity. When tomatoes sit in a jar for a period of time, it appears that their molecular structure changes; they become less acid-forming in the body. Therefore, eating jarred tomatoes appears to be the only healthy way to consume tomatoes.

It is very important to keep one thing in mind when considering the Cayce alkaline diet. When he prescribed the diet, there was not the food quality degradation problem that we have today. Not only do we suffer from processed and mass produced foods, but we also have genetically engineered foods and foods manufactured with carcinogenic preservatives.

Also important is the fact that Cayce suggested we avoid pork, even though he did claim that a few strips of bacon once in a while would not be detrimental to a person's health. In addition, raw tomatoes were not recommended, even though we find tomatoes listed in the Cayce alkaline diet. This is probably because they are only mildly acidic and likely permissible in creating a slightly alkaline environment. As we shall see in the cancer prevention diet, people with cancer should avoid tomatoes completely. This is because the Hoxsey diet attempts to put the pH level of our body fluids as high as possible, 8.0 if we can do it, while the Cayce diet wants our pH just over 7.0, or slightly alkaline.

As a general rule, the Cayce diet is a cancer prevention diet because it counteracts the effects of the high number of acid-forming foods we tend to ingest today. Most people should avoid having a highly acidic level in the blood. For somebody who has cancer, the Hoxsey diet is by far the diet of choice. If you have cancer, you need to shoot for 8.0!

The Cancer Recovery Diet

The Hoxsey Diet

The following dietary information comes directly from the BMC in Tijuana, Mexico, and has helped literally hundreds of thousands of people with cancer. I have listed all the categories of information on diet that a BMC patient receives at the first visit, and then expounded upon them so readers can better understand the benefits of such a program for health recovery.

During a visit to the Biomedical Center, a cancer patient's afternoon will be filled with discussions about X-rays, the condition of the cancer, and supplements and herbal prescriptions for the type of cancer. There will also be a lengthy segment on nutritional and dietary counseling. Staying on the Hoxsey diet is the most difficult aspect of Hoxsey therapy for most patients. However, those who do stay on the diet are more likely to be counted in the clinic's 80 percent success rate. This has been true not only for me but also for the 30-some people I've interviewed. The diet, in conjunction with the herbal medicines, is crucial to a patient's recovery.

Most BMC patients have success by staying on the diet for a five-year period. When I first went to the clinic, its program for Hodgkin's lymphoma was a four-year diet. The fifth year was three months on and three months off the diet, in order to prepare my immune system to attack carcinogens and processed foods without overtaxing it again. This is still up for debate among the doctors because it depends on my progress.

It is important to note that some people are told to stay on the diet for more than five years, depending on their progress. For example, Bernie Main, co-producer of the video *The Patient Experience*, contracted non-Hodgkin's lymphoma and was on the Hoxsey diet for nine years. This was about 15 years ago now. It turned out to be a wise decision, because recovery from lymphoma through traditional medicine is only 50 percent after five years, according to the most current statistics (which are based on five-year recovery studies).

In order to master the cancer recovery diet, we must become good label readers when we shop, as well as good natural food cooks. I must admit I was not a good cook when I began the Hoxsey diet, but four months later, my family's Christmas present to me was a chef's smock titled "Healthy Gourmet Chef." It was a sign of my becoming a fairly good cook with the ingredients I was allowed by the diet, which needed herbs and spices to activate flavors.

Now let's look at the Hoxsey diet. Its goal is to eliminate carcinogenic and toxic substances, foods that may cause our body fluids to drop below a pH level of 7.0, foods that have reduced nutritional value or reduce our immunity, and substances that render the prescribed herbal medicines useless. Each substance in the diet has been evaluated for its benefits and detrimental effects on somebody with cancer who is on the Hoxsey system of recovery. What follows is the Hoxsey diet and is completely in accordance with the dietary recommendations of the Biomedical Center in the year 2006.

Tomatoes

Tomatoes neutralize the herbal medicines and turn our body fluids acidic. Tomatoes are found not only in condiments and sauces, but also in dried powdered spice mixes. A small amount of dried powdered tomatoes is enough to tip the pH balance toward acidic. Italian food lovers may want to convert to linguini sauce and whole grain or spinach pastas. Hoxsey patients should watch out for tomatoes, because even restaurants often don't realize how many foods contain tomato products.

Alcohol

Alcohol neutralizes the herbal medicine tonics, making them less effective. Unfortunately, most herbal tonic manufacturers who make herbal tinctures use alcohol to suspend their herbs, because it is a less expensive and less volatile manufacturing process. The only other way to suspend herbs in a tincture is through another liquid called potassium iodide. However, according to herbal manufacturers I've interviewed, the extremely high temperatures that the tincture must reach to suspend the herbs often leads to combustion and fire hazards. As a result, the manufacturing process is considerably more expensive.

Liquid alcohol may be found in other products as well, such as vanilla extract. Those who drink alcoholic beverages must eliminate them. However, my research shows that red wine is very high in antioxidants, so it appears that on special occasions, "once in a blue moon," a glass of red wine may not hinder the process.

Not every doctor at BMC agrees with this statement, because most of them claim that alcohol neutralizes the tonic for approximately three days after it is ingested. This is three days of no blood purification, which leads to a decrease in the effectiveness of immune function.

Salt (Sodium)

The BMC physicians will examine patients' blood tests, which have either been done in their home town or are done at the clinic, to determine if the patients are consuming too much salt. The daily limit is 2,300 mg. which is generally about a teaspoon a day. If we consume too much salt, our body fluids turn acidic. If we consume too little, we will have a noticeable lack of energy. Table salt contains iodine, which is used in all processed foods, so we tend to get more than enough iodine in our diets. Blood tests at the BMC will determine sodium, chloride, and iodine levels. Being in the middle to low range of normal for these elements is ideal.

In the past, people ate salt without iodine and often became sickly, so salt began to be manufactured with iodine. But today many processed foods contain iodized salt, giving our bodies the iodine we need, so any added salt should be sea salt. In addition, some vegetables, such as celery, contain significant amounts of sodium. To gauge how much salt we need without the use of blood tests, the BMC recommends that we consume just enough to overcome the blandness of food.

Natural salt crystals, such as those harvested from the sea, increase our energy levels, increase vitality, and help protect against harmful electromagnetic fields (kinesiology tests showing these results are discussed in a previous chapter). It is best to replace all salt at home with sea salt, and also take sea salt or herbal seasonings when eating out. I often carry with me a small snack bag containing healthy seasonings.

Artificial Sweeteners and Sugar

The anticancer diet does not allow refined or processed sugar, which includes white bleached sugar and high fructose corn syrup. We should replace these things in all our foods with the following: sugar cane, raw sugar or sugar in the raw, honey, molasses, maple syrup, sugar cane juice, evaporated crystallized sugar cane juice, or organic sugar.

What makes natural sugar different from white processed sugar? Raw sugar is much healthier because it generally contains nutrients that processed sugar does not. White sugar is obtained by refining sugar cane crystals, removing the sugar cane juice flavor and therefore many important nutrients. White sugar is basically pure sucrose. Sucrose not only lacks the natural phytonutrients stripped from raw sugar during the bleaching process, but it also spikes blood sugar, which leads to an increase in the hypermetabolic rate of dividing cancer cells. The body needs the energy it gets from sugar, but whatever the body doesn't use as energy it converts to fat. When the blood sugar spikes with sucrose, it also tends to convert it into fat.

Unfortunately, sugar in the raw and other natural sugars are more expensive because of the law of supply and demand. There are very few places left in the world that grow and produce sugar in the raw. Processed sugar is much more plentiful, so it is less expensive. Most commercial sugar in the raw, or what is also called "turbinado sugar," comes from plantations in the Hawaiian island of Maui, where it is made by crystallizing natural sugar cane juice. Thus, the benefits of ingesting natural crystalline structured food is emphasized here again, as it is similar to sea salt crystals in the ability to strengthen the body and reduce the effect of electromagnetic devices on the immune system.

Fructose, which is fruit sugar (not high fructose corn syrup), and maltitol (derived from alcohol) may be used in small quantities occasionally. So may natural sweeteners such as stevia, which is derived from a cactus.

We must avoid all artificial sweeteners, coloring, and flavorings. Saccharine has been proven to be carcinogenic, and aspartame is dangerously toxic. Aspartame, or what has been trademarked as NutraSweet, has been reported to break down into other chemical compositions when heated. Several reports claim that when the temperature of this sweetener exceeds 85 degrees F, the wood alcohol content converts to formaldehyde and then to formic acid (a poison found in the sting of fire ants). Metabolic acidosis may result, and cases of methanol toxicity have been reported, which mimics multiple sclerosis and systemic lupus. This highly toxic chemical has also been reported to cause headaches, seizures, brain tumors, and various forms of cancer. Regardless of temperature, methanol toxins found in diet drinks further taxes the immune system of cancer patients, limiting their chances of recovery.

As mentioned in the introduction, in 1984 I met and spoke with one of the scientists involved in researching and developing aspartame. He told me that it should not have been approved for public consumption. Therefore, readers should beware of this highly toxic chemical.

Almost all synthetically manufactured artificial sweeteners are off limits, including sucralose, which is a refined sugar. However, an artificial sweetener named maltitol (an alcohol derivative) in small quantities on an occasional basis is permissible. Most valuable among sugars are the natural sweeteners, as they actually help rebuild our cell walls to fend off cancer, multiple sclerosis, and other diseases. They also give us beneficial phytonutrients and minerals.

Scientific Support for the Use of Natural Sugars

Natural sugars derived from fruits and vegetables contain highly valuable glycoproteins, which have recently been researched and deemed effective against a wide range of DNA-derivative diseases, including cancer. Glycoproteins are proteins that contain carbohydrates as part of their structure. Research shows that these carbohydrates change in individuals when they contract cancer. Such changes enable cancer cells to adhere to other cells in a process called metastasis, or the spreading of cancer. Altered glycoproteins have been found in intestinal, pancreatic, hepatoma, ovarian, prostate, and lung cancers.

Plants and other organic sources have been found to contain both polysaccharides and glycoproteins. Studies show that glycoproteins, which have mannose sugars on the surface, can activate macrophages, one of the most important cells involved in fighting cancer. The binding of mannose to cell surfaces also induces these cells to secrete substances that stimulate other cells within the immune system designed to kill cancer.

There are many other natural sugars that have demonstrated anticancer or antitumor activity. These sugars and the ones described above may be researched in *GlycoScience and Nutrition*, April 1, 2000, vol. 1, no. 14, published by Mannatech, Inc.

Mannatech manufactures and sells a powdered form of glyconutrients. Many people I've talked with seem to be getting results in recovering from a variety of DNA-derivative diseases. The primary concern I have in using glyconutrients is that some people with cancer who use them in place of consuming fruits and vegetables will not get the roughage necessary to combat cancers that are dependent on a high-fiber diet, such as colon cancer. However, research into glyconutrients provides impressive support for their use.

Natural sugars should be consumed by those who desire to kill their cancer, while processed sugar, which is stripped of glyconutrients during manufacturing, simply fuels hypermetabolizing cancer cells and should be avoided completely. Needless to say, there is much research showing the detrimental effects of processed sugar on normal healthy bodies, let alone those with a compromised immune system.

Liquids

The rule of thumb, according to the BMC, is that you must drink at least two quarts of liquid daily. If you can drink more, this is better. This is because liquids rid the body of toxins while hydrating it. Some cancer experts claim that dehydration is a primary causative factor in our contracting cancers. For the Hoxsey patient, it is imperative to drink a lot of liquids, because the medical staff at the BMC claims that the herbal blood purifiers they prescribe tend to dehydrate the body, if the minimal two quarts are not consumed.

Of this two quart requirement, Hoxsey patients are to drink one pint of diluted grape juice, white or red, with a pint of water or melted ice. Grape juice is excellent as an organ cleanser, thus assisting in proper immune function.

BMC patients take, as the foundation of their therapy, four doses of the herbal medicine tonic daily. I put two doses of herbal tonic (my afternoon and evening doses) into a quart-sized sports bottle, from which I sip all afternoon. I take my first dose of the herbal tonic with my morning beverage, and my last dose with my bedtime tea or spring water. First thing in the morning, last thing at night: this was easiest for creating a routine.

Most of my mornings start with fresh squeezing citrus juices. In my first year of recovery, this was true every morning. For quick production and ease in clean up, I use a hand juicer with a rotating spindle, which grinds halves of lemons, limes, oranges, grapefruits, and kiwis. To increase my nutrients, I remove the pulp strainer.

In my first year of recovery, instead of fresh squeezing my daily grape juice requirement, I bought large jugs of non-concentrated grape juice, such as the kosher brand Kedem, which is manufactured in New York and often used as a wine base. Kedem is the next best thing to fresh-squeezed grape juice. It can be purchased through many large discount stores such as Costco and Sam's Club, and some grocery stores through a special order.

It is not advisable to use juice concentrates in the first year of recovery, because of their age. Some juice concentrates are a year and a half old before they are unfrozen and released for consumption. Older concentrates begin to lose their nutritional value.

It is highly advisable in the first twelve months of recovery to consume fresh squeezed juice in the morning, and non-concentrated grape juice throughout the day. For the next four years of the five-year recovery period, we may consider switching to a concentrate—if our lives are not overtaxed with stress.

I decided to switch to grape juice concentrate after the first year, but continue to squeeze fresh citrus fruits almost every day (lemon or lime, grapefruit, orange, and kiwi). Lemons are very healthy for a wide variety of illnesses, but particularly for cancer; they have acidic properties that change the body fluids to a high level of alkalinity. Beware of store-bought lemon juices, however, which often contain the preservative sodium benzoate.

Kiwi has recently been found to have a number of health benefits. It is very high in antioxidants. However, the most impressive introduction to the food market is pomegranate juice, which is the highest antioxidant juice on the planet. Although it comes with a hefty price tag of about $10 per quart, it is a good replacement for wine sipping, which we can pretend we are doing if we are in the habit of drinking wine while socializing or eating. It is tart ,with a dry aftertaste like wine, and also costs about the same.

Other liquids that are recommended are spring water, herbal teas, green tea, various 100 percent fruit and vegetable juices, preferably freshly squeezed, and non-canned soups. Spring water improves our mineral content, which is very important because research shows that cancer patients can be deficient in zinc, selenium, and vanadium.

A Focus on Teas

Green tea is the most common health tea because it is high in antioxidants. One University of Southern California study found that women who drank about a half a cup of green tea daily cut their breast cancer risk by as much as 50 percent. Catechins, which are members of the flavan-3-ol class of bioflavonoids, are the polyphenolic compounds that provide the exceptional antioxidant activity in green tea that has proven to inhibit tumor formation and growth. In vitro studies have shown inhibited cancer cell growth in the following cancers: prostate carcinoma cell lines, human stomach cancer cells, human epidermoid carcinoma, human keratinocyte carcinoma, lung cancer cell lines, colorectal carcinoma cells, breast cancer cells, and virally transformed fibroblasts cells. Some studies also show that toxic concentrations of some chemotherapy drugs found in the liver and heart are reduced with powdered green tea.

White tea is the highest antioxidant tea on the planet. It is believed to be minimally processed, which gives it a major advantage over other teas. In one Oregon State University study, cancer-prone mice that ingested white tea developed 23 percent fewer tumors than those given green tea. It is difficult to find, however, so if you can't find it in local specialty shops that stock bulk teas, www.InPursuitOfTea.com or other web sites may be good resources.

Other teas that are medicinal include the following. *Brassica* tea is a green tea fortified with sulforaphine, a compound derived from broccoli. Each cup is comparable to the antioxidant protections of a three-ounce serving of broccoli. John Hopkins School of Medicine found it to be so valuable in their research, particularly for cancer, that their researchers patented it. It may be found at most health food stores.

Rooibos, referred to as *red tea,* contains valuable quercetin. Quercetin is an antioxidant that was used in earlier traditional medicine asthma therapies, and it too has been proven to inhibit cancer growth. Red tea comes from a flowering shrub in South Africa and can taste quite strong; it is better diluted with milk or soy milk.

Other medicinal teas include *peppermint* tea, which is good for stomach problems, heartburn, intestinal cramps, and aching muscles. *Ginger* tea is good for motion sickness, and *passionflower* tea may help manage anxiety, according to the *Journal of Clinical Pharmacy and Therapeutics. Valerian* tea is beneficial for mild insomnia, according to an article published in the *American Family Physician*; however, it is strongly recommended that it not be combined with alcohol or other sedatives.

Liquids to Eliminate

Black teas are the most carcinogenic teas, and should be avoided like the plague. The reason is that we Americans do not counter-balance our black tea consumption with green tea, as is traditionally done in Asia. Asia has lower heart disease and cancer rates, according to population studies, and it is believed that one contributing factor is the high consumption of soy products and green tea. Black tea comes from the same plant as green tea, the *Camellia Sinensis* tea plant, but green tea leaves are harvested earlier than black tea leaves. Black tea is often found in chai tea and is served as Chinese tea at Chinese restaurants. It also may be found in the most common restaurant or store-bought teas manufactured by large American commercial tea companies, and it makes up our popular beverage iced tea. Black teas are also fairly high in caffeine, which should be avoided.

All *carbonated beverages*—sodas, seltzer water, sparkling water, and beer—contain carbon dioxide, which evolves into carbonic acid as it is ingested. It will turn our body fluids acidic. In addition, sodas often have phosphoric acid, the active ingredient of toilet bowl cleaner, making them a greater detriment to our health. Phosphoric acid has been found in cigarette tobacco, another reason among many to quit smoking. Sodas also contain high fructose corn syrup, a processed sugar.

Caffeinated *coffee* should also be eliminated, not only because of the acid-forming qualities of coffee, but primarily because of the rest factor of the Hoxsey cancer recovery system. The high amount of caffeine in coffee does not allow us to recognize when we are tired. We need to be aware of when our bodies are asking us for a break, a nap, or more sleep. The concept of rest is very important to cancer recovery, because rest increases our resistances and strengthens our immune systems.

Even *decaffeinated coffee* should be minimized, because of its acid-forming qualities. The BMC says to drink only one or two cups daily. It should be only naturally decaffeinated coffee; this can be verified on the label. To obtain decaffeinated coffee, most coffee beans are stripped of their caffeine using a carcinogenic chemical called methylene chloride, which is a significantly less expensive decaffeination process. Because of this, most coffee shop chains, hotel chains, and other franchises tend to stock decafs that are not naturally decaffeinated.

The Swiss steam process in naturally decaffeinated coffees is more expensive to use. However, some commercial coffee manufacturers, such as the bulk coffee bean supplier found at most Kroger's, Millstone Coffee, Inc., have been able to keep their prices down because of the high amount of decaffeinated coffee they manufacture.

The Swiss steam process uses a safer chemical called ethyl acetate to strip the beans of their caffeine. Ethyl acetate is a naturally occurring substance found in foods such as apples, bananas, and pineapples. The solution is poured onto the beans and then drained off, taking the caffeine with it. Then the beans are steamed to rid them of the ethyl acetate. The trace amount of ethyl acetate left in the beans—less than ten parts per million—is so low you would have to drink 500 cups of naturally decaffeinated coffee in order to equal the amount found in one very ripe banana.

One further measure of safety may be to purchase organically grown, naturally decaffeinated coffees from your local heath food store. Organic coffee claims assert that it is grown without the use of pesticides.

Grains (breads, crackers, pastas, cereals, etc.)

The cancer patient must be careful to consume whole grains only, eliminating processed (white) flour. The whole grains are generally darker in appearance. My mother, who is a nurse, always said, "The whiter the bread the quicker you're dead." Bleached flour is the most detrimental, because in consuming it we consume some residual bleach for our immune system to wrestle with, a bad choice while it's trying to fight the battle of hypermetabolizing cancer cells.

All-purpose flour is processed as well, but without being bleached. It is not as harmful to the immune system, but is bad for the intestines, so it is not recommended. Remember that if you mix processed flour with water, it literally makes glue. When I was in kindergarten, we mixed flour and water to make a paste for gluing paper. Imagine what your intestines look like after you eat processed flour with a glass of water. Besides this, the simple carbohydrates found in white bread and pastas turn into sugar, which spikes blood sugar levels and increases the hypermetabolic rate of cancer cells. These carbohydrates also rapidly convert to fat cells, a disadvantage for recovering cancer patients.

This is why many of the latest diet fads include eliminating simple carbohydrates.

Whole grain breads, cereals, and pastas are the healthiest because they are not processed. Processing wheat, for example, takes the gluten out of the grain; gluten is a sticky mixture of very healthy proteins. Some people are allergic to gluten, however, and therefore cannot enjoy its health benefits. In general, though whole grains are very healthy for the digestive tract, helping us to be more regular and thinner. Beware of commercially bought grains in supermarkets, though, because most whole grain breads contain traces of vinegar, alcohol, and processed sugar or high fructose corn syrup. While the trace amount of alcohol is likely to evaporate in baked bread, the other two should be completely eliminated.

We should shop for cereals high in dietary fiber, but also be aware that many cereals contain artificial sweeteners and processed sugar, and some have unhealthy preservatives. We should consume whole wheat crackers only, and get our protein more from grains and legumes such as beans (soy, lima, pinto, garbanzo, etc.), lentils, and tofu, than from meat.

In general, the cancer patient should eliminate all white grains, such as white bread, white pasta, and white rice.

Nuts

Unsalted nuts and low-salt popcorn are recommended by the BMC. Edgar Cayce, during one of his readings, recommended that a few almonds be eaten each day to "thwart a tendency toward cancer." Many types of nuts (excluding peanuts), and in particular almonds, have been determined to contain valuable anti-cancer agents. The BMC recommends eating seven to ten almonds per day, or an equivalent amount of almond butter, because of their cancer-fighting properties.

The BMC says to never consume peanuts, peanut butter, or peanut products. Aflatoxins are produced by mold and fungus, which commonly grow in the peanut shell and in some seeds and grains when left where moisture can penetrate them. The increased incidence of certain cancers in Germany was attributed to molds and funguses found in grain bins susceptible to moisture. Aflatoxins, found in such molds and funguses, are highly carcinogenic. It is best to store seeds and grains in sealed dry containers. According to Harkness, FASCP, Brathman, M.D., and Kroll, Ph.D., authors of *Everything You Need to Know about Reducing Cancer Risk*, studies have linked aflatoxins to esophageal and liver cancer in many countries where contaminated foods are commonplace.

Almond butter, soy butter, and cashew butter are a healthier bet with all-natural fruit jellies to make a good old-fashioned nut butter and jelly sandwich. In addition, making a trail mix of various dried fruits and dry non-salted nuts, such as almonds, sunflower seeds, and pecans, is very healthy in the broader scheme of cancer recovery.

Fruits and Vegetables

The BMC recommends consuming all kinds of fruits and vegetables, preferably fresh or home grown, or commercially frozen. These are best eaten either raw or lightly cooked, preferably lightly steamed. Raw fruits and vegetables contain the highest amount of nutrients and anti-cancer enzymes. If store-bought in frozen form, then the clinic recommends that we read the label carefully for toxic or carcinogenic preservatives. All forms of fruits and vegetables are advisable—cruciferous are the best—and they should be part of every meal. Snacking on fruits and vegetables throughout the day is also very wise.

The American Cancer Society (A.C.S.) recommends that we eat a minimum of five servings of fruits and vegetable daily in order to prevent cancer. These foods are the best source of cancer-fighting vitamins and nutrients, minerals, fiber, phytochemicals, and antioxidants. They also provide extra energy, which is essential for those people whose habit is to rely on caffeine to be alert and productive. They are especially good for people with cancer, who commonly experience a significant lack of energy due to the illness.

Hoxsey patients must remember that canned fruits and vegetables are off limits due to age and to sodium and other preservatives.

Grapes have long been known to be valuable in cancer prevention. In my research into the Cayce readings, I found one case where grapes had been reported as a cancer cure solely due to Cayce suggesting a grape fast. I also found various sources suggesting that grapes help a variety of other illnesses. This bioflavonoid antioxidant helps with vision improvement, skin elasticity, and other regenerative cell activity.

Grapes are most beneficial to our immune systems, because their antioxidant qualities help in free radical reduction. Particularly in juice form, they are also liver and spleen cleansers; these organs are key to our immune function. The non-concentrated juice form is ultimately best, or fresh-squeezed grape juice.

One of the most beneficial aspects of grapes is the seeds, which contain powerful antioxidants. Imported grapes from Chile and Mexico may prove to be the best, because they are not genetically engineered and therefore still contain the seeds. For digestive purposes, the seed is most beneficial when chewed; however, it is very bitter. For this reason, many people prefer to swallow grape seeds whole or buy grape seed capsules.

Although juicing fruits and vegetables is beneficial, we should note the value of the dietary fiber in their membrane segments, which we get when we eat fruits and vegetables whole. Because of their high-fiber diet, the Chinese have a much lower incidence of colon cancer and heart disease than Americans, and of all the cancers, colon cancer statistically is linked to the highest number of fatalities in America. It is also important to note that the traditional Japanese diet contains soy products, which have specific anticoagulant and anticancer enzymes. The Japanese also regularly consume other culinary herbs and plants with phytochemicals containing extraordinary health benefits.

I was told at the BMC that fresh, dark green vegetables are particularly healthy for the cancer patient. I later discovered that broccoli and other cruciferous vegetables, such as kale, cauliflower, cabbage, brussels sprouts, and mustard greens, all have a valuable phytochemical called sulphoraphane, which stimulates a type of enzyme that, according to many studies, blocks the progression of cancer. Broccoli sprouts are therefore very good to eat on whole grain bagels and are available at health food stores.

Yellow and red onions are also beneficial. They contain allinase and selenium, both of which have important anti-cancer properties. Alfalfa sprouts contain the highest amount of enzymes of any food on the planet. In the category of fruit, papaya (especially its seeds) has the highest amount of enzymes. Many alternative medicine clinics promote phytoenzymes as the most important factor in cancer recovery. It is best to consult with an alternative medicine specialist who specializes in cancer recovery to make sure that the type of cancer you are fighting (if you have cancer) will benefit from phytoenzymes, which are enzymes derived from plant sources. Most cancers are stymied by phytoenzymes.

The fast track to dietary cancer prevention is to consume six to nine helpings of fruits and vegetables every day. How many of us do this? Not many people in the western world, I'm sure. For the cancer patient, it should be mandatory. When I shop, the produce department in the local grocery store is usually my first stop, then the health food aisle. Everything else is secondary. The local health food stores, particularly the larger, more economical ones, are on my weekly shopping trip as well.

Meat

The BMC's research indicates that the fat and some chemicals present in some meats, such as beef, cause the muscles to react to heat, thereby producing unhealthy chemical reactions. In fact, many of the chemicals used to produce cancer in laboratory animals are derived from burned meat fats. When beef and pork are exposed to high temperatures, it creates dangerous carcinogens called heterocyclic aromatic amines (HAAs). This is why the BMC recommends against grilling, particularly grilling beef (pork is off limits). However, many nutrition experts claim that moderate consumption of certain types of meat is generally a wise step in cancer prevention.

The Hoxsey diet suggests four servings of meat each week, in order to get the protein and amino acids we need to be healthy. The problem with meat is that our bodies become acidic when we digest it. It is inadvisable to completely eliminate meat from our diets, because then we must be sure to replace the amino acids and proteins our bodies generally require. Vegetarians are often deficient in protein and amino acids. To compensate, amino acids spray, which is found in most health food stores, can be used at home as a seasoning. Because of the recommendation for low meat consumption, the BMC also recommends that its patients consume vegetable proteins such as lentils and other beans. The Hoxsey diet contains the following meats.

Beef or wild game (once a week). We may have beef and other red meats no more than once a week, if it is corn-fed and, preferably, organically raised. Unfortunately, non-organic red meats often contain steroids. Farmers give their animals steroids to "beef them up," and antibiotics to reduce the sores caused by the steroids. Our overuse of antibiotics leads to our bodies becoming immune to them, when we may need them to save our lives. Mass production of meat often contributes to the problem. A good replacement for beef, which is available at some supermarket chains (such as Kroger), is organic buffalo. It tastes similar to hamburger, but even better. It is also less fattening.

Wild game is one of the healthiest meats to eat, because of the lack of pesticides, steroids, and antibiotics in it. In particular, venison (deer), rabbit, quail, buffalo, elk, and turkey are lean and without chemicals. The BMC recommends that we substitute game for beef, if possible. Unfortunately, most people in our society don't have access to wild game, and not just because they live in cities and don't hunt. Unfortunately, state laws don't even allow the sale of wild game. Therefore, it may be a good idea to request a favor from any hunters you know, if you aren't a hunter yourself.

Fish and poultry (three times a week). Hoxsey patients are allowed to have chicken and turkey up to twice a week, but preferably once a week, and fish twice a week. Farm-raised fish is excluded, particularly salmon, because dyes are often injected for coloring. Because of this, wild salmon, which can be found in Super Wal-Marts, is best. Organically raised poultry, as opposed to poultry from commercial farms, is also more healthy, but not required. Beware of pre-sliced packaged poultry, which generally contains carcinogenic preservatives such as nitrites and sulfites.

Occasionally we can have fish three times a week and fowl once a week, if we skip red meat and game that week, but eating this way regularly is inadvisable because of the mercury build up in some fish. In addition, some poultry may have high amounts of bacteria that our immune systems expend extra energy to fight, when that same energy can be used to fight our cancer. Poultry is also commonly fed chicken feed grown with pesticides. Remember that pesticide use is becoming less regulated over time, and has been cited by several credible sources, including the American Cancer Society, as a primary cause for the increased incidence of lymphoma.

Salmon, tuna, and mackerel were recommended by Cayce in several readings, and also recommended by nutritional cancer expert Julian Whitaker, M.D. They are particularly high in omega-3 and omega-6 essential fatty acids. Trout, sardines, and eel are also high in omega-3. These essential fatty acids are not only good for protecting against circulatory diseases, but omega-3 fatty acids in particular have also been shown to have significant antitumor activity. My personal choice, after discovering this, was to replace my weekly beef allowance with fish, but I needed to do some research first.

The Food and Drug Administration's advisory on mercury and fish consumption in March, 2004 got lots of media attention. According to A.C. Nielsen, sales of fish in cans and envelopes fell 9 percent in the 12 months after the advisory, which primarily singled out tuna. In the same year, sales of refrigerated seafood in the United States fell 2.1 percent.

The FDA and the Environmental Protection Agency first stated in 2001 that some fish have so much mercury that eating them was dangerous to the developing brain of a fetus. Mercury affects the migration of brain cells in fetuses, preventing signal transmission pathways from developing properly. Researchers also believe that high levels of mercury damage the autonomic nervous system, which tells blood vessels when to contract or relax and the heart how fast to beat.

The FDA recommends that pregnant women and young children not eat fish with high levels of mercury, such as shark, swordfish, king mackerel, and tilefish. Only one meal a week should be albacore, or white tuna, because its mercury levels are high enough that two servings are too much. Light tuna, which is darker than albacore, is a mix of tuna types that is lower in mercury and not subject to the recommendation. Larger, older, predatory fish have the highest levels of mercury, but fish that don't consume other fish, such as salmon, don't have the problem.

Since the 15th century, mercury in the environment has increased 200–500 percent, according to Elsie Sunderland, an EPA scientist. One of the largest sources today is burning coal. In 1998, the EPA estimated that U.S. coal-fired power plants emit about 50 tons of mercury into the atmosphere each year. In third world countries, coal is a primary source of energy. Meanwhile, the Bush administration has pulled the United States out of participating in the Kyoto Accord, an effort establishing world-wide preventive and corrective steps toward correcting pollution of this nature.

Mercury in smoke travels across the globe through a process called "atmospheric transport and deposition." It falls on water, is eaten by bacteria, digested, and turned into methyl mercury, which when ingested binds tightly to muscle tissue. Therefore, in each step of the food chain, methyl mercury is passed along. Tiny plankton are eaten by smaller fish, which are eaten by medium-sized fish, which are eaten by larger fish. Thus mercury is concentrated in predatory fish, which have consumed all the mercury in all the fish below it in the food chain.

Pork. The cancer patient must eliminate pork. It is highly acid-forming. People with a compromised immune system can't have any pork, pork skins (around sausages), or pork grease, which is commonly used in cooking. My family eats turkey bacon (without the nitrites/nitrates or sulfites/sulfates). We also replace sausages with soysages or soy derivative sausages, but be careful, because some of them contain a pork skin wrapping.

If you will recall, in an earlier chapter I talked to Paul, my friend who took my CT scans. He is also an osteopathic physician who does extensive research into alternative medicine and nutritional healing. He told me that pork cells under a microscope resemble cancer cells. We should also keep in mind that Jesus, a Jew, didn't consume pork either. In fact, he sent demons into a herd of pigs!

As a general rule, the four weekly servings of meat that a Hoxsey patient is allowed to eat should alternate among fish, poultry, and wild game. Because of this low consumption of meat, Hoxsey patients must remember to increase their intake of plant-based proteins in order to stay healthy.

Dairy

Cancer patients should have dairy products only occasionally and only in small amounts. If we are accustomed to drinking milk every day, we should reduce it to every two days. If we have been consuming cheese every day, we should reduce it to once every two days. However, aged cheese should be eliminated: such as cheddar, parmesan, and Swiss. As a general rule, we should avoid any cheese with a hard consistency, which tend to be aged. Aged cheese carries molds, which tax our immune systems.

Soft cheese is permissible, but again not on a daily basis. Soft cheeses that we may safely consume include mozzarella, American, havarti, low-fat cottage cheese, gouda, goat, feta, ricotta, and cream cheese. Occasionally jack and pepper jack (make sure the jalapeno peppers haven't been jarred with vinegar) are permissible. Soft cheeses that we cannot consume include blue cheese and Roquefort, because they contain unhealthy molds. All processed cheeses are permissible.

Natural yogurt may be consumed, but by "natural" the Hoxsey clinic means yogurt with only natural sugar (not refined sugar or high fructose corn syrup). For example, Stonefield Yogurt contains organic sugar.

The clinic's diet allows three to six eggs each week, if the patient does not have high cholesterol. The best way to cook the eggs is hard or soft boiled, because fried eggs may be hazardous to our health unless we pan-sear them with olive or grape seed oil.

Food Preparation

The anti-cancer diet involves cooking foods in such a way that they do not absorb extra fat or get burned in the process. Charred foods are carcinogenic, so if food gets burned in the process of cooking, at the very least the charred part should be scraped off; better yet, the whole piece of food should be thrown away. As a general rule, we should not eat grilled foods and we should never eat fried foods. It is best to eat steamed, stewed, baked, broiled, or boiled foods. These methods are the least carcinogenic.

Barbecued or grilled foods are not recommended, but they are not completely against the rules for recovery as long as the meat is extremely lean and is not charred. When grilling high-fat meat such as beef and pork, burning fat drips into an open flame and forms polycyclic aromatic hydrocarbons (PAHs), which have been proven to be dangerously carcinogenic. Dark brown or blackened toast also contains a variety of carcinogenic substances. We must avoid charred or burned food in every cooking process. In fact, burned fat and bread are typically given to laboratory animals to cause them to develop cancer.

Fried foods, as in deep fried, are definitely off limits. Any cooking method that involves enough oil so the food gets saturated with fat is unhealthy. Eating fried food is simply reckless for those prone to cancer and those with cancer. For people who are good conscientious cooks, we may risk pan-searing foods. I say good-conscientious cooks, because the amount of oil required to pan-sear or sauté the food in a pan is minimal. A conscientious cook would use just a tiny smidgen, or perhaps a smear of oil from an olive oil spray, to lightly coat pans or baking trays. Non-stick baking trays are a good idea. When it comes to oil, less is more (although a diet where fat is nonexistent is not healthy either). Now let's look at the healthiest oils to cook with.

Grape seed oil is one of the healthiest cooking oils. It is an essential fatty acid, containing no harmful trans-fatty acids, and can be heated to 485 degrees without becoming carcinogenic, unlike vegetable and other oils. It has a pleasant nutty flavor that brings out the taste in many foods.

Olive oil is another oil that may be heated to 485 degrees before turning carcinogenic. Virgin or extra virgin cold-pressed olive oil is by far the healthiest, and the most economical, healthy cooking oil.

Canola oil, which comes from a plant harvested in Canada (thus the name canola), contains the highest level of omega-3 fatty acids of any natural dietary substance, including fish and flax seed. However, it is not a good idea to cook with canola oil because it doesn't share the benefits of the non-carcinogenic properties, such as olive and grape seed does. In addition, if it is not cold-pressed, it is not as healthy. I would recommend only consuming it cold on occasion, perhaps on salads.

Eliminate *vegetable oil* from your diet. Because it is inexpensive, it is commonly used by restaurants (French fries, etc.) and commercial food manufacturers (in potato and corn chips, etc.). In addition, we should eliminate any other oils that may turn carcinogenic when heated. There is limited research, so if we are not sure about the heat range of an oil (the heat range is the temperature at which it becomes carcinogenic), we should avoid it. We should stay with the oils we are sure about: cold-pressed olive and grape seed oil. Cancer patients should certainly eliminate all hydrogenated or partially hydrogenated oils.

Microwave ovens are definitely off limits. Microwaves were banned in Russia, primarily because they reduce the nutritional value of food and promote illness. One short-term study showed pathological changes in test subjects after they ate microwaved foods. The changes included an increase in leukocytes, which indicated a significant stress was taking place in the body. A decrease in lymphocyte counts also occurred, an effect similar to what occurs in food poisoning. The subjects' total cholesterol levels increased, while blood iron levels decreased.

Cow's milk was also tested after exposure to microwaves; the tests showed:

a. increases in acidity and sedimentation
b. a change in the structure of fat molecules
c. a reduction of folic acid content
d. an increase in non-protein nitrogen

In addition, some microwaved foods have shown suppression of amino acid hydrolysis, and an amino acid conversion process proving to be toxic to the nervous system and poisonous to the kidneys.

The atomic structure of food, when it is microwaved, breaks apart, and the atoms bump into each other at such a rapid rate that it causes friction and thus heats the food. The logical truth is that it is not the same food with the same nutritional value coming out of a microwave oven as it was going in. (For more information on microwave ovens refer to chapter 7 which discusses traditional causes and treatments of cancer.)

Anticancer Culinary Herbs

Garlic is good for preventing cardiovascular diseases, but a high number of studies, many from Japan, also show a valuable anticancer effect. There was strong evidence showing a link between garlic consumption and a reduction of prostate and stomach cancers. Garlic contains allyl sulfur compounds, which slow or prevent the growth of tumor cells, particularly when it is eaten 15 minutes after the cloves are cut and exposed to the air. This is when allinase, the medicinal component in garlic, is at its highest potency.

Studies listed with the NIH show that powdered garlic and garlic extract are most effective against cancer when taken together. Cultures with a garlic-rich diet, such as China's, have a low cancer rate. On our family's shopping list is a large jar of minced garlic, or fresh garlic cloves of various types, which we use on a regular basis in food preparation.

Other culinary herbs with health benefits that the BMC recommends are: basil, thyme, rosemary, marjoram, dill, sage, tarragon, chives, mint, ginger root, cilantro, parsley, fennel, pepper, oregano, cinnamon, garlic, bay leaf, curry, cumin, paprika, ground mustard, nutmeg, and chili powder.

We grew many of these herbs in the mountains before we moved to the beach, but we still plan to grow many of them again, adding to the collection in our back yard.

Preservatives and Genetically Modified Food

The BMC says to eliminate all carcinogenic or toxic preservatives. These include monosodium glutamate (MSG), sodium benzoate, nitrites and sulfites. Monosodium glutamate is often found as a spice at the local grocery store, and it often is in store-bought rice dishes, sauces, and in foods at Chinese food restaurants. Sodium benzoate is often found in soy sauce, yogurt, and many other foods as a preservative.

Nitrites and sulfites are often found in store-bought meats, like packaged turkey, chicken, and bacon (of course, pork is off limits). Reading labels will eliminate from our diet most pre-sliced, packaged meats, forcing us to choose full roasts of fowl, for example, and then slice it ourselves. Nitrites and nitrosomines are widely known to be carcinogenic.

The FDA has tested many of these preservatives for their disease-causing potential. But often these tests don't take into account the quantities of these preservatives that Americans are likely to consume over time. Therefore the results can't be trusted in guaranteeing the preservatives' safety. They also don't test for combinations of these chemicals, which is how they end up in our diets. Nor do they test for small quantities of carcinogenic or toxic preservatives used over a long period of time and in certain environments with pollutants or specific forms of stress.

In the United States, we tend to eat a variety of foods with these preservatives in them. The widespread use of toxic or carcinogenic preservatives is one reason why Asia's rate of cancer is beginning to catch up to that of the United States. It is a good idea to reduce them if you are prone to cancer. If you have cancer, the BMC requires you to eliminate them from your diet.

Rest and Sleep

According to recent studies, our bodies naturally create the highest amount of antioxidants between 10:00 pm and 2:00 am during a normal sleep cycle. For many cancer patients, the worries of having the disease include the financial drain, inability to care for loved ones, and other things. These concerns can interrupt our sleep cycles and should therefore be discussed with BMC doctors, mental health professionals, a caring traditional oncologist, a minister, or an understanding relative or friend. Once these concerns are resolved, more sound sleep should ensue.

One thing cancer patients may need to learn is how to take care of themselves, rather than taking care of everybody else (more on this in the next chapter). Part of taking care of ourselves is resting when we need a rest. In other words, we need to learn to go to bed when we are tired and not try to stay awake to socialize or finish work. Particularly during the day, if we are tired, it may be time to sneak away to a quiet place and take a siesta (the Mexican word for afternoon nap). Perhaps the afternoon nap the Mexicans learned to take is a good recipe for health. We must learn to rest when the body asks for it.

According to research conducted in sleep clinics, the brain must enter into the delta wave state once or twice each night, or each sleep cycle, for one and one-half hours each time, for us to feel we have had a good night's sleep. Worrywarts tend to miss delta sleep, and this is unhealthy. Delta brain waves indicate a deep, restorative sleep.

Proper rest allows the body to repair, rebuild, and prepare itself for another day. It keeps our resistance high and our immune systems in top shape. It also helps us think more clearly and thus make sound decisions.

The Red Flags

Restaurants, Stress, Acidity, and Preservatives

Eating out is risky business. Because we are fighting against an early death, it is not advisable to eat out. However, on rare occasion, if we must eat out, we should check our alkalinity the morning after to discover if we accidentally ingested four of what I call the *sickening seven* substances, the four high acid-producers: pork, tomato, vinegar, and carbonated beverages. The entire sickening seven follows.

1. Pork
2. Tomato
3. Vinegar
4. Carbonated beverages
5. Alcohol
6. Processed flour
7. Processed sugar

I have tested acidic on litmus paper on only three occasions during the three years that I've been on the diet. The first time, I went to a Greek restaurant and ordered a Greek salad without the vinegarized olives and without the vinegarized dressing. I requested fresh lemon instead (not lemon juice, as bulk lemon juice in a bottle will always have sodium benzoate in it). When I ate the salad, I thought I tasted a trace of vinegar on it. I asked the waiter if there was vinegar on the salad and he said no, he didn't think so. However, when I checked my saliva the next morning, I was acidic. This is how I found out he was wrong. The truth is, many of those waiting tables don't really care, unless you tell them it's a life or death situation.

The second time occurred when I went out to eat sushi. I thought for sure I would be safe if I avoided the vinegarized ginger and the vinegarized horse radish in the wasabi (these can be made at home with lemon and ginger). But when I tested my saliva the next morning, I was acidic. I contacted another Japanese restaurant and discovered that vinegar must be added to the rice on all sushi rolls to get the rice to stick together for surrounding the fish. White rice was not forbidden by the BMC in 2003, but became a no-no by 2005.

The third time I was acidic was one Christmas time, when my teenage daughter was screaming and yelling at the family for several hours, beginning one night and going into the next morning. We were stuck in a hotel room preparing to visit my parents. Knowing it was wearing on us all, I tested my pH level and found that I was acidic. At that moment, the rest of the family left the motel room, with her yelling at us from the parking lot, and went shopping for a couple of hours. When we came back, we set a boundary on this kind of behavior by striking an agreement with her from the window of our van that she would get a ride to her grandparents only if she promised to act civil. *Stress will cause body fluids to turn acidic!* We will talk more about stress in the chapter on the mind-body connection.

A Sobering Note about Success and Failure

Three people of the approximate 30 I interviewed got themselves into big trouble by not following the Hoxsey diet. All three abandoned Hoxsey therapy and began using traditional medicine to try to save their lives. Some of the people I interviewed exhausted traditional medical efforts before turning to the BMC as the *court of last resort*, but most began Hoxsey therapy when they were diagnosed and it was their only form of treatment.

All three people (fictitious names are used) who failed on Hoxsey therapy explained to me that they followed the diet only for a short while, got results, cheated on the diet, and then left the BMC's care for traditional medicine. Otherwise, the Hoxsey method would have proven to be nearly 100 percent effective for the people I followed over the past few years. Here is how they failed.

1. Kathy, from the Midwest, had ovarian cancer and had done only the Hoxsey method (diet, herbal medicines, and supplements) through the Biomedical Center. She was in remission after four years. At the end of the fourth year, it was discovered that her ovarian cancer had returned, and she was in the process of committing to radiation therapy to save her life. How did this happen? I asked. Kathy admitted to me that she loved Chinese food and in the latter two years of the four she was on the program, she increasingly ate out at Chinese restaurants. The problem is that Chinese food is loaded with MSG, chicken fat, and carcinogenic sodium benzoate, which is found in all soy sauces (except the soy sauce replacement found in health food stores, Tamari sauce). She admitted to me she had cheated and wound up in trouble. When her U.S. oncologist recommended radiation, she checked with the doctors at the BMC. They approved it, making saving Kathy's life a priority over pushing Hoxsey therapy.

2. Then there's Joe. I contacted Joe, who had Hodgkin's lymphoma, before I even went to the BMC. He told me, "The Hoxsey program works; I know a girl who did it several years ago and she's still cancer-free. I just got sick of eating rabbit food." Joe followed the diet religiously for a year and a half, until he couldn't do it any more. In those one and a half years, Joe said the tumors in his mediastinum (the web of lymph nodes between our heart and lungs) had shrunk from several centimeters each, down to about one centimeter when he quit the program and did chemotherapy instead to finish out his treatment. This was about eight years ago (11 years ago as of this writing) and MOPP (a type of chemotherapy) was the method of choice. He experienced a return of cancer between years five and 13 from using MOPP, which can be common. His Hodgkin's lymphoma returned a second time now, and he was taking six months off to do more chemo. He claimed that chemo was easier for him, since he didn't feel too sick or lose his hair, as was the case for most.

3. I also talked to Susan, who had Hodgkin's lymphoma. She said that she was too young—only 16—to follow the diet when she contracted cancer and basically ate anything she wanted. Her lymphoma came back between

years five and six, at which time her doctor didn't like the size of the tumors in her mediastinum and recommended chemotherapy. She took it as a precautionary measure and she was in her forties when I interviewed her.

The three cases above represent the only ones I've discovered of all those I made contact with who failed using the Hoxsey system, and they failed because they couldn't follow the diet. Amazingly, I also interviewed some Hoxsey patients who did not follow the diet to the letter and were still cured. However, this is not recommended for a life-threatening illness. In my opinion, it doesn't take much to tip the immune scale. A good rule of thumb for those with cancer is: if you're going to do it, do it right, so you can "live long and prosper"!

As a general rule, because the Hoxsey diet is a low-fat diet, women will lose about 20 pounds on it and men will lose about 30 pounds. The pictures of me before and after the Hoxsey diet are dramatically different. I lost approximately 30 pounds and have kept it off. The diet and the supplements (which are described in the next chapter) make you feel good. In fact, if I forget my supplements and don't eat well, I feel my energy wane. Together, they also restore a youthful appearance. Many people have commented that it seems like the Hoxsey system has taken ten years off my age.

Author's before and after Pictures
(Before Cancer and after Committing to Hoxsey Therapy)

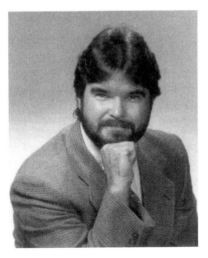

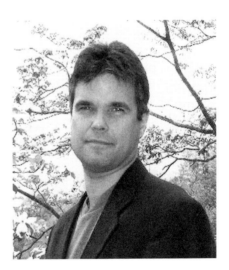

Taken in the summer of 1999
used for first edition/first book

Taken in the summer of 2004
used for recent book editions

Summary

In the seminars where I present this natural recovery system, people ask me what type of diet I would recommend for cancer prevention. I recommend the Cayce diet, the 80/20 program, which is a slightly alkaline diet. A slightly alkaline diet is healthy over a period of many years, and this type of diet makes some basic, conscientious eating habits relatively easy to follow. A slightly alkaline diet reduces the likelihood of succumbing to infectious bacteria and viruses, which are thought to be precursors to cancer.

For those who have a history of cancer in their genetics, I recommend a slightly higher alkalinity, by adding fresh-squeezed citrus in the mornings, which also boosts the immune system. I also recommend reducing or eliminating malted food products, the highest acid-forming foods. I have met some people who followed such a diet and lived to an older age than their parents, who had died of cancer. I also recommend some supplements, which I describe in the next chapter.

For people who have cancer, I recommend the Hoxsey diet. It is the most powerful anticancer diet available; it is the greatest complement to any comprehensive cancer therapy, particularly the herbal medicinal approach. The macrobiotic diet is very similar to the Hoxsey diet, and it too has a respectable reputation for success. If a cancer patient doesn't take herbal medicines, perhaps the macrobiotic diet would be second-best as a form of treatment. However, the Hoxsey diet has the longest track record of documented successes of any anticancer diet in the world.

Chapter 10

Supplements and Chinese Medicines

There are six categories of nutrients we need to sustain life. These are proteins, fats, carbohydrates, vitamins, minerals, and water. The first three provide energy. Vitamins, minerals, and water are vital to the proper regulation of the body's biochemical processes, including, but not limited to, the regulation of the immune system.

Vitamins are organic substances derived from living matter, such as plants and animals; minerals are inorganic substances that originate in the soil and end up in our food sources. All 13 vitamins are considered *essential* nutrients because they must be obtained from what we eat. Also essential are approximately 15–20 minerals and one oil (linoleic acid).

The water-soluble vitamins are stored in the body temporarily and get washed out regularly; therefore they need frequent replenishing. Vitamin C and the B vitamins are all water-soluble. Fat-soluble vitamins, which include A, D, E, and K, are stored by the body. Therefore they cannot as easily reach levels of deficiency, but they have the potential to build up to toxic levels. It is important to note that the body can make vitamin A from another nutrient called beta-carotene.

In this chapter, we will focus on supplements: their daily recommended doses, toxicity levels, and the doses that help bring deficient nutrient levels up to normal for either increasing immune function or killing cancer in vitro (in the body). In addition, we will discuss Chinese medicines, which, when used in conjunction with the Hoxsey herbs, add to the effectiveness of a comprehensive all-natural cancer therapy. I will also share the regimen that helped me in the process of my own recovery. All these concepts will fall under the category of the body's ability to kill its own cancer, which is at the foundation of naturopathic medicine.

Supplemental Nutrients and the Immune System

A good resource for the scientifically minded is a naturopathic textbook titled *Encyclopedia of Natural Medicine*, by Murray and Pizzorno. It shows that by increasing the intake of antioxidants vitamin C, vitamin E, zinc, selenium, and beta-carotene, we can prevent thymus gland involution and increase immune function, thereby preventing or correcting cancer. The thymus gland, located in the chest, is extremely important because, as mentioned previously, cancer involves a breakdown in the ability of certain lymphocytes and larger mononuclear cells designed to fight cancer cells.

Our immune system has multiple defenses, but once cancer cell immunity is compromised, the cancer cells, which regularly form within a normal human body, proliferate, increasing in size and territory. The thymus may be the most important component in our immune system, but it is susceptible to mental and physical stress overload. Therefore, its breakdown in efficiency has been linked to cancer and other illnesses. By increasing the nutritional antioxidants listed above, we may help strengthen and regulate the thymus gland and teach our immune response to once again detect cancer cells as foreign invaders.

These nutrient-based antioxidants are agents that deactivate *free radicals*. Also called oxygen-free radicals or oxidants, these are unstable molecules that can damage cell membranes and scramble cellular genetic information (DNA), starting a chain reaction that can often lead to the development of cancer. As mentioned previously, traditional science has proven that changes in DNA are at the root of cancer.

Free radicals are naturally produced in the body from normal cell metabolism, tissue injury, and from exposure to tobacco smoke, sunlight, X-rays, and other environmental sources. If any of these sources create specific changes in our DNA, cancer cells may be given a free ticket, so to speak, to grow out of control.

Researchers believe that cancer cells may generate a surplus of oxidants that send signals to the body that lead to uncontrolled cell growth, and that antioxidants block these signals. Therefore antioxidants, particularly in the form of nutrients, are very important for both cancer prevention *and* recovery.

"Control of signaling pathways involving oxidants may explain why some antioxidants appear to prevent development of certain cancers."
Keikobad Irani, M.D., of Johns Hopkins Hospital

In general, antioxidants vitamin C, vitamin E, zinc, selenium, and beta-carotene may be the most significant nutrients to take for preventing cancer or helping to eliminate it.

For cancer prevention, the recommended daily values listed on vitamin bottle labels may be sufficient. But if we are trying to cure a cancerous condition we may want to increase our supplemental intake, particularly with the water-soluble vitamins, which are safer in higher doses. As a preventative, vitamin E, beta carotene, and vitamin C provide the most effectiveness against the widest range of cancers. In addition, there are a multitude of other supplements (discussed later in this chapter) that have shown promising results in helping eradicate specific types of cancer.

Why Take a Multivitamin/Multimineral?

A *supplement* is something we take to supplement nutrients we should be getting from food. Anything that can be put in capsule form, instead of eaten in the raw, and is valuable to the cancer patient or cancer-prone person, will be categorized here as a supplement. In this category, I am also including things like culinary herbs, such as garlic, and also omega-3/omega-6s, macrominerals, and microminerals.

In recent years, several traditional scientific sources have been issuing statements to the public that it would be wise, particularly for Americans, to take a multivitamin in order to maintain an optimal state of health. This is because we Americans are not getting the vitamins and beneficial minerals we need from foods that the U.S. food industry offers us in our grocery stores. In other words, the average American consuming the average American diet is probably not getting the recommended daily allowance of vitamins and minerals recommended for optimum health.

A one-a-day multivitamin/multimineral is best, since many people forget to take the ones that are twice a day. Macrominerals and microminerals are especially important, because without them, certain vitamins and enzymes cannot function properly in the body. Some of them prevent or correct cancer. These are what is commonly lacking in our soil and therefore in our foods. An additional consideration is that exercise and perspiration naturally flush minerals from our bodies, so these need to be restored. When an athlete gets cancer, for example, it's not due to their lack of exercise, certainly, but due to mineral depletion. Therefore, in my opinion, a multivitamin/multimineral is essential for preventing cancer or assisting with a cancer cure.

It is important to consider that many multivitamin/multimineral supplements contain *macrominerals*, such as calcium, magnesium, manganese, zinc, and iron, but lack some important trace minerals, or what are also referred to as *microminerals*, such as vanadium and molybdenum, which have been known to neutralize carcinogens. There are about 87 known trace minerals, but finding a supplement with all 87 is probably impossible. Therefore, we should find a multivitamin/multimineral that contains some of the most important minerals, such as phosphorus, potassium, zinc, selenium, copper, chromium, and iodine.

Cell salts, which are also referred to as mineral salts, or tissue salts, are trace minerals that are at the foundation of every cell in our bodies. Without them, we would die, so they are therefore crucial to optimal health. These 12 essential cell salts are potassium sulfate, magnesium phosphate, sodium chloride, sodium phosphate, sodium sulfate, calcium phosphate, calcium sulfate, calcium fluoride, ferric phosphate, potassium chloride, potassium phosphate, and silica.

A broad-spectrum multivitamin/multimineral formula with the cell salts listed above would be ideal for cancer prevention and recovery. Other ways to obtain cell salts are to regularly consume sea salt or raw natural sugar, or take a coral calcium supplement, in addition to a multivitamin/multimineral supplement. This, in my opinion, would ensure we build up the levels of all the trace minerals. If taking mineral supplements, our multivitamin/multimineral from the local grocery store could suffice, provided it has at a minimum vitamin A, thiamin (B1), riboflavin (B2), niacin (B3), choline (B4), calcium pantothenate (B5), pyridoxine hydrochloride (B6), biotin (B7), inositol FCC (B8), folic acid (B9), cyanocobalamin (B12), vitamin C, vitamin E, and PABA.

Some scientific sources claim that natural vitamins are more effectively assimilated in the body than synthetically produced vitamins. For example, the B vitamins are so important to proper cell formation and cell longevity that if you have active cancer you may want to take these vitamins in a more naturally absorbable liquid form. Taking extra B vitamins in addition to the ones in a multivitamin is reasonably safe, since they are water soluble and need to be replenished. Yet it is worth reiterating that a diet rich in fresh fruits and vegetables will provide many of these. Cruciferous vegetables, for example, are particularly rich in various vitamins and minerals.

Vitamin Deficiencies

Through studies from the National Cancer Institute and other sources, we see that when people contract cancer—specific vitamin deficiencies have been found to exist in their bodies. This would lead to the safe assumption that those who contract cancer had specific vitamin deficiencies that existed beforehand. Science has proven this many times in population studies that show that deficiencies of specific soil nutrients indicate higher rates of certain cancers. Therefore, it is reasonable to assume that specific vitamin and nutrient deficiencies, particularly those that are antioxidant-based, such as vitamin A/beta-carotene, C, E, zinc, selenium, and coenzyme Q-10, will create an environment favorable to cancer.

For example, in Finland a study of 36,265 adults found that a diet low in vitamin E increased the overall cancer risk by 50 percent. Research is consistent in showing that women who live in southern states have a much lower rate of breast cancer than those who live in northern states. This is due to the vitamin D we absorb through the skin when exposed to sunlight; people in the south are exposed to more sun than those in the north.

In addition, some studies indicate that micromineral supplementation may be cancer preventive. For example, a low level of the micromineral molybdenum in soil samples in China was linked to a higher rate of esophageal cancer. In some places in the United States where molybdenum is absent from the drinking water, there was found to be a 30 percent increased rate of esophageal cancer. As a result, we can accurately assume that specific nutritional or mineral deficiencies lead to cancer.

This whole concept led me to wonder if we could develop a more elaborate blood test to discover our deficiencies to prevent illnesses before they happened. In the process of talking about this with some physicians who are personal friends, I discovered that a thorough blood test geared toward measuring our vitamin and mineral levels and determining our deficiencies is available but not covered by insurance. Therefore, it would require an out-of-pocket expense of up to $500. Some naturopaths offer testing at a more economical level, but the testing is not as thorough.

Further research led me to discover an affiliate of the American Holistic University, the American Association of Drugless Practitioners, which supplies its graduating naturopathic doctors with testing procedures that are more economical and able to identify many deficiencies. These tests include analyzing blood slide, hair, and saliva samples. They are relatively inexpensive (about $40 each), and can provide a general picture of the body's health condition relative to nutritional levels. In addition, iridology—the scientific study of the iris (the ring around the pupil)—has some important diagnostic capabilities. Iridology is a science that was discovered centuries ago, when illnesses were able to be documented in certain strands of the iris. Once traditional medicine became more advanced and deemed more reliable, iridology became less popular as a diagnostic tool. However, it is becoming more popular among natural health practitioners.

We need our insurance companies to focus more on naturopathic medicine and for our policies to cover the tests we need to prevent the epidemic of cancer, rather than funding temporary pharmaceutical antidotes. Someday, traditional medical science will be advanced enough in the areas of preventive and natural medicine to routinely offer and perform such a blood test. Until then, we will need to make sure we consume a healthy diet and some well-chosen supplements that reflect our genetic predisposition. In other words, if breast cancer runs in our family, we should be certain we take specific vitamins (listed in this chapter) that have been researched and found to prevent or rectify such a condition.

Studies have found that natural forms of nutrients, particularly in foods, tend to be more effective cancer preventatives and remedies than those in pill form. For example, foods high in beta-carotene have other carotenes that contribute to cancer prevention and recovery better than the beta-carotene supplement by itself. Therefore, if we have, or are prone to have, a specific form of cancer, in addition to store-bought supplements, we will also want to consume the appropriate foods high in the nutrients we need. However, we will not want to exceed RDAs, or what are considered to be safe levels.

Now let's ask ourselves how we got into such a state of deficiency.

Degradation of the Food Industry: The Cause

Have you ever asked yourself why home-grown fruits and vegetables taste so much better than most of the ones from the local grocery store? The answer is simple: the soil in the local garden has more nutrients in it. Also, unfortunately, mass-produced fruits and vegetables are commonly sprayed with toxic pesticides, while dangerous synthetic fertilizers are used in the soil, all in the name of producing more profitable crops. In addition, most mass-produced crops are picked before they are ripe. This is done so they don't rot during storage and transport, but this also reduces their vitamin and mineral content.

Here in the United States, where cancer rates are unusually high compared to the rest of the world, we consume a diet deficient in vitamins. This is a result of the depletion of beneficial minerals and microbes from the soil. The body is then left vulnerable to cancer.

Next, we must look at genetically modified produce, which every Hoxsey patient is warned against, because it's not only less nutritious, it's dangerous. Genetic engineering of food involves merging genes from plants, animals, viruses, and bacteria in ways that do not occur in nature. For example, the DNA from a cold-water fish such as a salmon may be spliced with the DNA of a tomato to make the tomato more frost resistant. Many scientists are very concerned about our limited amount of knowledge of the consequences that may result from genetic engineering. They worry that there may be irreparable damage some day to planet earth and the human life it sustains. They are worried that some modified viruses and bacteria may produce new diseases unknown to our immune systems. In addition, these transmutations may move into other organisms, such as those in our food chain.

The government allows genetically modified food, then pays farmers to reduce their yields while people are starving—all in the name of profit—and we are leaving ecology out of the picture. What happened to health being a number-one priority? How about the logic that if we aren't around, we can't enjoy the money?

No wonder we Americans need to take supplements to avoid deadly illnesses now. It's becoming more obvious that the rate of cancer is at epidemic proportions because of politics, greed, and personal irresponsibility. Over the last two centuries, medicine progressed in extending our life span, while the quality of our food and our environment declined. As a result, we've become more dependent on medicine, or corrective measures, rather than taking preventive measures such as proper diet, exercise, and a healthy environment. We now live in a society oriented toward corrective health, rather than preventive heath, and each of us is paying the price.

Enough said. Now let's move past frustration about the things we cannot immediately change, at least by ourselves. The primary point I am making is that preventive health today in America must include a healthy diet with supplementation, to make up for the nutrients, vitamins, and minerals that the food from corporate America often lacks. While cancer cells also drain nutritional resources from the body, cancer patients must consider rectifying their state of malnutrition by taking the antioxidant vitamins, minerals, and supplements discussed in this chapter. I did it, and now I'm here writing this book; readers can do the same, if needed.

Now let's look at the way I did it.

Supplements and Chinese Medicines I Used in My Recovery

The supplements and Chinese medicines I used in the first two years of my recovery, specifically intended to cure cancer, are listed below. In addition, I used other supplements for other health issues, which I've also listed. For easy referencing, the supplements and Chinese medicines are listed in alphabetical order.

Artemisinin (sweet wormwood). I discovered this Chinese medicine during a homeopathic consultation with Dr. Gutierrez at the BMC. He gave me an article titled "Chinese Herb Cures Cancer," from a newsletter published in Atlanta called *Second Opinion* (May 2002, vol. 7, no. 3), written by Dr. Robert Jay Rowan. Artemisinin is a derivative of the Asian herb sweet wormwood, also known as artemasia. Artemisinin is 300 times more potent than artemasia when manufactured by a California nutritional medicine company called NutriCology/Allergy Research Group.

The article described the shark cartilage era, when science mistakenly believed that shark cartilage showed promise in curing cancer. It went on to discuss how some cancer vaccine therapies tested were found to be effective. Later in the article, it mentioned how doctors Henry Lai and Narenda Singh, bioengineering professors at the University of Washington, tested artemisinin and found a 100 percent kill rate of breast cancer cells and leukemia cells in just hours, leaving normal breast cells and white blood cells unscathed. Furthermore, cancer cells did not build up a resistance to it, as is common with some chemotherapy drugs. These findings were published in the *International Journal of Oncology* (18; 767–773), 2001, by Efferth. Strangely enough, we didn't hear much more about this natural cure thereafter.

Here's a description of how it works in Dr. Rowan's own words published in the *Second Opinion Newsletter* referenced above:

> "…artemesia is a close cousin to oxygen therapy. Chinese researchers said the key to its effect was a peroxide linkage (two oxygen atoms hooked together) within the herbs active molecule. Remember our old friend hydrogen peroxide?
>
> All peroxides share a common feature. In the presence of free iron, they break down to form highly reactive oxygen-based free radicals. Malaria is a parasite (plasmodium) that infects the iron-rich red blood cell and accumulates iron. While the body avidly shields iron in a bound-up state (hemoglobin, enzymes, etc.), excess iron accumulates in the parasite, and the accumulation allows some iron to spill out of the bound state and become free. When the artemisinin products contact the iron-BOOM! A huge burst of free radicals is unleashed, virtually blowing up the cell harboring the free iron and destroying the parasite."

Oxygen therapy has been used successfully for a number of years, and it is not illegal in the United States when delivered by a physician who specializes in it. Cancer can only grow in the absence of oxygen, so when high levels of oxygen exist, it suffocates the cancer cells.

German scientist Otto Warburg, M.D., discovered many years ago that the lack of oxygen at the cellular level was at the cause of cancer. All cancer cells require a lack of oxygen in order to go through a process of fermentation, whereby they consume sugar and leave the by-product lactic acid, which creates an acidic environment, and the cycle continues. Since cancer cells require a lack of oxygen for fermentation to take place, high levels of oxygen are toxic to them. Dr. Warburg tested the absence of oxygen on embryonic cells and discovered that they divide at a hypermetabolic rate very similar to cancer cells. This discovery further coincides with Dr. Day's theory about the importance of getting enough fresh air and exercise, which helps our bodies get enough oxygen. Also, stress and anxiety, which limit breathing, over a period of time may limit our oxygen.

Many physicians use oxygen chambers to deliver oxygen therapies, in addition to ozone and hydrogen peroxide.

Dr. Hoang of Hanoi, Vietnam, used artemisinin for about 10 years with a group of family physicians who have achieved long-term remission in approximately 60 percent of 400 cancer patients. He claims that in his studies no type of cancer is unresponsive to artemisinin derivatives, and that all patients are responding and have at least stabilized.

Dr. Hoang recommends artemisinin treatment for a period of two years. It's proven to be non-toxic for this period of time, with no side effects expected. It should not be taken in direct combination with antioxidants, due to its oxygenating qualities.

I took the recommended dosage of artemisinin (500 mg twice a day) on an empty stomach for the first two years, with a three-month break in the middle. At times, I became nauseated. So the third year the BMC brought me down to 300 mg twice a day. It is fat-soluble, so I often took artemisinin with a cod liver oil gel cap, a flax seed oil gel cap, or with yogurt, to ensure I was absorbing and assimilating it.

Beta-carotene. Beta-carotene, from which our bodies can make vitamin A, and other sources of vitamin A, have been shown to reduce the risk of, or help rectify, cancers of the lung, stomach, esophagus, oral cavity and pharynx, endometrium, pancreas, and colon. Vitamin A has been shown to be significantly more effective in its natural form. This is because of the 500-plus other carotenoids and other nutrients present in natural combinations in many vitamin A-rich foods. The benefits of these carotenoids are still being researched. These natural combinations of carotenoids may help the absorption and assimilation of vitamin A, and therefore increase its value in cancer prevention and recovery.

The recommended daily allowance of beta-carotene has not yet been determined, but the RDA of vitamin A is 4500 IU. High levels of beta-carotene do not lead to vitamin A toxicity. An overdose of beta-carotene will lead to a yellowing of the skin, what is referred to as carotenemia. This condition is harmless and disappears rapidly after ceasing intake. However, increasing vitamin A to levels exceeding the RDA is dangerous, as this fat-soluble nutrient can to build up in the body and be lethal. For example, many years ago, whale meat was consumed by Alaskan natives in large amounts. Whale is high in vitamin A, and as a result scientists were finding large populations of specific tribes practically extinct.

The need for beta-carotene is easily met in a normal diet. Because of potential vitamin A toxicity, I made sure I filled my need through specific foods. (Keep in mind that heavy drinkers of alcohol, and smokers, show harmful effects from using beta-carotene, liver toxicity and increased incidence of lung cancer, respectively). I took no more vitamin A or beta-carotene supplements beyond what was in my multivitamin.

Concentrated amounts of beta-carotene are found in the following foods, going from higher to lower: sweet potato, carrots, spinach, mango, butternut and winter squash, papaya, cantaloupe, turnip greens, and mustard greens. Other foods high in this nutrient include broccoli, pumpkin, yellow corn, kale, apricot, and tomato. I eat many of these foods on a regular basis, except tomatoes, and I also take a multivitamin that contains 70 percent of my RDA of vitamin A (or 3500 IU), 29 percent of which is derived from beta-carotene.

Vitamins B6, B12, and B17. B vitamins are used by our bodies for cell formation and cell longevity and to make enzymes that battle cancer. These vitamins have been found to be deficient in cancer patients. B17 is the active ingredient of the popular cancer therapy known as laetrile therapy, which is derived from apricot seed extract. Laetrile has been studied by many researchers and found to be highly effective in tumor reduction activity (more later in this chapter).

It is a good idea to take an additional B complex vitamin. Some people prefer a liquid form because the body can assimilate it better that way. Because my multivitamin contains a variety of B vitamins, and I also had a diet rich in them, I decided to take a vitamin B complex only for the first two years. Thereafter, I took an E-B vitamin combination containing vitamins B6 and B12, the two in which cancer patients tend to be most deficient.

Bilberry Extract. Bilberry got its reputation from British bombers in World War II, who improved their night vision by taking this extract. It enabled them to see their targets more accurately in the dark. Bilberry is an antioxidant. With the daily eye exercises I do, it will keep me from wearing reading glasses as I pass through my forties, which is the primary reason I take it. This extract is a bioflavonoid antioxidant, which is the most potent type for reducing the possibility of cells building up on the cornea of the eye, the cause of age-related presbyopia.

I am in my mid-forties and currently have no need for corrective eye wear, and enjoy 15/20 or 20/20 vision, depending on the day I am tested. I take 1000 mg gel caps daily of bilberry extract and have done so for several years.

C Vitamins. Not all vitamin C supplements are equal. Some research shows that the average vitamin C supplement bought off the shelf is only absorbed at a rate of 20 percent, while 80 percent of Ester C (a particular form of vitamin C made by adding calcium and bioflavonoid to it) is absorbed and assimilated. Ester C is a powerful antioxidant. Studies show that vitamin C in high doses is associated with decreased risk of cancer. Dr. Ewan Cameron, M.D., a Scottish physician, proved that high doses of vitamin C inhibit the production of an enzyme that allows cancerous cells to infiltrate healthy tissues. At megadoses of 10 grams per day, his cancer subjects reported significant improvements in the quality of life and the rate of survival.

Numerous studies indicate that vitamin C-rich foods may prevent or help rectify cancers of the stomach, bladder, breast, cervix, colon and rectum, salivary gland, esophagus, larynx, pancreas, prostate, and lung, in addition to leukemia and non-Hodgkin's lymphoma.

This antioxidant strengthens the glue between cells, enhances immune function, and stimulates the formation of collagen—essentially encapsulating tumors and preventing them from spreading. It has been known to speed wound healing. Research also indicates that it enhances the effectiveness of certain chemotherapy drugs while reducing the toxicity of others. The BMC prescribes approximately 2000–3000 mg of Ester C for most cancers.

The RDA for vitamin C is 60 mg. Studies show that diarrhea may occur at daily levels of 4,000 mg. This nutrient is water-soluble, so it is relatively safe.

The first two years of my recovery I took 3,000 mg, because of research showing preventive and recovery benefits from increasing vitamin C. In my third year and thereafter, I took 2,000 when I felt healthy, then increased it to 3,000 mg if I caught a cold or my asthma kicked up. During the first two years, when I took 3,000 mg, I did not catch a cold or flu virus, which is astounding because I usually caught an average of one flu virus and about three cold viruses each year. I attribute this to my intake of vitamin ester C.

Coral Calcium (with magnesium and vitamin D). One of the highest populations of centenarians in the world (people who live to be 100 years old or more) was discovered in the island of Okinawa, near Japan. Coral calcium was identified as the key to their longevity and the lack of disease. It was discovered that their diet and life style was similar to people living in other parts of the region, but the water in the wells of these coral islands revealed a high concentration of calcium and many other trace minerals. This secret was discovered about two decades ago when a journalist sent by the *Guinness Book of World Records* interviewed the oldest living man, Shigechiyo Izumi, who lived on the island of Tokunoshima. He was 115 years old and had just retired 10 years earlier. Most people in the society lived past the age of 95, and even the very old were active and healthy.

All forms of calcium sold in stores are combined with magnesium and vitamin D, in order to increase absorption and assimilation.
Coral calcium also contains an estimated 70-plus trace minerals, including vanadium (V), and selenium (Se), both of which have significant anti-cancer

activity. It also commonly contains other minerals that support the immune system and organs. Such minerals are also effective with a variety of other diseases.

The RDA for calcium is 1000 mg for adults and 1,200 mg for people over 50. Most of us do not get this amount in our diets, so taking a supplement may be advisable. Research shows that an overdose of 2000 mg of calcium may inhibit the absorption of iron, zinc, and other minerals, in addition to causing kidney stones.

The BMC recommends that almost every patient take either chelated or coral calcium to get the benefit of increased energy. I was instructed to take 1000 mg of coral calcium daily. I found a coral calcium compound with 370 mg calcium, 9 mg vitamin C, 400 IU vitamin D, and 56 mg magnesium per serving (two capsules). I took six capsules per day, which I continued for several years.

Coenzyme Q10. This powerful antioxidant is an excellent cancer fighter, but somewhat more expensive than other supplements. It is a natural enzyme produced by the body during the normal sleep cycle. Those not getting good sleep may be deficient in it. NIH/NCI studies show that high doses of Coenzyme Q-10 (300 mg) had tumor reduction qualities in breast cancer patients. It is most active in mitochondria, the energy-producing aspects of all the cells in the body. According to Dr. Karl Folkers, the "father of CoQ-10," it is significantly effective in reducing and eliminating tumors in some cancer patients. In 1995, Folkers published a Danish study reporting tumor eradication in five patients with advanced breast cancer taking an average of 390 mg per day. CoQ-10, which is a fat-soluble vitamin, is best taken with fish oil, flax seed oil, yogurt, low-fat cottage cheese, or a meal, in order to increase its absorption.

CoQ-10 was found to be deficient in people with myeloma, lymphoma, and cancers of the breast, lung, prostate, pancreas, colon, kidney, and head and neck. Three breast cancer studies were listed on the NCCAM web site showing higher than normal recovery rates in people using a combination of traditional medical treatment, supplements, and CoQ-10. One woman even had full remission after cancer entered her liver. One study also showed that the chemotherapy drug doxorubicin had fewer effects on the heart when CoQ-10 was used.

The first year of my recovery I took 200 mg of CoQ-10, which was easy enough to find at my local health food store. For economic reasons, I later converted to a generic brand found at the local grocery store, still at 200 mg. At the beginning of my third year of recovery, I converted to 150 mg per day.

D Vitamins. Vitamin D has shown cancer-fighting capability in cancers of the breast, colorectal, pancreatic, and prostate. Studies show that women with breast cancer who have higher body stores of vitamin D (remember it is a fat-soluble vitamin) have a significantly longer survival rate. In addition, one study showed that women with exposure to sunlight lowered the risk of breast cancer by 20 to 40 percent or more. It is possible that just 10 to 15 minutes of direct sunlight (not from behind glass) each day will suffice in providing this protection.

The RDA is 400 IU for adults and 600 IU for people over 70. Vitamin D has the greatest risk of toxicity of all vitamins. Yet, it is necessary for the body to be able to absorb calcium. Excessive doses of 50,000 IU daily have been known to result in vitamin D poisoning, causing excessive calcium blood levels, kidney stones, appetite loss, nausea, weakness, constipation, and weight loss. Most receive their RDA from milk and dairy products, sunlight, and fortified breakfast cereals.

My multivitamin contained 400 IU vitamin D. With the coral calcium compound I took that contained another 400 IU, I took 800 IU of supplemental vitamin D per day.

DHEA (dehydroepiandrosterone) is naturally produced by our adrenal glands, which sit atop the kidneys. It is produced abundantly until the age of twenty-five, when it peaks in the bloodstream. It has anti-aging effects, similar to the popular human growth hormone (HGH) and melatonin. More importantly for our purposes, it blocks an enzyme known to produce fatty tissue and promote cancer cell growth.

One form of DHEA therapy involves using extracts from yams, which the body converts into DHEA. It has been known to improve a wide variety of illnesses and increase memory and the immune system; however, animal studies show that high doses of this supplement can lead to liver toxicity. For this reason, low doses are recommended, and only in conjunction with vitamins C and E and selenium, to prevent oxidative damage to the liver. Laboratory animal studies showed a 50 percent increase in longevity when given DHEA.

This supplement is recommended by the BMC for hormone-based cancers (breast, prostate, etc.). Within the first few years of my lymphoma diagnosis, I took 22.5 grams of DHEA daily, and continued thereafter, not only to reap its cancer prevention benefits, but also its youth-promoting qualities (stimulating estrogen and testosterone).

E Vitamins. Vitamin E is an effective fat-soluble antioxidant, which means we should take it with a meal. It has proven through multiple studies to be effective against cancer, particularly in preventing or eliminating prostate cancer.

A diet rich in vitamin E foods is associated with a lower risk of cancers of the colon, stomach, throat, mouth, prostate, esophagus, breast, skin, colorectal, and liver. A Finnish study of more than 36,000 adults showed that a diet low in vitamin E increased the risk of cancer by 50 percent.

Research shows that natural vitamin E is three times more potent than its synthetic form. In 1997, Japanese researchers discovered that 400 International Units (IU) of vitamin E was equivalent to 150 IU of natural vitamin E, when measuring absorption levels in the blood stream. Effectiveness ratings are compared as follows:

Synthetic vitamin E (dl-alpha-tocopherol) = 1.1 IU per mg
Natural vitamin E (d-alpha-tocopherol acetate) = 1.36 IU per mg
Natural vitamin E (d-alpha-tocopherol) = 1.49 IU per mg

Scientists believe that vitamin E may protect cell membranes and DNA from oxygen-free radicals. They've also discovered a significant boost to the immune system. In addition, many believe that vitamin E, together with other antioxidants such as vitamin C, vitamin A (beta-carotene), and selenium work, as a more powerful antioxidant team. Studies show a significant decrease in cardiovascular disease with 100 IU per day. A reduced incidence of fatal heart attacks was discovered with doses of 400–800 IU per day.

The RDA of vitamin E is 30 IU. Many health studies showed success at 440–800 IU, and up to 1000 IU can be taken without any adverse effects. I took a gel cap containing 400 IU of natural vitamin E in my first two years of recovery, in order to rectify a potential state of deficiency. I continued on this supplement for a number of years thereafter, not only because of its cancer recovery benefits but also for its youth-promoting capabilities. In year three and afterwards, most of the time I took a synthetic 400 IU vitamin E complex with vitamins B6, B12, and folic acid, in order to maintain adequate levels of these other nutrients.

Fish Oil contains omega-3 essential fatty acids, which are known to lower LDL (low-density lipoprotein), cholesterol, and triglycerides. Research shows that omega-3 lowers the rate of heart attacks, strokes, high blood pressure, arteriosclerosis, heart and kidney failure, and more. In addition, omega-3 has been shown to be cytotoxic; it kills cancer cells. Other research suggests that the DHA and EPA (docosahexanoic acid and eicosapentaenoic acid) in omega-3 fatty acids inhibit the growth and metastasis of tumors.

I consumed a lot of omega-3 through the Hoxsey diet's weekly allocation of fish. Swordfish and tuna have been found to contain significant levels of mercury, but cod does not. I was prescribed a Chinese medicine that was fat-soluble, meaning it was absorbed by the body much more efficiently when taken with some type of fat. As a result, I often took a gel capsule of cod-liver oil with my Chinese medicines, which increased my omega-3s.

Flax seed (lignans) and flax seed oil are good sources of omega-3 and omega-6, because they contain the plant-derived alpha-linoleic acid, but the body must work harder to convert this into essential fatty acids than it does the omega-3 and omega-6 found in fish oil. This may cause a further strain on a system already in a weakened state, such as having cancer.

Nonetheless, studies specifically demonstrate flax seed oil's anticancer activity against breast cancer. Low levels of alpha-linoleic acid in fatty breast tissues are associated with an increase in cancer invasiveness and its spread to other areas of the body. In addition, it is theorized that lignans in flax specifically protect against breast cancer by converting into phytoestrogens, which block the activity of the stronger estrogen found naturally in the body. For this reason, breast cancer patients may want to make flax seed and flax seed oil a regular part of their diet.

Flax seeds taste similar to licorice, and may be used to season foods. The oil should not be used in cooking, because it is easily damaged by heat and light. Flax seed oil is excellent in salad dressings. I use the oil on salads, take gel caps to help absorb the Chinese medicine, and occasionally use the seeds as a seasoning.

Folic Acid deficiency is one of the most common vitamin deficiencies in the world and has been linked to the contraction of colorectal, lung, and mouth cancers. And, taking it in sufficient quantities has been credited with the prevention of recovery from these same cancers. In particular, folic acid is an effective protection against cervical cancer, as well as cancers of the colon, lung, and mouth. A 1992 study directly linked folic acid deficiency to the contraction of cervical cancer.

Folic acid supplementation has been documented as reversing cervical dysplasia in women taking oral contraceptives, but a doctor's supervision is highly recommended.

The RDA of folic acid is 400 mcg. Studies with subjects using levels as high as 15 mg showed no adverse effects. However, folic acid can mask vitamin B12 deficiencies if taken in higher amounts. I limit myself to the folic acid content in my multivitamin, which is the RDA, to provide myself with adequate levels of this valuable nutrient.

Garlic Extract (allium sativum). I chose to take garlic extract, because recent studies in Japan reported good results in malignant tumor reduction. I found studies available through NIH indicating that a diet high in garlic, such as that of China, might reduce the proliferation of tumors in humans. When garlic extract and garlic powder were individually tested in laboratory experiments, there was no reduction in cancer cell growth. However, when the garlic extract was combined with garlic powder, there was a clear inhibition of tumor cell growth. This occurred at concentrations as low as 30 micrograms/ml.

Other research I found suggested that freshly-cut garlic is most effective against cancer when it is allowed to sit before it is cooked Allyl sulfur compounds in garlic, which slow or prevent the growth of tumor cells, are most potent when eaten 15 minutes after cloves are cut open, as in food preparation.

Other research suggests that the allinase in garlic extract may exhibit antitumor effects because of its ability to kill bacteria in the stomach that promote the formation of cancer-causing substances in the gastrointestinal tract. There was particularly strong evidence showing a link between consuming garlic and preventing prostate and stomach cancers. Some studies suggest that because garlic and onions are high in selenium, which they extract from the soil, this may be one reason for their impressive anti-cancer effects, particularly for men with prostate cancers.

I put myself on the highest store-shelf doses of garlic extract (500mg) and kyolic garlic (500 mg of the powdered form) that I could find. This resulted in my taking a garlic supplement dose of 1000 mg per day in the first two years. I've lowered this down to 500mg of kyolic garlic, since the manufacturing process guarantees that it is exposed to the air for an extended period of time, probably increasing the amount of beneficial allinase.

Ginkgo Biloba. This ornamental tree originated in China thousands of years ago. Now it grows in several places throughout the world. Its leaves are used as an herbal medicine. It not only serves as a good antioxidant, but also, more importantly, a good memory enhancer. It has been known to slow the progression of Alzheimer's disease. It increases blood circulation and oxygen supply to the heart and brain. Because of this, it is referred to as the "smart herb" of our time.

Since I lost some short-term memory after one treatment of chemotherapy, I decided to take ginkgo biloba. When I first got it, it was in a compressed pill form; it smelled fresh, so I was fairly convinced it would do the trick. After a few months, my memory was back to normal, except for the events that occurred within 30 days of the treatment.

Approximately two years later, I was eating dinner out with a friend of mine, who is a physician, and a friend of his, who is also a physician, and our wives. I mentioned that I had lost some memory from one dose of chemotherapy. They all agreed that unless the chemo was a miracle drug it wouldn't have cured me. Then one of the women told us that her sister had breast cancer and did chemotherapy and her personality had noticeably changed. One of the doctors told us that it was the intravenous steroids that people receive to reduce the body's rejecting the chemo drugs that causes the memory loss and personality changes.

It seems wise to take ginkgo biloba if you do any chemotherapy through traditional medicine, while keeping in mind that a rarely used, much milder form of chemotherapy is available at the BMC. When used in conjunction with the herbs and diet, it provides less shock to the body while still being effective.

I started taking 400 mg of ginkgo biloba every day in the beginning years of my recovery and plan to continue for many years to come.

Glucosamine. Glucosamine and glucosamine chondroitin compounded, are excellent joint care supplements, providing a joint rebuilding effect for people with degenerative joint disease and arthritis. These supplements improve movement and flexibility in joints, because they enhance the function of cartilage and joint fluid. MSM (methylsulfonylmethane), which is often combined with glucosomine or glucosomine chondroitin, is an effective anti-inflammatory that helps counteract both bronchial and joint inflammation. I take these supplements in various doses at various times, as joint pain arises from past injuries.

Grape Seed Compound. Grape seeds are highly potent antioxidants. Antioxidants first surfaced in the public eye as a great way to decrease free radical oxygen and thereby increase our immune system response, decrease colds, enhance youth, and more. This extract was suggested, when it first came out, as one of the most powerful antioxidant supplements. I started taking Grape Seed Extract Plus, an antioxidant blend, the first year and plan to continue for many years. I take one capsule a day. This extract should contribute to the family of antioxidants that cancer patients, and those prone to cancer, take on a regular basis.

One capsule of the Grape Seed Extract Plus that I take daily contains 15 mcg selenium, 50 mg grape seed extract, and a 130 mg antioxidant blend of green tea, citrus bioflavonoids, and bilberry.

Lymphoma Rx. Another prescription for Chinese medicine I was given is manufactured by Spring Wind Herbs, a Chinese medicine pharmacy in Berkeley, California (800-588-4883). The herbs in this powdered tea, which the company will put into capsules upon request for a minimal extra charge, are all harvested from Asia. They are:

Radix Asparagi	30g
Spica Prunellae	30g
Flos Lonicerae	24g
Radix Scrophulariae	24g
Radix Ampelopsis	12g
Rhizoma Paridis	12g

All are antibacterial but one, and many are antiviral and anti-inflammatory; some are antitumor. This is important because it appears from the research that I obtained that links between bacterial and viral infections and lymphoma are becoming well documented.

During most seasons of the year, I used it as a tea, but during the summer, I had it put into capsules. I took 2 grams of this compound each day for the first three years. Then, because the herbs in the Hoxsey formula had similar actions, and under the direction of the physicians at the BMC, I quit taking it. This occurred with the BMC documenting my making a significant recovery.

Multivitamins: Which One is Best?

I often get this question. My answer is that if you are eating a healthy diet, such as the Cayce or Hoxsey diet, then you don't need to worry about finding the best multivitamin on the market. You could get the basic low-cost multivitamin/multimineral available at your local grocery store and probably will do fine. This is what the BMC recommends, under the assumption that you are eating right.

However, most people are not eating like this. I tell people that their best bet is to get an all-natural vitamin if they have a poor diet, because their body is an all-natural biochemical machine, so it assimilates natural supplements better. In other words, if they want to use a multivitamin to make up for where their substandard diet falls short, considering that even a good, balanced and healthy diet is not providing everything it should, they should get an all-natural multimineral/multivitamin. There are plenty of them available at health food stores, on the internet, through reputable multi-level marketing companies such as Shaklee and more. The sources of these are virtually limitless.

One thing I like to caution people about, however, is to not get duplicate supplements. In other words, if you get a vision improvement supplement *and* take a multivitamin, you will probably exceed the RDA for vitamin A. Most vision improvement vitamins contain high amounts of vitamin A. This vitamin, and a couple of others, is not like vitamin C, where we can consume more than the RDA and our bodies will eliminate the excess. Vitamin C cannot build up to toxic levels in the body; however, vitamin A can.

I also recommend multivitamin/multimineral supplements for reasons mentioned earlier. As a general rule: good diet—generic multivitamin; poor diet—all-natural multivitamin. Research shows that natural vitamins are assimilated better, because higher concentrations in the blood are discovered after ingestion (as discussed earlier). Therefore, deficiencies are more likely rectified with natural vitamins. However, they are much more potent. As a result, it is advisable that individuals check with their naturopathic doctors or traditional medical doctors (if they can find one who is educated in nutrition), or perhaps their local pharmacist, to make sure they don't have a health condition that contraindicates the use of specific supplementation. Some multivitamins are not well balanced with RDA doses and can cause further health complications.

Papaya Seeds. As I read various natural health books, I recognized that papaya seeds are very high in cancer cell-inhibiting enzymes. These seeds were easier to find without processed sugar in them in Pharmacias Natural (natural pharmacies) in Mexico, because herbal and natural medicine is more popular there and more available to the public. I go on and off these seeds. I take them whenever I can locate them without processed sugar, or I buy papaya and scrape them out of the fruit and dry them, then add them to my pepper grinder. Papaya tastes much better in the southern states, particularly in South or Central America, as I discovered on my travels.

Pranosine/Isoprinosine (Metisoprinol). This pharmaceutically manufactured protein is antiviral. It is not approved for production in the United States. In Mexico and Germany, it is manufactured by pharmaceutical companies. Basically, it is a protein that brings the body into balance and supercharges the immune system. I was prescribed pranosine for winter time only, at which time I commonly caught multiple flus and colds and struggled with allergy-induced asthma, which was hazardous to my immune system.

It has helped me greatly. As I interviewed other Hoxsey therapy patients, I noticed that some were also prescribed pranosine for its antiviral and immune-boosting properties relative to the type of cancer they had. In my case, I used half a tablet (250 mg) and I don't recall contracting a viral infection since the 2002/03 winter season, which was several years ago.

Quercetin. The physicians at BMC monitor all the medicines we take in order to discover if there are any conflicts with the herbal medicines they prescribe, or particularly with hormonally-based cancers (i.e. prostate, breast, uterine, etc.). In addition, for asthmatics, arthritics, and other patients who have hyperactive immune disorders, they attempt to balance the immune function with natural medicines. They recommend the elimination of immune suppressors such as steroids.

In my case, I was taking steroid inhalers to reduce my hyperallergic response to dust in the winter. I was told at the BMC that these immune suppressors needed to be eliminated. I located a book I owned called *The Pill Book*, by Bantam Books Publishing, and I identified the actions of synthetic drugs to counteract asthma and attempted to duplicate these actions with natural remedies. From there, I researched some of my naturopathic books and found that quercetin, which is a powerful antioxidant in its natural form, was used in synthetic forms by traditional medicine years ago to treat asthma, not as a bronchial dilator but as a bronchial anti-inflammatory.

One of the most pure forms of supplemental quercetin is the one by NutriCology, a product by the name of Quercetin 300. The literature about it states, "shown to reduce the production of prostaglandins and leukotrienes, which are thought to play a much larger role in promoting inflammation than histamine...strengthening mast cells in the release of histamine, potentially inhibiting that activity." During my research, I also found some evidence that quercetin was an effective antioxidant in the prevention of cancer.

I was able to reduce my asthma attacks by taking 300 mg of quercetin two to three times a day during the winter season, for a total of 600–900 mg/day. I also used ionizing air cleaners, which helped, then moved to the beach, which practically took care of the problem altogether.

Selenium. I have uncovered literally dozens of studies that indicate that selenium deficiency is involved in causing many cancers. I have also found many studies showing the benefits of taking selenium to restore DNA and cure cancer.

Researchers have found a selenium deficiency in the blood of many people with various cancers, particularly breast cancers. States with the lowest levels of selenium in the soil are the following:

Washington, Oregon, California, Wisconsin, Illinois, Iowa, Michigan, Ohio, Pennsylvania, West Virginia, New York, Vermont, New Hampshire, Maine, Massachusetts, Rhode Island, Connecticut, New Jersey, Maryland, District of Columbia, and Florida. With the exception of West Virginia, all are considered to have high rates of breast and other cancers.

In a study presented by Larry Clark, Ph.D., of the Arizona Cancer Center, it was indicated that supplemental selenium could reduce cancer death rates by as much as 50 percent. This study was conducted with 1,312 cancer-prone patients, where 50 percent took a daily dose of 200 mcg of selenium, and the other half took a placebo. Of those who took the selenium, there was a 37 percent lower cancer rate, and of those who contracted cancer, there were 50 percent fewer deaths from the cancer. The results were so convincing that researchers stopped the study early to give those in the placebo group who had contracted cancer the actual selenium supplement.

The antioxidant nutrients vitamins A and E are shown to activate selenium, making it more potent against cancer cells. Essentially, selenium is such a powerful antioxidant that it helps to quickly repair free radical damage to cells. This damage to cellular nuclei is at the root cause of cancer. Thus, antioxidants are generally a good prescription for repairing a cancer patient's DNA.

Gerhard Schrauzer, Ph.D., a chemistry professor at the University of California's Revelle College, is known by some as the leading selenium researcher. He believes that selenium prevents cancer partly by inhibiting cell division long enough for a carcinogen-damaged cell to repair its chromosomes.

John A. Milner, Ph.D., of the University of Illinois, transplanted cancer cells into healthy mice, then injected a group of these mice with selenium salts. After six weeks, 100 percent of the unsupplemented mice were bloated with tumors, but the supplemented mice were healthy and tumor-free. In *Science,* Dr. Milner was quoted as saying "Complete inhibition of tumor development was observed..." and selenium protected the mice for three weeks after supplementation stopped.

My multivitamin had adequate amounts of selenium in it, as listed on the container. I took the RDA, and sometimes, particularly in my first year of recovery, I would also take an additional selenium supplement, which would put me slightly above the RDA.

Selenium should be an essential supplement for cancer patients, as it actually causes cancer cells to self-destruct before they replicate, preventing further tumor growth. It also assists the body in producing other antioxidants that help in cancer prevention. It appears that for most people, taking 200 mcg of selenium daily, particularly if you are genetically predisposed to cancer, is a safe and effective dosage. The most bioavailable form is high-selenium yeast.

The RDA for this nutrient is 70 mcg in men and 50–55 mcg in women. Many studies showed anti-cancer results starting at 200 mcg daily. Doses up to 350 mcg daily are generally believed to be harmless, but at 750–1000 mcg daily, toxic effects, such as GI and central nervous system distress and loss of hair and nails, have been reported. Selenium absorption is reduced in the presence of heavy metals or high doses of vitamin C.

I often took an extra 100 mcg in the first year of recovery, because of the selenium I was already getting in my multivitamin and my antioxidant compound (Grape Seed Plus). By the third year, I simply relied on the selenium in my multivitamin to do the trick. My diet is also high in selenium, derived from garlic, onion, and other things. I also take a daily garlic supplement, which contributes to my selenium quota.

Yew Tree Needle Tips (Taxus brevifolia). The yew tree originates in Scotland and is possibly Europe's oldest tree. Yew trees have a long life span. The Fortingall yew in Glen Lyon is purported to be about two thousand to nine thousand years old. This species of tree is believed to have existed 200 million years ago. Native Americans have long used parts of the tree for its medicinal cures, calling it "the chief of the forest." The tips are a popular remedy for headaches, cystitis, neuralgia, colds, flus, fungal and bacterial infections, rheumatism, sciatica, kidney problems, lung problems, and of course, cancer.

In 1962, the U.S. Department of Agriculture funded a search by the National Cancer Institute to find any plant that may help cure cancer. On the committee was botanist Dr. James Duke and Kurt Blum, who tramped through Washington state's Gifford Pinchot National Forest looking for any plants that looked intriguing. Kurt Blum is credited with spotting the bright red berries on the Pacific yew. On behalf of NCI, the committee sent samples of the berries, bark, and roots of the tree to the Wisconsin Alumni Research Foundation laboratories with other natural plant samples thought to be medicinal.

Two years later, when it was thought the yew had cancer-killing properties, samples were sent to Research Triangle Institute in North Carolina, where the natural medicinal component of the yew, taxanes, was discovered by two scientists, Dr. Monroe Wall and Dr. Mansukh C. Wani. Taxanes was later researched and documented to be highly effective against tumor cells. Although Dr. Duke was on the team of researchers that originally discovered yew tree needles, pharmacology researcher Dr. Wani is credited with its discovery and its popularization as the chemotherapy drug Taxol.

Its curative properties are derived from its ability to gum up the functioning of the microtubule apparatus, a process involved in the rapid cell division in abnormal cells. Rapid cellular division is the lethal factor in all forms of cancer. Taxanes have proven to destroy abnormal cells by binding to the microtubules. This action paralyzes cell division, thus inhibiting the growth of abnormal cells such as cancer cells.

As one of the most powerful antioxidants on planet earth, yew tree extract effectively eliminates free radicals and oxidation, and also potentially assists in repairing the body's DNA by triggering a process called *apoptosis*. Apoptosis aids in the necessary death of cells, removing cells whose DNA has been damaged and making way for new cells.

Taxol is the bioengineered synthetic form of the Pacific yew and is patented by the pharmaceutical industry. Although it is highly cytotoxic to ovarian and breast cancer tumor cells, it is also highly toxic to other systems of the body. The synthetic version has gotten rave reviews in traditional medicine for its effectiveness in treating many forms of cancer.

At first, the yew's bark was used. But since it takes 100 years before the tree can be harvested, and it takes at least three trees to treat one cancer patient, extinction became a concern. Illegal harvesting became rampant and resulted in a lot of waste; poachers were taking the bark off the trees that were easiest to reach. Now, after government regulation, yew twigs and needles are being harvested for natural yew caps and its synthetic sister Taxol in a manner safer for the tree's survival.

The BMC generally prescribes yew tree needle caps for many of its patients. Doing this in the doses they prescribe won't make you sick (anemic, hair falling out, nauseated, etc...), as most chemotherapy drugs do. Furthermore, since the caps have about 1/50th the strength of its synthetic counterpart, they are relatively safe to take over a long period of time. If one were to take it alone, rather than as part of a comprehensive alternative medicine cancer therapy program, then it probably wouldn't have much impact on cancerous conditions in the body. But as part of a comprehensive natural recovery program such as the Hoxsey system, it greatly contributes to recovery. The BMC often prescribes yew tree needles for cancers of the blood (lymphoma, leukemia, etc.), breast, ovarian, lung, and more.

I have taken yew tree needle capsules containing just the tips, which are the most potent, since my first visit to the BMC. I was prescribed to take it for a full five years. I take three capsules, at 300 mg per capsule, three times a day.

Zinc (zinc oxide). Zinc is a powerful antioxidant that assists in thymus gland function, and therefore increases our immune response to foreign invaders, such as cancer cells. It also enhances sperm counts in men, and therefore may increase libido over time. This may be important for cancer patients who desire to be sexually intimate, because sexual intimacy is shown to dramatically decrease when someone contracts cancer and enters treatment.

I took zinc supplements the first year of my recovery. I felt I noticed a difference when I combined the zinc with DHEA (a testosterone-promoting supplement), in my desire to be intimate. My wife and I also noticed that our friendship got stronger during the long periods of time that we weren't intimate, which primarily involved the first few months after I was diagnosed. Oddly enough, this was also highly advantageous to the development of our relationship.

Sequential Timed Doses

All BMC patients receive literature describing how to take the herbal and Chinese medicines that are prescribed. Chinese medicines need to be taken on an empty stomach, while it is best to take all the other herbal medicines and supplements that are part of the Hoxsey program with a meal.

With the help of the BMC, I constructed a daily oxygenation and subsequent antioxidant routine. I oxygenated my bloodstream first thing in the morning, and then took antioxidants at breakfast and lunch to reduce any excess free radicals in my bodily systems. At bedtime, I took oxygenators again so that my bloodstream would be oxygenated throughout the night, when natural antioxidants are secreted by the body. I always took the artemisinin on an empty stomach with a small amount of healthy fat (usually cod liver oil or yogurt), because it is fat soluble, which means fat is necessary for its absorption. I also took my other Chinese medicines first thing in the morning and last thing at night, because all Chinese medicines are prescribed for an empty stomach.

Besides cheating on the diet, one of the other ways people become part of the 20 percent who fail to recover is to forget to take their medicines. This may be a challenge for many older patients, who make up the majority of people who contract cancer due to the breakdown of the immune system that often occurs with age.

What follows is a list of my routine of vitamins, herbs, and supplements that I settled on for the first two years of my recovery.

Morning (on an empty stomach)

Chinese medicine tea	2 grams
Artemisinin (to oxygenate)	500 mgs
Cod Liver oil (or 2 TB yogurt)	1 gel cap
Yew tree needle tips	900 mg
Black tonic	2 oz
Glucosamine/MSM*	500/500 mg
Coral Calcium Compound	500 mg

With Breakfast

Multivitamin/Multimineral	1 tablet
Ginkgo biloba	400 mg
Grape seed compound	50 mg
Natural Vitamin E	400 IU
Ester C	1000 mg
DHEA	12.5 mg
Kyolic Garlic	1200 mg
Vitamin B complex	varied
Zinc	varied
Quercetin (winter)*	300 mg

With Lunch

Coral Calcium Compound	500 mg
Bilberry Extract*	1000 mg
Ester C	1000 mg
Black tonic	2 oz
Yew tree needle tips	900 mg
Co Q-10	200 mg
Ginseng Royal Jelly Plus*	752 mg
Quercetin (winter)*	300 mg

With Dinner

Black tonic	2 oz
Quercetin (winter)*	300 mg
Coral Calcium Compound	500 mg

At Bedtime (on an empty stomach)

Chinese medicine tea	2 grams
Black tonic	2 oz
Yew tree needle tips	900 mg
Artemisinin (to oxygenate)	500 mg
Flax Seed oil (or 2 TB yogurt)	1 gel cap

*Indicates use for health issues other than cancer, even though many of these are antioxidants that are effective against cancer.

Keeping Scheduled Doses

I took the advice of Carol and Bernie Main, the video producers who were cured of lymphoma and pancreatic cancer by the Hoxsey method, and put three of my four doses of black tonic in a large liter-sized cup with a straw, which lasted throughout the entire day. In the cup was grape juice on ice, and sometimes other juice combinations as instructed by the BMC. I generally took my evening dose of black tonic with my evening dose of Chinese medicine tea. A pill box designed for separating a week of supplements and Chinese medicines into four daily doses proved a valuable purchase from the local drug store for keeping on track of all the supplements required for a natural recovery.

Summary

Scientific studies show that the natural forms of nutrients found in food are superior to supplemental forms. Therefore, second to consuming the proper diet, supplements that are manufactured and sold in a more natural state are going to be more effective for cancer prevention and recovery.

It is important that the cancer patient take multiple antioxidants and supplements, because we started with a deficiency before contracting the illness, and furthermore the illness leads to more malnutrition by its very nature. Malnutrition results in infections and organ failure and is a common way that people die from cancer. Cancer cells break down glucose in the absence of oxygen, generating lactic acid in the process, which, with other toxins, is taken up by the liver. The liver strenuously converts the lactic acid back to glucose, which energetically feeds the cancer cells—and the cycle continues until it is stopped.

Essentially the cancer patient's immune system needs to be whipped into shape to be able to fight this thing. His or her DNA needs to be repaired with the help of antioxidants. And his or her liver and other organs need to be cleansed of toxins using the herbs recommended in this book, so the organs that regulate the immune system can become more efficient, efficient enough to put a stop to this thing!

The BMC prescribes certain supplements for certain types of cancers, but taking the wrong supplements for hormonal cancers can cause more harm than good. Certain enzymes and hormonal systems need to be blocked with certain forms of supplements, in order to inhibit or reverse the growth of specific types of cancer cells.

I do not recommend that cancer patients experiment with various alternative medicine approaches, unless they are engaged in a comprehensive recovery therapy through a reputable naturopath, physician, or clinic *and* such experts agree that trying these things may be advantageous. It is strongly advisable to discuss supplemental prescriptions with experts, such as the physicians at the BMC. This is particularly important for those who have a hormonal cancer. It is unwise for people with cancer to experiment with their lives!

It is important to remember that consuming high amounts of specific nutrients mentioned in this chapter in foods circumvents the need for them in supplements. Keep in mind that many nutrients are fat-soluble. So if these nutrients are consumed on a consistent basis, adding the supplemental form of such nutrients may be toxic. For this reason, it is important to have a good naturopath, nutritionist, or one of the holistic oncologists at the BMC to regulate supplement intake.

And last but not least, the most absorbable forms of nutrients are natural forms—the ones found in foods and natural vitamins. Even with this, people may be depleted in certain macro and microminerals, because of soil deficiencies, so the best advice is to "supplement wisely."

Remember that supplements, drugs, and herbs can all interact with each other. This is a good reason to see a good naturopathic physician or allopathic physician who is willing to do such research for you, in order to rule out potential unhealthy side effects from these interactions. A good book that may help these professionals, available at the American Holistic University on-line bookstore, or perhaps other sources on the internet, is *The A-Z Guide to Drug-Herb-Vitamin Interactions*, by Lininger, Gaby, Auston, Batz, Yarnell, Brown, and Constantine.

There are many sources for the studies I mention in this chapter, many of which readers may research further through the books and web sites I list in the reference section at the end of this book. One of my favorite sources for supplemental education for the general reader is *Reducing Cancer Risk*, by Richard Harkness, Pharm., FASCP.

Naturopathy is the study of how to put the bodily systems back in balance in order to restore health, as compared to traditional medicine's more invasive approaches. With this in mind, the book *Encyclopedia of Natural Medicine*, by naturopathic doctors Murray and Pizzorno, is my favorite source for gaining a more scientific understanding of the roles that organs, glands, and nutrient-based antioxidants play within the intricacies of our immune system. All three books mentioned are good reads for alternative health professionals.

Once we select the right herbs, foods, and supplements, our next step (the next chapter) involves looking into the "right attitude" and the all-powerful, mind-body connection.

Chapter 11

The Holistic Approach

As a mind-body therapist and researcher for more than a decade, I was able to access and utilize effective mind-body interventions to help in curing my own cancer. In this chapter, we will focus on one of the three causes of cancer in the causative triangle mentioned previously: lifestyle. Lifestyle and stress are often key factors in the breakdown of the immune system when a person contracts cancer.

However, using only mind-body interventions in an effort to obtain a cure would be feeble and dangerous. This would be similar to praying to God as the only form of treatment, giving God an ultimatum: either heal us directly through a spiritual intervention, or let us die, which in most cases could be considered a form of suicide.

This form of thinking reminds me of a popular story. A flood came and a man crawled on top of his roof as the water rose. He was determined that God would save him. A boat came by and asked him if he wanted a ride to dry land, and he declined, saying, "No thanks, God will save me." He prayed some more and a helicopter offered to pick him up and he claimed again that God would save him, declining the help. The water rose, he drowned, and went to heaven. There he asked God why he didn't save him even after he prayed so fervently. God said, "I sent you a boat and a helicopter. What else did you want?"

I must say that as a result of prayer, I was sent helpful dreams and spiritual visitations by loved ones. More importantly, I was sent key people from the Health and Rejuvenation Center at the Association for Research and Enlightenment, which eventually led to my discovering the BMC. They have been the answer to my prayers. Prayer and the mind-body connection should not be the only form of treatment, but they are important catalysts in the larger scheme of recovery. Spiritual messages, dreams and signs helped clarify my choices so I could make better decisions about the therapies I needed to obtain a cure.

Nonetheless, do not underestimate the awesome power of the mind-body connection in this immune-based disease we call cancer. It is wise to use such interventions to increase our chances for success. I am happy there is a natural cancer cure, 80 percent successful, available to us, but why not make that 100% by using our minds? If the mind is a major contributing factor to the breakdown of the immune system and our contracting cancer, then conversely it also has the ability to reverse the process by restoring our immune function.

"There is solid evidence that the course of disease in general is affected by emotional distress...We may learn how to influence general body systems and through them modify the neoplasm which resides within the body...As we go forward...searching for new means of controlling growth both within the cell and through systematic influences...we can widen the quest to include the distinct possibility that within one's mind is a power capable of exerting forces which can either enhance or inhibit the progress of this disease."

Presidential address to the American Cancer Society in 1959, by Pendergrass (three years before the Hoxsey clinics were shut down).

In order to understand the role of the mind-body connection, we will first look at the role personality plays in our recovery, relative to beliefs, values, and attitudes.

The Cancer Personality

If you read enough books on the mind-body approach, you may find in them a description of the "cancer personality." There are personality characteristics that seem to be consistent from one cancer patient to the next. They include:

Excessive or unresolved fears
Excessive or unresolved anger
Feelings of helplessness over an important life stress
The loss of a spouse or important loved one
Tendency to put others' needs over our own

The people I met who are cancer survivors are some of the most selfless, conscientious people I've encountered. They tend to care for others and often put the needs of the people they care about ahead of their own. They are other-oriented, but are often easily disappointed because others do not put the same effort into their relationship as the cancer patient does. And research shows that if they lose a loved one, they often find it difficult to go on living. Essentially, most are some of the nicest, most beautiful people you'll ever meet.

Another group of people who contract cancer are those who carry too much repressed anger and fear, which often affects their overall approach to life's circumstances. According to Bernie Siegel, M.D., author of *Love, Medicine, and Miracles*, cancer patients have often suffered from childhood traumas, where they develop these personality characteristics. Dr. Siegel recommends art therapy to get at the roots of these unconscious memories. In addition, counseling, either ministerial or professional, can be effective for uncovering the causes of irrational perceptions. It can also explore current life concerns for the purpose of obtaining an objective view of things.

When people feel helpless to change something, this can affect their recovery. In one study with breast cancer patients, when a woman felt that a stressful life event was beyond her control, the likelihood of relapse was found to be statistically greater. In general, women, more often then men, base their happiness on their relationships with the people close to them. This may be true for many family-oriented men as well.

According to Dr. Douglas Brodie, of Reno, Nevada, many cancer patients studied were found to internalize their cares, concerns, and problems. For this reason, he says that the carefree, extroverted individual is far less likely to contract cancer than the caring introvert. In one 30-year study involving medical students, those who were characterized as "loners" and hid their emotions behind a bland exterior were 16 times more likely to contract cancer than those who expressed their emotions and took active measures to relieve anger and frustration.

Dr. Brodie also says that people who develop cancer are generally plagued by depression, indecision, hopelessness, low self-esteem, chronic fatigue, anxiety, grief, loneliness, or isolation, because these things depress immune function and increase susceptibility to cancer. His view is that "excessive levels of stress combine with the underlying personality to promote the immune deficiency which allows cancer to thrive."

Having experienced a recent loss is another very important factor. Studies by Goldfarb, cited in *Visualization: The Uses of Imagery in the Health Professions, P. 210, 2005, by Korn & Johnson*, showed that a high percentage of cancer patients had lost an important emotional relationship just prior to developing a neoplasm (cancer). A primary component to such occurrences involved the cancer patient being unable to find an effective outlet for the psycho-emotional energy.

Developing a network of support is very important to recovery. Stanford psychiatrist David Spiegel demonstrated that women with breast cancer who attended a weekly support group lived twice as long as those who did not. Although I personally did not attend support groups, I spoke with and visited regularly with other Hoxsey patients, family members, and friends. The topic of my overcoming my illness was always on the agenda and all were free to comment on the medicinal, spiritual, or psychological aspects of my recovery. This was a healthy personality characteristic I chose to adopt after I became ill.

Selecting the "Right Doctors"

As I interviewed all the doctors, staff, and the director of the BMC, they all mentioned one commonality in getting better: the single most important factor to curing this disease is a person's attitude. Research shows that the cancer patient's relationship with their physician is directly linked to the outcome of therapy. Studies show that patients have a smoother recovery with an empathetic physician who has good rapport and informs the cancer patient of the nature of their condition. The physicians at the BMC are obviously aware of this fact because they maintain excellent rapport with their patients and keep us well informed. As a general rule, I haven't found many kind, compassionate, and caring oncologists in the medical profession in the United States. Many appear to be detached from their patients, overworked, and very scientifically-minded. They stick with the facts, but if the facts don't look good, particularly if they're losing a patient, they may not share all the facts with him or her. They often don't treat the patients as equals in understanding the disease. They also often don't have enough time to do this. According to Dr. Siegel these social aversions are due to the unresolved pain oncologists tend to carry from losing a substantial number of their patients to the disease. This is not always easy for BMC physicians, either.

I remember a woman with cancer who was at the BMC for the first time. She was carrying a lot of anger. In the waiting room, she and her husband didn't socialize with the other patients, who are typically laughing, sharing, and supportive of each other. She took her anger out on the staff and doctors, who were directly affected, because this personality type is rarely encountered there and they leave themselves unguarded. As a result, the clinic staff met in private to discuss her attitude. I was not part of these discussions; however, it was obvious the staff was directly affected by her misdirected anger. I left that day feeling bad for the people at the BMC and aware that empathy is a two edged-sword.

It is important for me to mention here that I was very fortunate in that my American oncologist was deeply spiritual and compassionate. I was able to freely share my spirituality relative to my life and my disease, and the alternative medicine approaches I'd chosen. We also are both writers, and this contributed to our friendship. I was fortunate that he was willing to run legal and political risks inherent in ordering oncological tests and following my progress. Many American physicians would have not only scolded and belittled such patients for choosing "a death sentence," but would have also refused to see them any longer. For my local support, I truly feel blessed.

For those with cancer, I recommend that they choose their physicians wisely. The physicians at BMC are among the most knowledgeable in alternative medicine approaches, because this is what they've specialized in for the past eighty years. My American oncologist repeatedly said, "I don't know anything about alternative medicine." The physicians at BMC have seen just about everything connected to alternative cancer therapies, and they are willing to tell you about their experiences with live human subjects, straight up, with no hidden agenda. They are willing to explain all your X-rays and discuss the progression or regression of your disease. Then they will offer you hope out of the successes they've had with the tens of thousands of patients on the Hoxsey program, or they'll have you consider other alternatives that can save or extend your life.

Whether it's a traditional physician or an alternative medicine professional, or both, an empathetic physician who is willing to share spiritual concepts, be open and honest with us about progress, and yet is supportive of our decisions, is paramount to our recovery.

The Role of Spirituality

Many physicians in the United States avoid the topic of spirituality, yet the doctors at the BMC include it in their therapy under lifestyle counseling. They are not trying to convert people to a specific religion, however. As I've always told my students when teaching mind-body therapies, it's not a patient's religion that concerns us, as long as it is working for them; it is their individual sense of spirituality that we need to examine. In other words, how do they practice or cultivate their relationship with God? Do they attend a church, practice meditation, or pray? A religion is a group of people with similar enough beliefs that they practice their spirituality together.

A study conducted by the University of Michigan in Ann Arbor found that people who attended church services lived longer than those who did not. It may be concluded, then, that belonging to a faith community contributes to longevity. The researchers compared church services betterment to health to the process of quitting smoking and being involved in a regular moderate exercise program.

Spirituality is extremely important to a cancer patient's ability to release stress to a higher power. The health benefits of stress relief alone make this a worthwhile practice. In addition, God will not only help us find peace, but also will assist us with a healing, if it is in our destiny. Therefore, prayer is very powerful. Bernie Siegel mentions this in his talks and writings, citing an important blind study that proves the power of prayer. Of two groups of people who had cancer, one group was put on an extensive prayer list, while the other was not. The group that was prayed for lived, on average, 10 years longer and showed spontaneous healings. For this reason, according to Dr. Siegel, it is advisable to get on as many prayer lists as possible.

During the most difficult months of battling this disease, one of my daily reads was a book called, *God's Promises: For Your Every Need,* compiled by Dr. A.L. Gill. It contains passages from the Christian Bible, grouping them by common human thoughts and emotions. For me, since I grew up Christian and became more eclectic with age, my Christian roots became ever so important to my recovery. It was an individual choice, as it is with each cancer patient, to use what seems to best foster my relationship with God.

As I glance at the old tattered cover on this book even now, as it stares at me from one of the many book shelves towering in my home, it holds a power of its own. When I see it, it reminds me how God gently carried me through each stage of my recovery, like a parent taking a young child by the hand and showing him or her how to perceive life and what to do that day, one day at a time, one moment at a time. Every action, and every word, is heightened in our awareness when we are facing a life-threatening illness. My copy of Dr. Gill's book was published in 1995 by Word Publishing. How it ended up on one of my book shelves and in my hands, I'll never know. All I know is that it was there when I needed it, which is how things work on this journey, if we are keeping awake and watching for them.

My parents said they were praying for me every day at the daily church services they attended. My sisters said the same thing. In addition, I talked to the campus minister about my illness, and he came to my home one day. I told him about all my major life stresses, the things I wanted to change in my life, or in myself, and the unfinished business I had, so I could clear my conscience. His father had recently passed away from cancer, so he had a reference point for this type of exchange. In addition, he seemed to have more compassion than my primary minister. Our meeting involved a lot of sharing on that sunny afternoon, and it ended with the two of us holding hands in prayer. At this point, I don't even remember what was said, only that it was a significant moment in my walk with God through the revolving doors of my recovery.

There were other ways God reached me, and I reached out to him, which I mentioned in the first three chapters of this book. In general, we must feel that God is present during our suffering. We must invite this presence into our lives and make a connection through both direct and metaphorical means—perhaps through prayer, dreams, dream journaling, meditation, and other spiritual rituals. We must recognize, too, when God is speaking through others. We must establish a phone line to the heavenly place of existence and then be a good listener to discover what God wants from us during this unique journey. While we fight to survive, we must consider what my traditional oncologist said: "There are many people who die with great virtue, as they finish their business on the earth with an uncanny level of nobility and simply move on to the next world."

Many survivors teach those around them how to value life enough to fight for it, and not take it for granted. We teach people to enjoy it more, as we live more in the moment. We also teach people to think more about where we are all headed when this journey ends. We teach faith, hope, humility, and more. Many cancer patients, after recovery, will often claim that the disease was the best thing that ever happened to them, because it taught them how to live.

The Holistic Approach

A holistic approach to cancer recovery is what many cancer patients request of their health care practitioners and health systems today. Holism is the process of recognizing that the body, mind, and soul affect each other. Holistic methods involve incorporating the whole human being into the recovery process. Using holistic methods, which is what the BMC emphasizes, is essential for a cancer patient's recovery process, because this particular disease is due not only to environmental or genetic factors, but also lifestyle and the will of God.

The mind's ability to handle life's challenges, and the spiritual values of an individual, directly affect the ability to ward off stresses, and therefore the immune system's ability to ward off intruders. The mind and immune system both need to rebuild themselves so we may truly become a survivor.

One attitude that may help in recovering from this adversity, or any adversity, is reflected in the saying, "What doesn't kill you will make you stronger." But if the mind is so integral to the process of recovery, we must ask ourselves, What is the *right attitude?* Until we achieve a solid remission, each day may represent a roller coaster ride, where the cancer patient is on a roller coaster ride from doctor to doctor, clinic to clinic, and exam to exam. It can seem that everybody is playing the game called "hot potato," as ideas get tossed back and forth from one expert to the next. In the mean time, the clock is ticking. We are in a unique race against time to stop this thing from taking over our bodies. Meanwhile there are many people on the sidelines cheering us on to maintain the *right attitude.*

What is the *Right Attitude?*

Discovering the right attitude was tricky for me. I describe in Part One of this book my experience when I got a CT scan, and how the X-ray technician reminded me how important it is to have the right attitude. Because I was having a bad day, the statement hit my emotions. I choked out the words, "What is the right attitude?" Eventually, I did find the answer to this question all on my own.

When I asked, "What is the right attitude?" it was because I'd been exposed to a wide variety of theories on the subject without any experience. Later, I talked to many people with cancer, people who'd survived cancer, and various health care practitioners. I analyzed their opinions, tested them, and then ended up being able to accurately define what felt *right* for me. Here is what I discovered.

Let Go. Things are never as bad as they seem. We may panic over a situation, or get upset about things in a relationship that seem they will never change. But the fact is that if there is love in that relationship, then it will evolve on its own. Love is the greatest teacher. If a little thing out of our control does not work out to our expectation, we have to say, "so what?" It's usually not as bad as the heat of the moment paints it out to be. We must not be emotionally attached to outcomes. If God closes one door, he'll open another. If things don't go the way we intended, then they were never meant to be.

Be Optimistic. Pessimists often think of the worst case scenario, when in fact it rarely ever happens. Instead, we will be much healthier focusing on the best case scenario. Things always work out in the end, and every end has a new beginning. Most of us can look back and admit that everything that has occurred in the past has generally worked out for the best. In addition, focusing on our goals is not only statistically healthier; doing it means we are more likely to achieve them. Every cancer patient should have at least one goal they want to achieve after recovery that they hadn't achieved yet. Mine involved a vacation in Alaska, and then moving to the ocean, where I would be happier and healthier.

Living in the Moment. Many cancer patients come to realize, more than the average person, that our clocks are ticking. We're here today and gone tomorrow. I always thought it would be best to leave this world quickly, but when I got cancer, I realized that something beautiful had happened. I was able to say the things to my loved ones that I'd never had the chance to say before. I began living as if I were dying, and there is no greater gift from recovery. It gives us precious moments in time when words move through the air and into the soul, where they last forever. The moments we express our love are precious. We do what my wife and I call "heart speak." This is where we speak from the heart. Yesterday and tomorrow are less important than the present moment. We still plan, but we do it more grounded in who we are now and what we are feeling or sensing. Living in the moment is about learning more about who we are and learning who our loved ones are, because we are sharing ourselves more.

The Concept of "More." The concept of more states that regardless of how much money we make or have, human nature will always make us want more...the bigger house, the newer car, the better job, and so on. The truth is, we never have enough money. This is true of anybody, whether or not they have cancer—although statistically, one of the greatest concerns of a cancer patient is finances, since many Americans who contract cancer can't pay all their bills. There's a lot wrong with the American capitalist-based health care system. Too many people don't have health insurance and even those who do often go bankrupt after getting a life-threatening illness. But it is best to focus on what we can do about our situation to improve our financial picture. We need to learn how to cut back on expenses and keep our head above water until we make it to the five-year mark. It's best to come up with a plan for making payments and liquidating things we don't need. Admittedly, my career suffered. Many people heard I had cancer and the attendance levels at my seminars went down. I had to refinance my home, with cash out to pay bills, until things got better. We do what we need to do, but at least we have our lives after we recover from this thing; and life is good! We will always have the house payment, or the car payment, so once we make the decision about how we will meet our health bills, we need to let the worries go and just do the best we can. In the process, we need to put our health first, be thankful we have it right now, re-budget, and do more of the things we enjoy that don't cost much.

Reevaluate. Those of us with a life threatening illness often reevaluate our lives. Are we in a career where we are doing what our passion is? Do we enjoy going to work, or is it a real chore? How can we change our job tasks or careers, reduce expenses, and make it all work? The cars, the new home, are they really worth it? We can't take them with us in the end anyway. If they are doable, fine, but if not, maybe we should trim the fat. How will we shift our values to create a lower stress level, let go of the things we can't change, and be more detached when attempting to change the things we can? Can we let go and let God? These concepts and others are what we need to ponder when we think about what will increase our joy and reduce our burdens. We may find that what we do doesn't define who we are. We should be prepared to sever the things that *tax* our mental and emotional energy, and engage in more of the things that *give* energy back to us.

Be Honest with Feelings. I remember attending a holistic cancer recovery seminar with Dr. Bernie Siegel in a large auditorium. It was sponsored by a local hospital. The thousand-plus participants included medical professionals, medical students, and patients and their families. I found so much value in the things he discussed that I later wrote a paper on them for one of my doctoral courses. He said, "If we say no to ourselves, we say no to our body." This was in relation to expressing our emotions. We must learn to express our thoughts and feeling to the people we spend time with. We must learn to express our needs in a way that they become an absolute, that our thoughts and emotions are not taken for granted. With this, we better take care of ourselves, and therefore our health, because nobody knows how to do this for us better than we do. Even if somebody did know better, they cannot do it for us. Expressing our thoughts, feelings, and needs are key components to recovery. Many cancer patients are very kind, flexible people, but it's better to tell people "no" when we feel stretched too thin.

Minimizing and Maximizing. Perception and attitude are powerful things. It is extremely important for us to learn how to minimize the effects of stress and maximize the joy we receive from the good moments that pass through our lives every day. For example, minimizing may be done by recognizing that bitter people who yell at you in public are either lacking in spirituality, are not coping with personal problems in their lives, or haven't yet softened from life's sufferings—or in fact they may have hardened from them. It is sad to see people struggling to the extent that they feel the need to yell at other people. We must learn healthy detachment, how we can get our messages across without being emotionally invested in them. As for maximizing our experience, it may be that a new bird started coming to the bird feeder, or somebody called whom you hadn't heard from in a while. It may come from a simple stroke of unconditional love from the family cat when he pushed against your legs. We need to "carpe diem," which in Latin means "seize the day" or "seize the moment." It is important that we know how to live in the moment and enjoy the moment. In other words, it is important that we open our hearts up to positive people and situations and the bright moments in a day. If we are too far down in the ditch, attitudinally, we will miss them. We need to embrace the good as our primary reality, and accept the bad with faith and hope.

Pick Battles Carefully. How do you know if a conflict is weighing on you in an unhealthy way to the point where you should jump ship or give up the fight? The best way is to see if you are losing sleep over it. If you are, then you should consider giving up the fight so that it literally doesn't kill you. Cancer patients desperately need sleep to recover. Another way is to measure your pH level. If our pH level is acidic, we've allowed something to bother us, which we should either eliminate or learn to tolerate better. Watching the news can be unhealthy. We can't solve the whole world's problems. In fact, solving the ones in our personal lives tend to be challenging enough. Can we sidestep personal problems, or just tell somebody that we choose not to participate in the game anymore? Perhaps it's a loved one, and we need to tell that person that we love them but we can only handle a one- or two-day visit, at a maximum. Other people often don't know what's best for us, so it is up to us to inform them. If we think a battle is worth fighting, we would probably be most effective, and certainly more healthy, if we do it non-emotionally. If we get upset with somebody or with a situation, then so be it; we should let it all hang out at that point. Yet we should not allow ourselves to get to that point very often. We should be "slow to anger like (our) father in heaven." In addition, we should accept forms of support from friends, neighbors, relatives, or anybody who wants to help us. Kindness can boost our energy so we may face life's challenges better.

Make Time for Yourself. I can honestly say that before I contracted cancer I didn't make the proper time for myself. By proper, I mean that I was always trying to make sure everybody in my family was happy and on track with their responsibilities, while I juggled my own career, hobbies, and personal time. I did this to the extent that I really didn't take time for myself as much as I needed. If everybody else was happy, I was happy—that is, before I got sick. Now I still take the father role seriously, and I'm good at it, but I also have my own life, which is equal to or greater in value to me. I am a person who loves nature, music, fishing, camping, travel, and time away from it all. In fact, one of the first things my wife and I did, only one month after I was diagnosed, was to buy a time share at a resort. We listened to the presentation, and even though I was very worried about our finances, my wife and I took money out of savings and did it, for one reason: we would be forced to take a vacation, once a year, just the two of us, and in a place we could get pampered with four- or five-star service. This was something we would have never dreamed of doing before getting sick. Now we love it. It was one of the best decisions I ever made. You should set goals that you will accomplish after your recovery that involve just you, and nobody else, what you want to come into your life that brings you joy, and which are not contingent on other's state of mind.

Goal Setting. Goal setting is essential to recovery. Those with cancer should set up recovery goals, to experience the things in life they've always wanted to do. Research shows that lifestyle changes often precede a solid remission, and goal setting, in my opinion, is a way of telling our bodies that we are going to live past the current health crisis, that the body needs to respond to *our* time line and not anybody else's. I remember a story about a man who contracted cancer. He owned his own family business. His doctor gave him only months to live, so he quit the family business and started traveling. As he reached a great sense of freedom from his family stresses, he experienced a spontaneous remission and later attributed it to his change in lifestyle. He never went back to the family business. He lived well past his death date, the date his oncologist predicted his patient would die. Statistics indicate, remarkably, that many people die on that exact day, which proves the power of the mind in this disease. I have a friend from India who swears that both of her parents, when they became ill, told their loved ones the date they would die, and they did die on that date. We can now note the importance of setting goals for our bodies after recovery. Mine was a trip with my wife every year to pamper ourselves; it was also a chance to get away from our family business and just be friends and lovers. Another goal I set was to take an Alaskan cruise, something I would have saved for retirement, but I thought, "Who am I to predict how long I will live?" So I took money out of savings and did it. In fact, I am writing this very segment as we are pulling up to the port at Juneau, the capital of Alaska! I also have many post-recovery career goals, such as on-line courses in holistic medicine, other books I want to write, and opening a holistic health center in my home town. My wife and I also set a more distant goal of taking a windjammer cruise in 2008, on our 25th anniversary. Annual spiritual retreats for my family and me are on the agenda again. More goals included moving to the beach—which we have done—so I can write near the calm waters of the sound. We must keep in mind that goal-setting is not just a mental concept. A recent discovery science has made shows there are neuroreceptors in every part of the body, not just our brains! All things considered, it is important to keep our bodies thinking they need to *go the distance.*

People who are survivors do things that make them healthier in mind, body, and soul. Even if it is our time to leave this world, at the very least the attitudinal shifts outlined above will help us find peace in the process—but more likely will assist us with a cure if we put our minds to it.

Advice for Excessive Stress

As discussed in the chapter on diet, an overload of stress causes the body fluids to turn acidic. It wasn't until late in my first year of recovery that I realized the importance of this concept. I tell in Part One a story about how an incident with our daughter, when she was having problems, caused my pH level to turn acidic. That was when I knew that I needed to take responsibility for *myself* and my health, as well as for my family. I continue to strive to do this. As of the writing of this book, we have ongoing issues we are working on with our daughter, even though she is now in college; and it creates a challenge to balance the values of cancer survivorship with being an effective father.

The point is that stress causes an acidic response that we must gauge within ourselves. If we are getting upset about something, we must deal with it by effectively expressing our views and move through it quickly, so that we can focus on something more positive as soon as possible. Focusing on the things we are thankful for in our lives can create a sense of gratitude, and gratitude can help us find a healthy level of detachment.

Once, when I had a legal issue involving my daughter, I sent an e-mail to Dr. Gutierrez at the BMC, asking him whether I should pursue it with the help of meditation and detachment, or if I should just abandon it. My number-one goal was to maintain a good state of mental and physical health. His response follows:

> "...(the best medicine) for stress is, of course, meditation; and the best of all, 'Let it be' philosophy. What has to be, will be, and there is nothing we can do about it. We are only lonely ships in this vast ocean, and we bump against one another every once in a while; and our voyage is too short to waste in the dark side of the ocean."

According to Dr. Lawrence Taylor, M.D., of Chula Vista, California, a total change in attitude is necessary for a cancer patient to fully recover from cancer. His anti-cancer attitude includes these primary components:
1. Hopefulness, optimism, and life-affirming
2. Assertiveness regarding one's own needs.

When people are happy and joyful, their bodies produce endorphins, and this makes them feel good. Endorphins are the body's natural painkillers, but they also contribute to the synthesis of DHEA by the adrenal glands. DHEA stimulates the thymus gland, a crucial component of the health of our immune system (the value of DHEA is also discussed in the previous chapter). The immune system is restored with faith, hope, and feelings of happiness.

Attitude adjustment is particularly important for the cancer patient, because research proves, time and time again, that the mind directly affects the body.

My Methods of Mind-Body Cancer Therapies

Years ago, during my doctoral studies, I was exposed to research documented by O. Carl Simonton and Stephanie Matthews-Simonton. The Simontons maintain that cancer patients should comprehend that they can use their minds to alter the development and course of the disease. In particular, they report a significant number of remissions of advanced metastatic cancers. They published multiple articles and books showing a significant increase in recovery rates for those cancer patients who practiced a combination of meditation, self-hypnosis with positive suggestions toward recovery, and positive imagery, such as tumor reduction visualization and future life goals. Stress relief was also a primary focus (releasing stress during self-hypnosis exercises by imagining the exhaling of it from the mind and body), while bolstering an attitude of a will to live.

In a monumental study conducted by the Simontons about twenty years ago with 134 cancer patients, 100 went into solid long-term remissions, and even the 34 who died lived much longer than expected.

In the process of studying both the Simontons' and the Bernie Siegel's approaches, and with my own experiences with clients and then myself, I developed a mind-body cancer recovery methodology that became highly effective with cancer patients in my private practice. From this, I got wonderful results. The approach has five essential steps.

Mood Charting and Communication
Regressive Healing
Dream Induction
Customized Anti-Cancer Imagery
Future Life Goals Imagery

Mood Charting and Communication

The first thing I tell my new clients who have cancer is that they need to grade their mood at the end of the day and mark it on a calendar for all their loved ones in the household to see. This is a means of expression, and it leaves nobody guessing as to how the cancer patient is feeling. A+ is the best day a person can have and F- is the worst. Essentially, by becoming more aware, the family becomes more supportive and understanding of each other and the cancer patient's body responds more favorably to treatment. In fact, many family members are very accommodating in creating a more peaceful environment, which helps keep the body fluids more alkaline and restores its immune system.

In my case, my family didn't have to guess at my mood. I became extremely expressive and my wife also converted to expressing what was important to her. In addition, my children became supportive and expressed their concerns, spiritual beliefs, and desires for my healing as we prayed about them together almost every evening.

In addition, the entire family benefited from counseling, particularly my daughter. But I must say that the first two counselors we worked with made things temporarily worse. My daughter convinced the therapist that we were the problem and we became outsiders in the process, not knowing what was going on in the therapy sessions because we were excluded by the therapist. My daughter became even angrier. We fired that therapist and found another one, who proved to be impotent; after two sessions he said, "This family is creating a lot of anxiety for me."

But three was a charm. The third therapist was very intuitive with all of us as we did family counseling. She understood each person's issues well, helped each of us take responsibility, and we made tremendous progress in our interactions with one another, which was a big help. In addition, I could say what was in my heart and mind without interruption, and it was taken more seriously and seen as being important to my path toward recovery.

Effective communication is important to cancer patients, but it isn't always accomplished with the various personality types that exist in a family, since each person is unique and responds differently to a crisis, such as a serious illness. If communication among family members cannot effectively take place in person, mediation or counseling is often helpful. Second-best may be to write letters to let loved ones know how you feel, if you have cancer. After expressing your views, however, you must be willing to *release* specific people and situations that have been bothering you.

Regressive Healing

This method, which is usually our first hypnosis session, is where I put a person under hypnosis and instruct his or her unconscious mind to reveal the cause of the illness. People often go back to what the sociologist Charles Massey refers to as a *Significant Life Experience* (SLE). For the sensitive cancer personality, this may have something to do with being left by a spouse, or having abandonment issues as far back as early childhood. In my case, my teenage daughter got into a lot of trouble and threw the family into a tizzy and sometimes I lost my ability to communicate constructively. Family issues are strong triggers for illnesses, but it varies for each individual.

Once an individual with cancer discovers the events that reduced the immune system's ability to respond to foreign invaders, such as cancer cells, we can reframe and release the emotional content in their memories so the memories no longer bother them. Sometimes this results in moving through our past unforgiveness, negative emotions and perceptions that are lodged in past memories. Sometimes a regressive hypnotherapy session involves finding the parts of ourselves we lost in a memory and getting those parts back. Regressive hypnotherapy can include soul retrieval, an ancient healing art originating from Native Americans and Alaskan natives. During the process, the person seeking the healing finds positive parts of themselves that he or she lost at the time of contracting an illness, which for the cancer patient can be very effective in healing his or her illness. After going through soul retrieval, the client feels much more whole.

For example, in the beginning of my healing journey, I had a soul retrieval done on myself by a hypnotherapist I trusted, who was also working with Sloan-Kettering Hospital's oncology department at the time. He put me back into a memory that occurred just before I contracted cancer. The memory involved disappointments and a loss in my ability to trust others. After the process I felt more whole, with a prevailing sense of peace.

In addition to this mind-body intervention, it was beneficial for me when I saw a minister of my denomination for the process of forgiveness. This proved to be another step on the climb to my recovery.

Dream Induction

This step I only perform in cases where the client suffers from insomnia, which may also cause other problems such as mood swings and loss of appetite. As in most cases, the client's subconscious mind is trying to work out unresolved stresses that may have something to do with worries over their future, or the future of their families.

The procedure is that I put a client under hypnosis and then ask them to recall the dreams that are waking them up and often keeping them awake. The dream appears in their mind's eye and they recall it with a high level of revivification (reliving). In other words, because they are in a relaxed state of mind, their imagery is clearer and they practically relive the dream as we reinterpret it. This allows for nightmare resolution, and therefore a much better night's sleep, which also allows the cancer patient to rest, as the BMC recommends to boost our energy levels.

In my case, I seemed to sleep well after I did a soul retrieval, so I did not need dream induction. However, there was a time just before I contracted the illness when the combination of my asthma and stress led to a very ineffective, broken sleep pattern.

Customized Anti-Cancer Imagery

Imagery is a very powerful step toward killing cancer cells, reducing tumors, and more. Customizing imagery, or having a cancer patient choose the image that will be most effective in altering their disease, is most effective. In my case, I thought that because sharks don't get cancer, if I imagined sharks swimming in my blood and attacking the tumors, they would shrink. I remember the first CT scan that showed improvement. I was told by the radiologist, "It appears that your tumors are sagging, like cherries on a cherry tree wrinkling from a frost." This is essentially the effect we cancer patients want. This occurred in June of 2003, about the time my whole mind-body approach became more spiritual to encompass God. I changed my self-hypnosis imagery from a safe place in nature to an unconditionally loving light that emanates from where God exists. From there, I could begin feeling the warmth and purity of his love, and how it flowed through me and enveloped me.

In the process of doing this white light meditation, I would imagine that all my tumors were melting like a penetrating light from the sun melting ice cubes. I felt stronger about this than the shark imagery I used in the past. I knew it was helping with my healing.

Future Life Goals Imagery

Once a cancer patient does enough healing of the past, it is imperative that he or she focus on what kind of life they want in the future. This life is not about others, but about ourselves, and how we choose to live it. And it's about our relationship to God. If we have love or romance, it's icing on the cake, or in other words, something to be thankful for.

Cancer patients have a tendency to base their happiness on the contentment of their loved ones. If others are happy, then they are too. If others are not, they are not either. This is a roller coaster ride we must not allow ourselves to be on anymore, if we are going to get better permanently. Instead, what I like to do with my clients is have them go into a state of relaxation and imagine themselves years in the future enjoying their favorite activities, or experiencing something that is a goal they set for themselves. For me, it was trip to Alaska on the third year of my recovery, and a windjammer cruise on my 25th anniversary, which would be the fifth year of my recovery. I also imagined living in the Outer Banks of North Carolina, a vacationer's paradise where I would write often; and I imagined writing this book and achieving even more success as an author in the holistic health field.

Years ago, I saw a client who had throat and lung cancer. He could barely make it up the flight of steps to my office when I first saw him, because he came in tied to an oxygen tank, pale and gray. He wasn't eating or sleeping, and looked like he had gotten off his death bed to see me as a last resort.

After I did a session on dream induction to release a nightmare, he started sleeping again. His second session involved regressing him back to the day his physician told him he may never drive or engage in independent outdoor activities again. After reframing what was said, the client believed he had a future of independence, and he started eating again. The last thing we did was work toward creating future life goals imagery. He chose to imagine himself driving a truck by himself, and going fishing and hunting again, the two activities that were most important to him.

We taped hypnotic relaxation followed by these concepts on a self-hypnosis tape, which he listened to for several months. He became a long-term survivor, or what is referred to by oncologists as an exceptional patient. One day he came to visit me, and with a deep level of gratitude said, "I don't know if it was the hypnosis that helped me; to tell you the truth I don't even know if I was under hypnosis, but whatever you did really helped me get my life back, so I came here to thank you." Tears rolled down his face. This was one of the greatest tithes I did during the history of my private practice, because this particular client was on a sliding scale due to the financial challenges of the illness.

In order to fully recover, we must keep future goals fresh in our minds. We need to teach the body what we want it to do.

The above is just a brief synopsis of my methods for creating the right mind-body climate for the body to be able to heal itself. I could give readers several case histories describing how these methods helped a wide variety of my clients, but that would take another book. I have a wealth of information gleaned from the vast sea of healing arts I've studied over the years, but we simply don't have space for it here. To cancer patients, however, I want to emphasize that most if not all of the steps above can be accomplished with the help of ministers, counselors, hypnotherapists, meditation instructors, or by helping yourself, when you, or you and your loved ones together, are ready for the process. There are also many things you can do on your own, which will be explained in the next chapter.

An Unusual Mind-Body Side Effect of the Tonic

There is an unusual mind-body effect that many patients of the BMC using Hoxsey therapy have reported in my interviews. Once the patient starts using the herbs, they occasionally have the digestive cleansing effects mentioned previously. But they also seem to re-experience the emotions they had around the time they became ill, particularly if there was a major life stress that occurred just before the illness. I also encountered this effect, which motivated me to work on my issues and become more expressive during the healing process.

I asked myself why this was so consistent from one Hoxsey patient to the next and came up with a hypothesis. If the herbs we were taking were cleansing our organs, balancing our immune systems, and normalizing our bodies' health systems, it is because they are in natural harmony with nature. These natural medicines are more in harmony with God, because God created nature. And if we contract cancer because our minds and bodies are out of harmony with nature, then it is highly likely that the herbal medicines we are taking are putting us back into alignment with nature or God. During the process, anything that stands between us and God is revealed. We experience a mental and emotional purification while our minds and bodies return to a more natural state of homeostasis.

These herbs are the same ones that the horse at Harry Hoxsey's grandfather's farm intuitively knew to eat to cure its cancer. Most of us are aware that animals have a sixth sense that is much more acute than any human sense. For example, just before the tsunami hit Indonesia in 2004, devastating the coast lands and killing thousands of people, the animals were reported to have fled the coastal areas to move inland. This, in my opinion, was how the horse knew which herbs to eat.

It is important to note that these are the same herbs that Edgar Cayce, while in his enlightened state of mind, was told by God would cure cancer.

It makes me wonder: when will we all come to an understanding that nature can heal us? We simply need to trust what God gave us, the herbs, our minds and hearts, and the Holy Spirit. We need to trust that together, with God, the resources on the planet, and those in ourselves, we have the ability to heal ourselves of this illness.

Summary

An Overview of Anti-Cancer Psychology

Cancer patients must consider the type of life they want for themselves. We must ask ourselves the question, "What kind of career purpose does God want for us? What kind of marriage or relationship does God want for us? What kind of relationship should we foster with our children so they become more independent and allow us to become more independent, while trying to keep connected by love? What do I still want to see or do, with hobbies, travel, and recreation?"

I had to realize that the new home and the new car are just toys that we temporarily play with while we're alive on earth. I began to realize that owning land was just an illusion; in actuality we are just temporary stewards. Someday others would inhabit our homes, and our cars would become junked metal that would return to the earth. My kids, my wife—they too would evolve into other beings with or without my influence. God knew this before he even put us all together.

I had to let go and let God. I can only do so much as a father and a husband, and how good a job I do was probably foreseen by God before I even took the job. I needed to learn to appreciate that whatever life my wife and kids lead is unique to them on their own journey here. They are each on a unique path; we are just sharing certain segments along the way.

There's a popular country song called, "Live Like You Were Dying." It describes how a man found out he had contracted cancer. As he reviewed his X-rays with the doctors, he made the decision that he would do everything in life he hadn't done before and wanted to do, such as sky diving, etc. It is a very good song for the exceptional patient, or for anybody who takes life for granted. It indicates the beauty of people with or without cancer who live like they are dying. None of us knows when our hour will come. If all of us lived like this, the world would be a much better place. I believe this is the gift that the cancer patient receives: the awareness that we are all here for a limited time, so we need to make the best of it.

Putting the Holistic Approach into Perspective

The holistic methods I describe in this chapter are not meant to be a panacea for the process of cancer recovery. Spiritual healing and mind-body interventions are most successful as part of a comprehensive cancer recovery system, such as the Hoxsey therapy. They are not meant to be *the* method of recovery by themselves. When I interviewed former Hoxsey patient and videographer Carol Main, she told me that her attitude was adjusted toward getting better, but she didn't do any mind-body therapies. She trusted the Hoxsey system and did everything the doctors at BMC told her to do, and she credits the herbs and diet as the primary sources of her recovery.

Nonetheless, as we explore the research (described above) by the Simontons and Bernie Siegel, we must conclude that mind-body therapies should not be underestimated in cancer recovery. Dr. Gutierrez has stated may times when interviewed, "Possibly the most important thing is a patient's attitude." He claims that if patients using the Hoxsey method believe they are going to get better, they generally do. If the patient has a negative attitude toward the treatment program, or toward life in general, the staff at the BMC notices that this particular patient's chance of getting better is diminished.

This is why the attitude of the staff and patients at the BMC is always so positive. In contrast to a traditional oncologist's office, laughter, hope, friendship, outward affection, encouragement, and faith are common themes. Success stories are often shared in the waiting room while testimonials in the guest book are commonly read.

The patients at the BMC quickly come to realize that there truly is an alternative, all-natural treatment that has cured tens of thousands of people, and it won't make you sicker or give you more cancers. It was put here by God for us to discover. All we need to do is talk to others in the waiting room who are getting results, watch the testimonials on the video taped documentaries, or read the testimonials in the visitor's registry to come to the realization that we are on the road to recovery!

Chapter 12

Mind-Body Interventions

Self-Hypnosis and Meditation

Hypnosis is a relaxed state of mind that enhances the mind-body connection and also fosters a connection with our higher power, or God. Hypnosis *is* a state of guided meditation, in which, after entering into a state of relaxation, that which we think about becomes more real. It also expands our awareness about our illness and adds to our healing resources.

In chapter one of my first book, *Clinical Hypnotherapy: A Transpersonal Approach*, I classify all altered states of consciousness (ASC) as forms of hypnosis. These include meditation, transcendental meditation, biofeedback, imagery, guided imagery, visualization, yoga, and other forms of hypnosis. Of all of the altered states of consciousness studied, hypnotherapy and self-hypnosis proved to be the most efficient and effective in reducing stress and increasing health.

The ability to use hypnosis and meditation to affect our health should not be underestimated. By using chanting and other forms of self-hypnosis, I've seen people walk on fire, commonly stepping onto a bed of coals measuring 1,400 degrees Fahrenheit. I've also seen people demonstrate unusual levels of physical strength, such as full body catalepsy. This is where a thin, tall 100-pound woman's neck and heels were put on two chairs while she imagined she was a park bench. Then a 150-pound person sat on her. She supported the weight of herself and the other person without a problem.

Using Scripts

Well aware of the power of hypnosis and its ability to cement the mind-body connection, I committed to practicing imagery every day by using self-hypnosis and meditation. As I said earlier in the book, I started by using safe-place meditation with shark imagery. Eventually, however, I felt the white light meditation with ice cubes imagery was the most effective.

Two healing scripts, *emotion-based mind-body* and *reducing the effects of chemotherapy and radiation*, were created by Mark McGahee, a student in my professional hypnotherapy certification courses. When he found out I was sick, he explained that he was working with a cancer clinic in Richmond, Virginia, where he'd had good success with these scripts, so he made a self-hypnosis recording of the first one for me. When I got well, he gave me permission to use them in my books. I created a third script, the *healing bridge,* from an idea I heard about at one of Dr. Siegel's seminars. All the other scripts are completely original.

The safe-place meditation with shark imagery, or the white light meditation with ice cube imagery, should be used specifically for the purpose of tumor reduction. If you are battling cancer, and you feel that another image is more effective, you should feel free to use the safe place nature meditation and healing imagery script, where you may instead create an image that you feel more strongly about. With that script, the key is to imagine something that fits how you view your body's ability to heal itself. We need to give our body the message it needs to supercharge our immune systems and beat this thing we call cancer.

The suggestive therapy script near the end of the chapter is patterned after weight-loss hypnosis using suggestive therapies. By implementing suggestive therapy, I've seen literally hundreds of pounds melt off some of my hypnotherapy clients, so I know suggestive therapy works. It helps people create and maintain the willpower to say *no* to the foods that are unhealthy for us, and say *yes* to the foods that are healthy. The script for staying on the Hoxsey diet was designed from the suggestions the clinic published in the year 2006. These suggestions are the same ones that are discussed in chapter nine, "The Anti-Cancer Diet."

Readers should use the script they feel will benefit them the most. They can read through the scripts ahead of time, and then gauge their emotional response by being intuitive, by going with their gut feeling, you might say. Then readers can make their selection.

The easiest way to obtain the benefits from these holistic imagery practices is to record them in your own voice, or have somebody else record them who you feel has a pleasing voice. Then listen to them at bedtime or first thing in the morning. These down-times are easiest for creating the new habit of listening to recordings. I use morning time when it's a meditation I want to stay conscious of, and I use bed time when it's a suggestive script I want etched deep into my subconscious mind. At bedtime, we will often fall asleep to the recording and the suggestions go into our unconscious mind, where they can be more effective in creating new attitudes and sometimes deeper healing effects.

It is best in the beginning to record these scripts verbatim. Later, well-practiced self-hypnosis enthusiasts may adjust the scripts to suit their individual needs. The following scripts contain all the images that I used effectively for my own recovery.

White Light Meditation

(Start the recording device here.)

Meditation

Separate your hands and feet and put your back into a comfortable position that it can stay in for a long period of time. Close your eyes and allow yourself to imagine a beautiful light emanating from the highest source in the universe...the brightest, highest, most pure light from the most beautiful and peaceful place. You know where this place is and can draw this light to you. You can feel yourself being drawn into the light as well. This light stands for everything that's good in life and beyond, such as unconditional love, peace, serenity, tranquility, and pure relaxation. Experiencing this wonderful light is your birthright, as you are from this place. Now you may safely unite with the vibrations of the light.

Allow this beautiful light to flow through every part of your being. As it flows through you from head to toe, allow it to completely relax every muscle. As it begins to flow through the forehead, feel that area simply relax. It automatically flows through the facial muscles and continues to flow down over the temples and through the front of the neck...at the same time down the back of the head, neck, and shoulders. Allow gravity to pull the shoulders down into their natural position. The mind may wander and drift or it may become drowsy and foggy. Whatever happens is completely natural; you'll still hear the relaxing sound of my voice, which is soon to become a comfortable feeling in the background. My words will soon blend together and flow into your mind naturally, so you'll be free from having to listen to the words because the subconscious will recognize what they mean anyway. Imagine that the mind is like a big whirlpool full of thoughts that have been swirling around, and now you can pull the plug and let those thoughts just drift and drain away.

Allow the white light to continue to flow through the arms and out the hands. The breathing becomes a shade deeper. With each more relaxing breath, feel the body resting with a safe, deeper, more peaceful sense of relaxation. As the white light flows down through the back, all the muscles and tendons wrapped around the vertebrae unwind and the back settles into its natural position automatically. As it flows through the center of your being, notice that the light within you grows brighter and brighter. The part that has come from the light from within your center is now filling you and then emanating from you, as it intensifies. Feel your light surrounding you now with the light from the highest source. The light continues to flow through the waist, knees, ankles, and out through the toes. You and the light are one now...flowing within the same higher vibration.

Awakening Procedures

And now I'm going to count back from five to one and when I reach the number one, you can then normalize.

 Five...You'll remember everything you have experienced.
 Four...Very satisfied with the (changes that have taken place).
 Three...More in touch with the room around you.
 Two...The mind and the body are returning back toward normal.
 When you imagine the number *One*...in your mind's eye within the next minute, you'll become wide awake, refreshed, and feeling good.

(Turn off the recorder here.)

Safe Place Meditation

(Start the recording device here.)

Meditation

Separate your hands and feet and put your back into a comfortable position that it can stay in for a long period of time. Close your eyes and allow yourself to imagine a safe place in nature where you've been before or plan to be in the future; or you may just create it within yourself. Brighten up the color and notice how clear it is and how good it feels to be there. Notice the things that are moving about and how peaceful and wonderful the mood is. Hear the sounds of nature now, as they get a little louder. You may feel the warmth of the light in the sky, and the coolness of a gentle breeze. There may be a familiar scent in the air...a few clouds drifting gently across the sky, a sky that goes on forever, and a bright light that reaches you shining down between the clouds...allowing you to feel warm and relaxed. This light stands for everything that's good in life, such as love, peace, serenity, tranquility, and pure relaxation.

Allow this light to flow through you, relaxing every muscle fiber, cell, and tissue. As it flows through you from head to toe, allow it to completely relax each muscle group. As it begins to flow through the forehead, feel the stress lines simply spread apart. It automatically continues to flow through the eyes as the thread muscles behind the eyes simply unravel and the eyes get heavier. The white light automatically continues to flow down over the temples and through the front of the neck...at the same time down the back of the head, neck, and shoulders. Allow gravity to pull the shoulders down into their natural position. The mind may wander and drift or it may become drowsy and foggy. Whatever happens is completely natural; you'll still hear the relaxing sound of my voice, which is soon to become a comfortable feeling in the background. My words will soon blend together and flow into your mind naturally, so you'll be free from having to listen to the words because the subconscious will recognize what they mean anyway. And the mind simply unwinds like a big spring...letting go. As the sun rises on one side of the earth and sets on the other, each day is similar to the next with common themes. Each day has learning lessons of its own, regardless of the ups and downs, moods, stresses...it has nothing to do with this. This is just pure, simple relaxation. All fears, guilts, and self-blame are released. Problems, pressures, and stresses built up through time are useless and unnecessary.

Allow the white light to continue to flow through the elbows, wrists, and out the fingers. You may notice a tingling sensation in the hands, which further shows you're beginning to relax as the bodily functions are slowing down. The breathing becomes a shade deeper; with each more relaxing breath, feel the body rest more firmly against the pads that you're lying on or sitting against. As the white light flows down through the back, all the muscles and tendons wrapped around the vertebrae unwind, and the back settles into its natural position automatically. The light flows through the waist, knees, ankles, and out through the toes, pushing out all stress, concerns, worries, in the form of tension or tightness, which may have been locked up in the body and are useless to us now. Feel the nerves dimming, like dimming the lights. And with each beat of the heart, which you're naturally more in touch with from becoming relaxed in this way, allow yourself to go deeper into relaxation. Feel all the muscles and tendons droop and hang on the bone structure, loose and limp.

Awakening Procedures

And now I'm going to count back from five to one and when I reach the number one, you can then normalize.

Five...You'll remember everything you have experienced.

Four...Very satisfied with the (changes that have taken place).

Three...More in touch with the room around you.

Two...The mind and the body are returning back toward normal.

When you imagine the number *One*...in your mind's eye within the next minute, you'll become wide awake, refreshed, and feeling good.

(Turn off the recorder here.)

Safe Place Meditation with
Healing Imagery

(Start the recording device here.)

Safe Place Nature Meditation

Separate your hands and feet and put your back into a comfortable position that it can stay in for a long period of time. Close your eyes and allow yourself to imagine a safe place in nature where you've been before or plan to be in the future; or you may just create it within yourself. Brighten up the color and notice how clear it is and how good it feels to be there. Notice the things that are moving about and how peaceful and wonderful the mood is. Hear the sounds of nature now, as they get a little louder. You may feel the warmth of the light in the sky, and the coolness of a gentle breeze. There may be a familiar scent in the air...a few clouds drifting gently across the sky, a sky that goes on forever, and a bright light that reaches you, shining down between the clouds...allowing you to feel warm and relaxed. This light stands for everything that's good in life, such as love, peace, serenity, tranquility, and pure relaxation.

Allow this light to flow through you, relaxing every muscle fiber, cell, and tissue. As it flows through you from head to toe, allow it to completely relax each muscle group. As it begins to flow through the forehead, feel the stress lines simply spread apart. It automatically continues to flow through the eyes as the thread muscles behind the eyes simply unravel and the eyes get heavier. The white light automatically continues to flow down over the temples and through the front of the neck...at the same time down the back of the head, neck, and shoulders. Allow gravity to pull the shoulders down into their natural position. The mind may wander and drift or it may become drowsy and foggy. Whatever happens is completely natural; you'll still hear the relaxing sound of my voice, which is soon to become a comfortable feeling in the background. My words will soon blend together and flow into your mind naturally, so you'll be free from having to listen to the words because the subconscious will recognize what they mean anyway. And the mind simply unwinds like a big spring...letting go. As the sun rises on one side of the earth and sets on the other, each day is similar to the next with common themes. Each day has learning lessons of its own, regardless of the ups and downs, moods, stresses...it has nothing to do with this. This is just pure, simple relaxation. All fears, guilts, and self-blame are released. Problems, pressures, and stresses built up through time are useless and unnecessary.

Allow the white light to continue to flow through the elbows, wrists, and out the fingers. You may notice a tingling sensation in the hands, which further shows you're beginning to relax as the bodily functions are slowing down. The breathing becomes a shade deeper; with each more relaxing breath, feel the body rest more firmly against the pads that you're lying on or sitting against. As the white light flows down through the back, all the muscles and tendons wrapped around the vertebrae unwind, and the back settles into its natural position automatically. The light flows through the waist, knees, ankles, and out through the toes, pushing out all stress, concerns, worries, in the form of tension or tightness, which may have been locked up in the body and are useless to us now. Feel the nerves dimming, like dimming the lights. And with each beat of the heart, which you're naturally more in touch with from becoming relaxed in this way, allow yourself to go deeper into relaxation. Feel all the muscles and tendons droop and hang on the bone structure, loose and limp.

Therapy Script

As you relax further and further you'll begin to mentally shift your body with your imagination. You can create a metaphor now in your mind's eye that represents increased healing. You will be creative now and choose whatever comes to mind and focus on this image that represents increased healing for you. (Pause.)

Now brighten up the colors in the mind's eye and notice how much more clear the image appears... (Pause.)

Notice all the details you hear in the image and then turn up the volume so that you may experience these with more detail....(Pause.)

Now, imagine the feelings of increased healing. Notice the inward and outward feelings and sensations...(Pause.)

Now take some deep breaths. Inhale and hold a little while... and then exhale... Inhale again with a deep breath... and then exhale again. Repeat this several times until the sensation of stretching the chest and neck muscles begins to disappear, and these areas become naturally relaxed. Inhale... Exhale... Over and over, until deep breathing feels relaxing, refreshing, and very natural. As the chest cavity expands, you will notice that inhaling a large amount of air takes less and less effort. Notice how your posture improves from exercising your lungs. You sit straighter, you stand straighter. As you breathe deeper each day, your heart and lungs are healthier, working with less effort to send oxygen to every cell and tissue in the body. More oxygen going to the part of the body in need of rebuilding, restoring, and healing... remembering to breathe regularly and deeply, feeling more energetic, as you have more oxygen to your muscles, cells, and tissues with increased circulation, rapidly repairing.

This unique image is changing the body; it's training the body to respond to your thoughts now. You are overcoming any obstacles to healing with this image. You may notice that you think of this image often while you are in your room, your office, at your neighbor's home, your local shopping areas. You think of this image often because you want to have the healing occur more often. Your body wants you to do it. You give it that satisfaction, that natural satisfaction to your body now, because you deserve to improve it to the fullest level of health. Your body relaxes more deeply afterward. You feel more relaxed, less stressed, you forgot all about stress. You breathe out all your stress.

Breathing deeply...relaxing. Breathing deeply and relaxing. You have more energy available and you like yourself more this way. You are more aware of your body's needs and you are satisfying it more often, even if it's just minutes at a time.... You are allowing it to move more, breathe more, and heal more.

The body is responding, feeling better. You feel more balanced in mind, body, and spirit. You're taking care of your physical vehicle now and you have more value in your life. You're simply feeling good. You like your imagery adjustment technique. You like it, as changes seem to happen. You feel great.

Awakening Procedures

And now I'm going to count back from five to one and when I reach the number one, you can then normalize.

Five...You'll remember everything you have experienced.

Four...Very satisfied with the (changes that have taken place).

Three...More in touch with the room around you.

Two...The mind and the body are returning back toward normal.

When you imagine the number *One*...in your mind's eye within the next minute, you'll become wide awake, refreshed, and feeling good.

(Turn off the recorder here.)

Safe Place Meditation with Healing Bridge Imagery

(Start the recording device here.)

Safe Place Nature Meditation

Separate your hands and feet and put your back into a comfortable position that it can stay in for a long period of time. Close your eyes and allow yourself to imagine that you're approaching a beautiful beach on a bright sunny day, where the ocean seems like it goes on forever. Brighten up the color and notice how clear it is when you add all the details—and how good it feels to be there. Feel the sand being the perfect temperature as it form-fits your feet. You may softly lie down in the sand or walk on the surf and listen to the waves as you watch them roll in toward you. There's a sailboat in the distance whose mast is teeter-tottering, back and forth. You hear the birds calling to one another, and the scent of the ocean mist is familiar in some way. The breeze is slightly cool, but the sun is nicely warm.

A few clouds are drifting gently across the sky, a sky that goes on forever and the bright sunlight that reaches you shining down between the clouds allows you to feel warm and relaxed. This light stands for everything that's good in life, such as love, peace, serenity, tranquility, and pure relaxation.

Allow this light to flow through you, relaxing every muscle fiber, cell, and tissue. As it flows from head to toe, allow it to completely relax each muscle group. As it begins to flow through the forehead, feel the stress lines simply spread apart. It automatically continues to flow through the eyes as the thread muscles behind the eyes simply unravel and the eyes get heavier. The white light automatically continues to flow down over the temples and through the front of the neck...at the same time down the back of the head, neck, and shoulders. Allow gravity to pull the shoulders down into their natural position. The mind may wander and drift, or it may become drowsy and foggy. Whatever happens is completely natural; you'll still hear the relaxing sound of my voice which is soon to become a comfortable feeling in the background. My words will soon blend together and flow into your mind naturally, so you'll be free from having to listen to the words because the subconscious will recognize what they mean anyway. And the mind simply unwinds like a big spring...letting go. As the sun rises on one side of the earth and sets on the other, each day is similar to the next with common themes. Each day has learning lessons of its own, regardless of the ups and downs, moods, stresses...it has nothing to do with this. This is just pure, simple relaxation. All fears, guilts, and self-blame are released. Problems, pressures, and stresses built up through time are useless and unnecessary.

Allow the white light to continue to flow through the elbows, wrists, and out the fingers. You may notice a tingling sensation in the hands, which further shows you're beginning to relax as the bodily functions are slowing down. The breathing becomes a shade deeper; with each more relaxing breath, feel the body rest more firmly against the pads that you're lying on or sitting against. As the white light flows down through the back, all the muscles and tendons wrapped around the vertebrae unwind, and the back settles into its natural position automatically. The light flows through the waist, knees, ankles, and out through the toes, pushing out all stress, concerns, worries, in the form of tension or tightness, which may have been locked up in the body and are useless to us now. Feel the nerves dimming, like dimming the lights. And with each beat of the heart, which you're naturally more in touch with from becoming relaxed in this way, allow yourself to go deeper into relaxation. Feel all the muscles and tendons droop and hang on the bone structure, loose and limp.

Therapy Script

In a moment, I want you to imagine two worlds, the one that you are in right now, and one that represents healing. You will need to exercise your imagination to be able to create these worlds within yourself as we do this meditation. The first world is the one that you have now. I want you to close your eyes and allow your mind to become light so that it rises up above your body now. Notice that your mind can float above the room and you can imagine everything down below through your mind's eye. As you float higher, you can float above the building, while still being able to see yourself and your room getting smaller and smaller down below. And as you float higher, into the clouds of the sky, you can locate anything and anyone on it from up there, higher, lighter, and floating. Now as you float above this earth, you are going to notice a translucent planet earth next to this one. In that world, everything is perfect and you are healed, and everything around you is just the way you want it.

There is a bridge that connects the two worlds that you can see. Float over the bridge now... You are going to land on the bridge on this side of the present earth for now. As you look at the bridge before you, notice what it is made of. Step onto the bridge and you will notice how it feels; you will hear voices or other sounds behind you, but there are even more interesting ones before you in the world of health and balance. It's very interesting over there, because you don't know for sure just how it will be there. It's more different over there than we would normally think it to be sometimes. So start walking across the bridge and you will notice a light beam at the end of the bridge, which you must walk through. When you walk through it, you will notice a feeling in the body and all the problems in the body simply disappear. The light has eliminated its problems. As you come out through the other side, you have a perfectly healthy body...a perfectly healthy body. Some things on this planet are very similar as before, but some have changed here in many ways; first you will walk down the street to your house... notice as you walk down the street what the neighborhood looks like.

You come across your house now. Notice how it looks on the outside. It's just perfect for you. It's perfect on the inside as well; everything is in harmony and balance as you walk up to the front door and step inside. You look around and you can tell that there is something synchronistic to where everything is just right. It feels great to be in this home. Everything is perfect there. Now you can sit down and relax in a favorite chair and/or go to a favorite room. There, you will notice that you feel a complete peace. You stay there for a little while because it feels like you have come home... you feel a tranquility and peace... Then you realize that it's time to go into another room of the house, which will transport you into a purpose; it may be a purpose you are familiar with, then again it may be a purpose that is completely different from the one you are familiar with. This purpose supports your home and loved ones, but it seems easy and perfect for you. It is something you simply enjoy doing. You really enjoy doing it…so as you step into that room you are really enjoying this thing that you do. You really like it. It's interesting, challenging, and you know that people simply enjoy it. On the planet of balance and healing, everybody you talk to respects and enjoys what you do, because it offers you and others value. You really like it there...

And now you are going to float above that world, into the sky above the home and purpose down below; higher and lighter as you float above that world you can see anything or anyone and everything and everyone is just fine there, as a very bright light from above continually shines upon everything. You will float back into the current world, taking the body, feelings, thoughts, and realizations back into the present moment. You are coming back with all of it and you will be spending a moment in each day understanding what it will take to bridge the two worlds. These ideas will pop into your mind and you will simply know what they are from a creative resource. When you come back into the present moment, you have a beautiful sense of well being. When you open your eyes within the next minute, you will feel wonderful.

Awakening Procedures

And now I'm going to count back from five to one and when I reach the number one, you can then normalize.

> *Five*...You'll remember everything you have experienced.
> *Four*...Very satisfied with the (changes that have taken place).
> *Three*...More in touch with the room around you.
> *Two*...The mind and the body are returning back toward normal.

When you imagine the number *One*...in your mind's eye within the next minute, you'll become wide awake, refreshed, and feeling good.

Safe Place Meditation with
Emotion-Based Mind-Body Healing Script

(Start the recording device here.)

Safe Place Nature Meditation

Separate your hands and feet and put your back into a comfortable position that it can stay in for a long period of time. Close your eyes and allow yourself to imagine a safe place in nature where you've been before or plan to be in the future; or you may just create it within yourself. Brighten up the color and notice how clear it is and how good it feels to be there. Notice the things that are moving about and how peaceful and wonderful the mood is. Hear the sounds of nature now, as they get a little louder. You may feel the warmth of the light in the sky, and the coolness of a gentle breeze. There may be a familiar scent in the air...a few clouds drifting gently across the sky, a sky that goes on forever, and a bright light that reaches you shining down between the clouds...allowing you to feel warm and relaxed. This light stands for everything that's good in life, such as love, peace, serenity, tranquility, and pure relaxation.

Allow this light to flow through you, relaxing every muscle fiber, cell, and tissue. As it flows through you from head to toe, allow it to completely relax each muscle group. As it begins to flow through the forehead, feel the stress lines simply spread apart. It automatically continues to flow through the eyes as the thread muscles behind the eyes simply unravel and the eyes get heavier. The white light automatically continues to flow down over the temples and through the front of the neck...at the same time down the back of the head, neck, and shoulders. Allow gravity to pull the shoulders down into their natural position. The mind may wander and drift, or it may become drowsy and foggy.

Whatever happens is completely natural; you'll still hear the relaxing sound of my voice, which is soon to become a comfortable feeling in the background. My words will soon blend together and flow into your mind naturally, so you'll be free from having to listen to the words because the subconscious will recognize what they mean anyway. And the mind simply unwinds like a big spring...letting go. As the sun rises on one side of the earth and sets on the other, each day is similar to the next with common themes. Each day has learning lessons of its own, regardless of the ups and downs, moods, stresses...it has nothing to do with this. This is just pure, simple relaxation. All fears, guilts and self-blame are released. Problems, pressures, and stresses built up through time are useless and unnecessary.

Allow the white light to continue to flow through the elbows, wrists, and out the fingers. You may notice a tingling sensation in the hands, which further shows you're beginning to relax as the bodily functions are slowing down. The breathing becomes a shade deeper; with each more relaxing breath, feel the body rest more firmly against the pads that you're lying on or sitting against. As the white light flows down through the back, all the muscles and tendons wrapped around the vertebrae unwind, and the back settles into its natural position automatically. The light flows through the waist, knees, ankles, and out through the toes, pushing out all stress, concerns, worries, in the form of tension or tightness, which may have been locked up in the body and are useless to us now. Feel the nerves dimming, like dimming the lights. And with each beat of the heart, which you're naturally more in touch with from becoming relaxed in this way, allow yourself to go deeper into relaxation. Feel all the muscles and tendons droop and hang on the bone structure, loose and limp.

Therapy Script

Now one of the things you will train your subconscious mind to do in the days ahead is how to release the stress, anxiety, and fear you have associated with the cancer and to allow the various therapies you are undergoing to be successful. By doing this, you will greatly enhance their effectiveness. You will become relaxed and in balance with the world around you and will let go of all anger and fear associated with your condition. As you become more and more relaxed you will have the strength and confidence to reach the goal you have set for yourself to be cancer-free. Your body will work to kill and eliminate any cancer cells by allowing the therapies to be very effective. As you follow the therapeutic protocols, all healthy cells will be protected by a special coating, while all cancer cells anywhere in your body will be hypersensitive and will be killed off. Not a single cancer cell will survive. Your immune system is greatly enhanced and will help your body to eliminate and kill all cancer cells still present, if any, today and in the future, forever. Your love and acceptance of your own strength will allow you to mobilize your natural healing process to recover quickly and completely from all therapy.

Now you know that this is a time for recovery and healing. The more you allow your mind and body to relax, the more rapidly and completely the recovery and healing will be. You can now allow yourself to permit your body to nurture itself and adjust and thus come into balance to enhance your body's natural healing process. Your desire to recover, heal, and return to a normal life enables you to gain the inner strength and energy within you to meet your goals. You have much to give and much to accomplish in your life. As you participate in your therapies, your ability to relax will enhance the healing process and receptivity to the words of your care-givers and loved ones. They will be speaking to you and their words will be easily understood by you to enhance your healing process and your body's acceptance of the treatments you are undergoing.

Now as you listen to the relaxing sound of my voice, realize that you have the ability to release all cares, fears, worries, or other negative thinking. Right now all your cares, fears, worries, and negative thinking will just drift away. Now I want you to imagine that you are near a large body of water. You may hear the water as it splashes against the shore. You may feel the coolness of a soft breeze off the water as it blows against your skin. You notice a boat nearby. Now I want you to put your thoughts and feelings of self-doubt, being scared, your excessive worry about the cancer, feelings of helplessness, being overwhelmed, not believing in yourself and feelings of frustration on that boat; and allow it to drift off into the distance, off farther and farther away; so far and so distant that you can barely notice it. Allow it to be just a dot on the horizon. However, you do not let the boat totally disappear because you may choose to retain these feelings and retrieve them if you need them. You can always bring the BOAT back. But right now you have no need for these feelings. As you let them go, you gain a sense of peace and calm flowing within your body.

You can now allow yourself the pleasure of watching those feelings drift further and further away into the horizon. Notice that you do not allow them to entirely disappear, so that if you want those feelings back, they will be there. But right now, you have no need for those feelings, so allow them to go off towards the horizon.

Now you are achieving a peaceful, calm attitude with no anger or fear of the future. You move instead to the acceptance and continuation of life. You may want to make changes in your life in the weeks or months ahead and this is wonderful, but for today you are focused only on being healed and happy and relaxed, fully accepting of the love of God, your family and others who love you deeply.

Each day as you listen to this recording, you reaccept the suggestions that are included in this exercise. They are becoming more and more a part of you. Even though you may not consciously remember all of them, they will remain within your subconscious mind and will continue to be more effective than ever before. You will permit yourself to accept the suggestions in this exercise because you want to be cancer-free. And because you want to feel stronger, more in control, relaxed, healthier, and more vigorous. Your desire to be cancer-free, to be strong, and to take control of your life is so great that it easily allows you to accept the suggestions.

Each time you do this exercise, you will feel more alert, refreshed and relaxed, calm, bright, sharp, physically better, emotionally better, mentally better, and spiritually better than you have felt in a long time. These feelings of well-being will remain with you longer and longer with each time you listen to this recording. You truly feel more positive about yourself and the world in which you live. You look at things with a greater amount of faith that everything has a reason, and it will all work out in the end and you will be cancer-free. You feel a higher force, a spiritual force, at work in your life, which facilitates and supports the faith you have. You make a difference in the areas you can, and release the rest. You feel more relaxed in each and every way. You feel wonderful now, self-empowered, more in control. Everything is working out more naturally during the course of your life now and you are able to see yourself cancer-free, participating in all the activities you enjoy. You're living more peacefully and naturally and are more relaxed than ever before. Now take a moment to feel and visualize yourself happy, content, at peace with life with a perfect cancer-free body.

Awakening Procedures

And now I'm going to count back from five to one and when I reach the number one, you can then normalize.

    Five...You'll remember everything you have experienced.

    Four...Very satisfied with the (changes that have taken place).

    Three...More in touch with the room around you.

    Two...The mind and the body are returning back toward normal.

    When you imagine the number *One*...in your mind's eye within the next minute, you'll become wide awake, refreshed, and feeling good.

(Turn off the recorder here.)

Safe Place Meditation and
Script for Reducing the Effects of
Chemotherapy and Radiation

(Start the recording device here.)

Safe Place Nature Meditation

Separate your hands and feet and put your back into a comfortable position that it can stay in for a long period of time. Close your eyes and allow yourself to imagine a safe place in nature where you've been before or plan to be in the future; or you may just create it within yourself. Brighten up the color and notice how clear it is and how good it feels to be there. Notice the things that are moving about and how peaceful and wonderful the mood is. Hear the sounds of nature now, as they get a little louder. You may feel the warmth of the light in the sky, and the coolness of a gentle breeze. There may be a familiar scent in the air...a few clouds drifting gently across the sky, a sky that goes on forever, and a bright light that reaches you shining down between the clouds...allowing you to feel warm and relaxed. This light stands for everything that's good in life, such as love, peace, serenity, tranquility, and pure relaxation.

Allow this light to flow through you, relaxing every muscle fiber, cell, and tissue. As it flows through you from head to toe, allow it to completely relax each muscle group. As it begins to flow through the forehead, feel the stress lines simply spread apart. It automatically continues to flow through the eyes as the thread muscles behind the eyes simply unravel and the eyes get heavier. The white light automatically continues to flow down over the temples and through the front of the neck...at the same time down the back of the head, neck, and shoulders. Allow gravity to pull the shoulders down into their natural position. The mind may wander and drift, or it may become drowsy and foggy. Whatever happens is completely natural; you'll still hear the relaxing sound of my voice, which is soon to become a comfortable feeling in the background. My words will soon blend together and flow into your mind naturally, so you'll be free from having to listen to the words because the subconscious will recognize what they mean anyway. And the mind simply unwinds like a big spring...letting go. As the sun rises on one side of the earth and sets on the other, each day is similar to the next with common themes. Each day has learning lessons of its own, regardless of the ups and downs, moods, stresses...it has nothing to do with this. This is just pure, simple relaxation. All fears, guilts, and self-blame are released. Problems, pressures, and stresses built up through time are useless and unnecessary.

Allow the white light to continue to flow through the elbows, wrists, and out the fingers. You may notice a tingling sensation in the hands, which further shows you're beginning to relax as the bodily functions are slowing down. The breathing becomes a shade deeper; with each more relaxing breath, feel the body rest more firmly against the pads that you're lying on or sitting against. As the white light flows down through the back, all the muscles and tendons wrapped around the vertebrae unwind, and the back settles into its natural position automatically. The light flows through the waist, knees, ankles, and out through the toes, pushing out all stress, concerns, worries, in the form of tension or tightness, which may have been locked up in the body and are useless to us now. Feel the nerves dimming, like dimming the lights. And with each beat of the heart, which you're naturally more in touch with from becoming relaxed in this way, allow yourself to go deeper into relaxation. Feel all the muscles and tendons droop and hang on the bone structure, loose and limp.

Therapy Script

Now one of the things you will train your subconscious mind to do in the days ahead is how to release the stress, anxiety, and fear you have associated with the cancer and to allow the radiation therapy to be successful. By doing this, you will enhance the effectiveness of the radiation therapy which you are undergoing. You will become relaxed and in balanced with the world around you and will let go of all anger and fear associated with your condition. As you are more and more relaxed you will have the strength and confidence to reach the goal you have set for yourself to be cancer-free. Your body will work to kill and eliminate any cancer cells by allowing the radiation therapy to be very effective. As the radiation is absorbed into your body, all healthy cells will be protected by a special coating, while all cancer cells anywhere in your body will be hypersensitive to the radiation and will be killed off. Not a single cancer cell will survive. Your immune system is greatly enhanced and will help your body to eliminate and kill all cancer cells still present, if any, today and in the future, forever. Your love and acceptance of your own strength will allow you to mobilize your natural healing process to recover quickly from all therapy.

Now you know that the time at home and in the hospital is for recovery and healing. The more you allow your mind and body to relax, the more rapidly the complete recovery and healing will be. You can now allow yourself to permit your body to nurture itself and adjust and thus come into balance to enhance your body's natural healing process. Your desire to recover, heal, and return to an active life enables you to gain the inner strength and energy within you to meet your goals. As you have your radiation treatment, your relaxation will enhance the healing process and receptivity to the words of your doctor and the radiation technicians. They will be speaking to you and their words will be easily understood by you to enhance your healing process and your body's acceptance of the radiation.

Now as you listen to the relaxing sound of my voice, realize that you have released all cares, fears, worries, or other negative thinking. Right now all your cares, fears, worries, and negative thinking will just drift away. Now I want you to imagine that you are near a large body of water. You notice a BOAT nearby. Now I want you to put your thoughts and feelings of self-doubt, being scared, your excessive worry about the cancer, feelings of helplessness, being overwhelmed, not believing in yourself, and feelings of frustration on that boat and allow it to drift off into the distance, off further and further away; so far and so distant that you barely notice it. Allow it to be just a dot on the horizon. However, you do not let the boat totally disappear because you may choose to retain these feelings and retrieve them if you need them. But right now you have no need for them. As you let them go, you gain a sense of peace and calm flowing within your body.

You can now allow yourself the pleasure of watching those feelings drift further and further away into the horizon. Notice that you do not allow them to entirely disappear, so that if you want those feelings, they will be there. But right now, you have no need for those feelings, so allow them to go off towards the horizon. These feeling will be there if you want them back or want to be in touch with them.

Now as you enter the place in the hospital where they will do the radiation therapy and are sitting or lying down waiting for the therapy to begin, you can permit your body to become very relaxed by simply closing your eyes and taking a very deep breath, which will cause you to immediately become very relaxed and give you a peace of mind that the therapy will be very effective. It is possible that there may be other noises in the area. These noises will not disturb you; instead they will simply act as a signal to deepen your relaxation and receptivity to the radiation therapy. You know that your body will work to kill and eliminate any cancer cells by allowing the radiation therapy to be very effective. As the radiation is absorbed into your body, all healthy cells will be protected by a special coating, while all cancer cells anywhere in your body will be hypersensitive to the radiation and will be killed off. Not a single cancer cell will survive. Your immune system is greatly enhanced and will help your body to eliminate and kill all cancer cells still present, if any, today and in the future, forever. Your love and acceptance of your own strength will allow you to mobilize your natural healing process to recover quickly. After the radiation therapy is complete, you will open your eyes and be wide awake, feeling relaxed and happy with an optimistic attitude because you know that the therapy was so successful. Time will pass quickly and pleasantly during your therapy. As each day goes by and you listen to this recording, your positive attitude will continue to enhance the healing process and the body's acceptance of the radiation.

Now you are achieving a peaceful, calm attitude, with no anger or fear of the future. You move instead to acceptance and the continuation of life. You may want to make changes in your life in the weeks or months ahead and this is wonderful, but for today you are only focused on being healed and happy and relaxed, fully accepting of the love of God, your family and others who say they love you deeply.

Each day as you listen to this recording, you reaccept the suggestions that are contained on the recording. They become more and more a part of you. Even though you may not consciously remember them, they will remain there in your subconscious mind and they will work better and more effectively than ever before. You will permit yourself to accept the suggestions in this exercise because you want to be cancer-free. You will allow yourself to accept the suggestions because you want to feel stronger, more in control, relaxed, healthier, and more vigorous. Your desire to be cancer-free, to be strong, and to take control of your life is so great that it easily allows you to accept the suggestions contained on this recording.

As you listen to this recording daily, you will feel more alert, refreshed, and relaxed, calm and refreshed, bright, sharp, physically better, emotionally better, mentally better and spiritually better than you have felt in a long time. These feelings of well-being will remain with you longer and longer with each time you listen to this recording. You truly feel more positive about yourself and the world in which you live. You look at things with a greater amount of faith that everything has a reason, and it will all work out in the end. You feel a higher force at work in your life, spiritually, which also facilitates the amount of faith you have. You make a difference in the areas you can, and release the rest. You feel more relaxed in each and every way. You feel wonderful now, self-empowered, more in control. Everything appears to work out more naturally during the course of life now. You're living more peacefully and naturally and are more relaxed than ever before.

Now take a moment and visualize, hear and feel yourself with a perfect cancer-free body.

Awakening Procedures

And now I'm going to count back from five to one and when I reach the number one, you can then normalize.

> *Five*...You'll remember everything you have experienced.
> *Four*...Very satisfied with the (changes that have taken place).
> *Three*...More in touch with the room around you.
> *Two*...The mind and the body are returning back toward normal.
> When you imagine the number *One*...in your mind's eye within the next

minute, you'll become wide awake, refreshed, and feeling good.

(Turn off the recorder here.)

Ocean Meditation for
Tumor Reduction Using Shark Imagery

Ocean Meditation

Separate your hands and feet and put your back into a comfortable position that it can stay in for a long period of time. Close your eyes and allow yourself to imagine that you're approaching a beautiful beach on a bright sunny day, where the ocean seems like it goes on forever. Brighten up the color and notice how clear it is when you add all the details—and how good it feels to be there. Feel the sand being the perfect temperature as it form-fits your feet. You may softly lie down in the sand or walk on the surf and listen to the waves as you watch them roll in toward you. There's a sailboat in the distance whose mast is teeter-tottering, back and forth. You hear the birds calling to one another, and the scent of the ocean mist is familiar in some way. The breeze is slightly cool, but the sun is nicely warm.

A few clouds are drifting gently across the sky, a sky that goes on forever and the bright sunlight that reaches you shining down between the clouds allows you to feel warm and relaxed. This light stands for everything that's good in life, such as love, peace, serenity, tranquility, and pure relaxation.

Allow this light to flow through you, relaxing every muscle fiber, cell, and tissue. As it flows from head to toe, allow it to completely relax each muscle group. As it begins to flow through the forehead, feel the stress lines simply spread apart. It automatically continues to flow through the eyes as the thread muscles behind the eyes simply unravel and the eyes get heavier. The white light automatically continues to flow down over the temples and through the front of the neck...at the same time down the back of the head, neck, and shoulders. Allow gravity to pull the shoulders down into their natural position. The mind may wander and drift, or it may become drowsy and foggy. Whatever happens is completely natural; you'll still hear the relaxing sound of my voice which is soon to become a comfortable feeling in the background. My words will soon blend together and flow into your mind naturally, so you'll be free from having to listen to the words because the subconscious will recognize what they mean anyway. And the mind simply unwinds like a big spring...letting go. As the sun rises on one side of the earth and sets on the other, each day is similar to the next with common themes. Each day has learning lessons of its own, regardless of the ups and downs, moods, stresses...it has nothing to do with this. This is just pure, simple relaxation. All fears, guilts, and self-blame are released. Problems, pressures, and stresses built up through time are useless and unnecessary.

Allow the white light to continue to flow through the elbows, wrists, and out the fingers. You may notice a tingling sensation in the hands, which further shows you're beginning to relax as the bodily functions are slowing down. The breathing becomes a shade deeper; with each more relaxing breath, feel the body rest more firmly against the pads that you're lying on or sitting against. As the white light flows down through the back, all the muscles and tendons wrapped around the vertebrae unwind, and the back settles into its natural position automatically. The light flows through the waist, knees, ankles, and out through the toes, pushing out all stress, concerns, worries, in the form of tension or tightness, which may have been locked up in the body and are useless to us now. Feel the nerves dimming, like dimming the lights. And with each beat of the heart, which you're naturally more in touch with from becoming relaxed in this way, allow yourself to go deeper into relaxation. Feel all the muscles and tendons droop and hang on the bone structure, loose and limp.

Therapy Script

Now I want you to imagine there are sharks swimming in your bloodstream. These sharks are your friends. Notice that they represent your healing color. As they swim, they are searching for cancer cells, because this is what they eat. They feed on tumors and cancer cells. They've located where yours are in your body now, and they are starting to feed. You may feel a tingling sensation as they eat and chew…eating up the cancer cells in your body. They gnaw on all your tumors, several sharks at once, eating them up, gnawing, chewing, and continuing to devour them, Devouring them until they are all gone (pause). Now take the next few minutes to let this happen within your body…(long pause).

Awakening Procedures

And now I'm going to count back from five to one and when I reach the number one, you can then normalize.

> *Five*…You'll remember everything you have experienced.
> *Four*…Very satisfied with the (changes that have taken place).
> *Three*…More in touch with the room around you.
> *Two*…The mind and the body are returning back toward normal.
> When you imagine the number *One*…in your mind's eye within the next

minute, you'll become wide awake, refreshed, and feeling good.

(Turn off the recorder here.)

White Light Meditation with
Melting Ice Cube Imagery for Tumor Reduction

(Start the recording device here.)

White Light Meditation

Separate your hands and feet and put your back into a comfortable position that it can stay in for a long period of time. Close your eyes and allow yourself to imagine a beautiful light emanating from the highest source in the universe...the brightest, highest, most pure light from the most beautiful and peaceful place. You know where this place is and can draw this light to you. You can feel yourself being drawn into the light as well. This light stands for everything that's good in life and beyond, such as unconditional love, peace, serenity, tranquility, and pure relaxation. Experiencing this wonderful light is your birthright, as you are from this place. Now you may safely unite with the vibrations of the light.

Allow this beautiful light to flow through every part of your being. As it flows through you from head to toe, allow it to completely relax every muscle. As it begins to flow through the forehead, feel that area simply relax. It automatically flows through the facial muscles and continues to flow down over the temples and through the front of the neck...at the same time down the back of the head, neck, and shoulders. Allow gravity to pull the shoulders down into their natural position. The mind may wander and drift, or it may become drowsy and foggy. Whatever happens is completely natural; you'll still hear the relaxing sound of my voice which is soon to become a comfortable feeling in the background. My words will soon blend together and flow into your mind naturally, so you'll be free from having to listen to the words because the subconscious will recognize what they mean anyway. Imagine that the mind is like a big whirlpool full of thoughts that have been swirling around, and now you can pull the plug and let those thoughts just drift and drain away.

Allow the white light to continue to flow through the arms and out the hands. The breathing becomes a shade deeper. With each more relaxing breath, feel the body resting with a safe, deeper, more peaceful sense of relaxation. As the white light flows down through the back, all the muscles and tendons wrapped around the vertebrae unwind and the back settles into its natural position automatically. As it flows through the center of your being, notice that the light within you grows brighter and brighter. The part that has come from the light from within your center is now filling you and then emanating from you, as it intensifies. Feel your light surrounding you now with the light from the highest source. The light continues to flow through the waist, knees, ankles, and out through the toes. You and the light are one now...flowing within the same higher vibration.

Therapy Script

Now I want you to imagine that your tumors are like ice cubes. The spiritual light surrounding you is very healing and life-giving. It's also very warm. Now imagine that the light is penetrating the ice cubes, and as it does so, it begins to melt the outside of the ice cubes. The hot white light is now melting the ice cubes further as it shrinks them down. The outer layers of the tumors just drip away, and they get smaller, and smaller. Feel the ice cubes melting from the white light penetrating them. This higher loving light continues to melt the ice cubes down further and further as they continue to shrink (pause). Notice how this continues to happen as you just bask in the light (long pause).

Awakening Procedures

And now I'm going to count back from five to one and when I reach the number one, you can then normalize.

Five...You'll remember everything you have experienced.

Four...Very satisfied with the (changes that have taken place).

Three...More in touch with the room around you.

Two...The mind and the body are returning back toward normal.

When you imagine the number *One*...in your mind's eye within the next minute, you'll become wide awake, refreshed, and feeling good.

(Turn off the recorder here.)

White Light Meditation for Obtaining Spiritual Guidance

(Start the recording device here.)

White Light Meditation

Separate your hands and feet and put your back into a comfortable position that it can stay in for a long period of time. Close your eyes and allow yourself to imagine a beautiful light emanating from the highest source in the universe...the brightest, highest, most pure light from the most beautiful and peaceful place. You know where this place is and can draw this light to you. You can feel yourself being drawn into the light as well. This light stands for everything that's good in life and beyond, such as unconditional love, peace, serenity, tranquility, and pure relaxation. Experiencing this wonderful light is your birthright, as you are from this place. Now you may safely unite with the vibrations of the light.

Allow this beautiful light to flow through every part of your being. As it flows through you from head to toe, allow it to completely relax every muscle.

As it begins to flow through the forehead, feel that area simply relax. It automatically flows through the facial muscles and continues to flow down over the temples and through the front of the neck...at the same time down the back of the head, neck, and shoulders. Allow gravity to pull the shoulders down into their natural position. The mind may wander and drift, or it may become drowsy and foggy. Whatever happens is completely natural; you'll still hear the relaxing sound of my voice which is soon to become a comfortable feeling in the background. My words will soon blend together and flow into your mind naturally, so you'll be free from having to listen to the words because the subconscious will recognize what they mean anyway. Imagine that the mind is like a big whirlpool full of thoughts that have been swirling around, and now you can pull the plug and let those thoughts just drift and drain away.

Allow the white light to continue to flow through the arms and out the hands. The breathing becomes a shade deeper. With each more relaxing breath, feel the body resting with a safe, deeper, more peaceful sense of relaxation. As the white light flows down through the back, all the muscles and tendons wrapped around the vertebrae unwind and the back settles into its natural position automatically. As it flows through the center of your being, notice that the light within you grows brighter and brighter. The part that has come from the light from within your center is now filling you and then emanating from you, as it intensifies. Feel your light surrounding you now with the light from the highest source. The light continues to flow through the waist, knees, ankles, and out through the toes. You and the light are one now...flowing within the same higher vibration.

Meditative Script

Now imagine that your mind can simply float up toward the bright light...floating higher and higher. And as you continue to allow your mind to travel up into the light, you may notice a number come to your mind. The number you hear, see, or feel is the number of spirit guides or angels that are there to assist you. Notice any other details about them...(pause). Now, completely blank your mind so that you may hear their message for you at this time. Just blank you mind now, and trust what comes...(long pause).

Awakening Procedures

And now I'm going to count back from five to one and when I reach the number one, you can then normalize.

Five...You'll remember everything you have experienced.

Four...Very satisfied with the (changes that have taken place).

Three...More in touch with the room around you.

Two...The mind and the body are returning back toward normal.

When you imagine the number *One*...in your mind's eye within the next minute, you'll become wide awake, refreshed, and feeling good.

(Turn off the recorder here.)

Hypnotic Suggestive Therapy for
Staying Committed to the Hoxsey Diet

(Start the recording device here.)

Safe Place Nature Meditation

Separate your hands and feet and put your back into a comfortable position that it can stay in for a long period of time. Close your eyes and allow yourself to imagine a safe place in nature where you've been before or plan to be in the future; or you may just create it within yourself. Brighten up the color and notice how clear it is and how good it feels to be there. Notice the things that are moving about and how peaceful and wonderful the mood is. Hear the sounds of nature now, as they get a little louder. You may feel the warmth of the light in the sky, and the coolness of a gentle breeze. There may be a familiar scent in the air...a few clouds drifting gently across the sky, a sky that goes on forever, and a bright light that reaches you shining down between the clouds...allowing you to feel warm and relaxed. This light stands for everything that's good in life, such as love, peace, serenity, tranquility, and pure relaxation.

Allow this light to flow through you, relaxing every muscle fiber, cell, and tissue. As it flows through you from head to toe, allow it to completely relax each muscle group. As it begins to flow through the forehead, feel the stress lines simply spread apart. It automatically continues to flow through the eyes as the thread muscles behind the eyes simply unravel and the eyes get heavier. The white light automatically continues to flow down over the temples and through the front of the neck...at the same time down the back of the head, neck, and shoulders. Allow gravity to pull the shoulders down into their natural position. The mind may wander and drift, or it may become drowsy and foggy. Whatever happens is completely natural; you'll still hear the relaxing sound of my voice, which is soon to become a comfortable feeling in the background. My words will soon blend together and flow into your mind naturally, so you'll be free from having to listen to the words because the subconscious will recognize what they mean anyway. And the mind simply unwinds like a big spring...letting go. As the sun rises on one side of the earth and sets on the other, each day is similar to the next with common themes. Each day has learning lessons of its own, regardless of the ups and downs, moods, stresses...it has nothing to do with this. This is just pure, simple relaxation. All fears, guilts, and self-blame are released. Problems, pressures, and stresses built up through time are useless and unnecessary.

Allow the white light to continue to flow through the elbows, wrists, and out the fingers. You may notice a tingling sensation in the hands, which further shows you're beginning to relax as the bodily functions are slowing down. The breathing becomes a shade deeper; with each more relaxing breath, feel the body rest more firmly against the pads that you're lying on or sitting against. As the white light flows down through the back, all the muscles and tendons wrapped around the vertebrae unwind, and the back settles into its natural position automatically. The light flows through the waist, knees, ankles, and out through the toes, pushing out all stress, concerns, worries, in the form of tension or tightness, which may have been locked up in the body and are useless to us now. Feel the nerves dimming, like dimming the lights. And with each beat of the heart, which you're naturally more in touch with from becoming relaxed in this way, allow yourself to go deeper into relaxation. Feel all the muscles and tendons droop and hang on the bone structure, loose and limp.

Therapy Script

You want your body fluids to be alkaline, so your cancer is eliminated. You want to reduce toxins and carcinogens in foods, so your cancer is eliminated. You want to eat healthy fruits, vegetables, and grains so that you restore your health back to normal. Now, perhaps even with the help of God or spirit, from this day forward, you are going to be acutely aware of the foods you select to eat. For the sake of living, and perhaps your loved ones, you are going to make healthy choices everywhere you go, because you are bound and determined to extend your life. You will be well aware of the ingredients in foods you buy, foods at home, foods at the few restaurants you visit, and at the grocery stores where you shop. You will concentrate on reading labels and healthy choices that will *save your life*.

These labels will show you what to avoid, such as unhealthy preservatives, including benzoate, nitrites, and sulfites. The thing your mind singles out to eliminate will also be any foods containing tomatoes, pork, vinegar, alcohol, processed sugar, and processed flour. White, bleached sugar, rice, and flour are off-limits. They would make you feel bad if you consumed them. Beware of condiments, most of which contain acetic acid or vinegar. Other foods that you will be repulsed by will include deep-fat fried foods and fast food, farmed fish, and high fructose corn syrup. You don't like food dyes or artificially colored foods, as it is the same as pouring ink into them, which is sickening.

Other sickening foods include sodas, peanuts, hardened-aged cheeses, and hydrogenated or partially hydrogenated oils. You also eliminate prepackaged snacks and meats, which contain MSG and high levels of sodium. Salty foods taste very bitter now, so you are reminded to avoid them. Too many sweets, even with the permitted natural sugars, make your stomach queasy.

Electronics are avoided or altered for your safe use. For example, if you work at the computer, you will wear crystals, or use a radiation shield to filter out the radiation. In addition, if you use a cell phone, you will use a wired ear piece so you do not have to touch the phone itself when talking. And neither you, nor anybody else who cooks your food, will be permitted to cook your food in destructive, food-altering microwave ovens.

Now, you can take a deep breath, a breath of fresh air and relax… because you've promised yourself a new way of life, not just in letting stress roll off your back, like water off a duck's back, but you are committed to cultivating a new diet within your mind and within your life. This new diet will save your life. You will find that you desire healthy foods now everywhere you go. Because it's a life or death situation, you remain completely committed to the following foods, and, possibly, to your own amazement, they even taste better. They certainly leave you feeling better as they boost your immune system and fill the nutritional deficiencies in your body.

These attractive, healthier foods that you really enjoy include delicious whole grains, such as brown rice and whole grain breads, cereals, and pastas. You may find the best bread at a health food store, or make it at home with your bread maker. You find you enjoy unsalted nuts and seeds, particularly when combined with moderate quantities of dried fruit. You will find yourself craving fresh fruits and vegetables of all kinds on a daily basis. Each week you will consume only moderate amounts of healthy meat. You will not consume more than three servings of fish, or two servings of fish and one serving of poultry. Occasionally, you will substitute these with organic beef or wild game. You will enjoy all sorts of beans and grains, and brown rice, wild rice, and basmati white rice. You enjoy moderate amounts of soft cheeses and dairy foods, such as organic yogurt, mozzarella, ricotta, yogurt or soy cheeses, and kefir cheese. You will get your protein from beans each week, if possible, and eggs, three to six per week, if desired. Low-fat milk, buttermilk, and cottage cheese are also appetizing.

The oils you buy and consume will include virgin olive, grape seed, hazelnut, almond, and sesame seed. You may also eat butter and sweet butter, if they appeal to you. You will find that you enjoy cooking with olive oil, natural sugars, and occasional sea salt. The sweeteners you buy and enjoy eating will be honey, raw sugar, turbinado sugar, demerara, molasses, natural maple syrup, sucanat, and stevia. You will limit your sodium intake to one teaspoon of salt, or 2300 mgs, per day. Almonds and almond butter may be appetizing on a regular basis. You enjoy all types of herbs and seasoning that are without powdered tomatoes and sugar. Fresh culinary herbs are very healthy and appetizing; they make your foods taste better. You may even find you enjoy cooking with spices and herbs, such as basil, thyme, rosemary, marjoram, dill, sage, tarragon, chives, mint, ginger root, cilantro, parsley, fennel, pepper, oregano, cinnamon, garlic, bay leaf, curry, cumin, paprika, ground mustard, nutmeg, and chili powder.

When it comes to liquids, you will be thirsty on a daily basis, consuming two quarts of liquids daily, which creates an attraction for spring water, filtered or reverse osmosis water, decaffeinated herbal teas of all types, and freshly squeezed fruit and vegetable juices, while eliminating acid-based tomato juices. In addition, you will drink grape juice daily, fresh grape juice when possible. You can dilute the grape juice with ice, or 50 percent water, and enjoy the purification qualities to your body, as the liquids you consume cleanse your mind and body, and because you are eating right, you can relax and simply let go, knowing you've done your best and it's up to God for the rest. Now you can relax, as the new eating habits are adopted quickly and easily with a little effort, and you find you enjoy them. Perhaps, to your own amazement, with a little effort you find you even enjoy the new eating habits more, because they leave you feeling healthy, thinner, more attractive, and with more energy. You like your new lifestyle now, so you can relax… You are doing the right thing, so you'll find you're more relaxed every day, as these suggestions and habits become more natural with each passing day.

Awakening Procedures

And now I'm going to count back from five to one and when I reach the number one, you can then normalize.

> *Five*…You'll remember everything you have experienced.
> *Four*…Very satisfied with the (changes that have taken place).
> *Three*…More in touch with the room around you.
> *Two*…The mind and the body are returning back toward normal.
> When you imagine the number *One*…in your mind's eye within the next

minute, you'll become wide awake, refreshed, and feeling good.

(Turn off the recorder here.)

The Effects of Altered States of Consciousness

There are a wide variety of effects we may feel physically and mentally that indicate we've entered into an altered state of consciousness. These include: feeling a complete sense of calmness and peacefulness, feeling heavy or weightless, feelings of detachment or numbness, rapid eye movement, slowed respiration and heart rate, and more. From using meditative forms of relaxation, we enter into alpha or theta brain waves and begin to build a bridge between the mind and body.

In addition, if we practice the spiritual meditations, we may actually encounter God's presence. Sometimes we can ask questions, such as what our healing color is, what we need to do to get better, or what the purpose of our illness is. Provided we are able to blank our minds, at least intermittently, we may receive messages from God or God's messengers. Those who are more open-minded, you might say, or those who open their minds, are more likely to receive spiritual guidance.

Summary

These meditations are essentially a crash course in self-hypnosis, yet they still offer the same benefits to all readers, whether they are practiced self-hypnosis enthusiasts, regular meditators, or beginners of the art. The reason is, whether an expert or a beginner reads them, the scripts are just as effective. It may be advantageous for a person seeking healing to work one-on-one with a hypnotherapist. In this case, the hypnotherapist can customize the script to the cancer patient's needs, which may increase results. However, some research also shows that self-hypnosis and meditation is more effective than any other hypnotic therapy, because it's self-designed.

For anyone who wants a better understanding of self-hypnosis, and wants to become proficient in the art, I recommend a book called *Self-Hypnosis: Creating Your Own Destiny*, by Henry Leo Bolduc. Another book will provide you with a full library of scripts, but has less explanation on how to use them; this is one I wrote called *Script Magic: A Hypnotherapist's Desk Reference*. Though designed for hypnotherapists, many self-hypnosis enthusiasts have reported using it successfully as well.

A valuable shortcut to all these methods would be to obtain and listen to the professional anti-cancer CDs that I recorded in my own voice (1996 hypnotic voice of the year award). These include quality nature sounds and musical backgrounds. See the resources section for ordering information.

A Note to Clinicians

In addition to the recommended CDs, clinicians, such as guided imagery professionals, hypnotherapists, or counselors who specialize in cancer recovery may consider obtaining another book I wrote, *Script Magic: A Hypnotherapist's Desk Reference, Second Edition*. The book has the scripts in this chapter, in addition to many other scripts for stress, anxiety, sleeping well, and more.

Disclaimer

Those who use these scripts use them at their own risk. The publisher, the author, their affiliates, and the bookstores where these scripts and CDs are obtained, cannot be held responsible for any adverse effects that are claimed by those who use them. Self-hypnosis is the art of suggestion, and the responsibility to accept such suggestions lies in the hands of the self-hypnosis practitioner. They can either accept such suggestions or reject them. It is dangerous to listen to any self-hypnosis recordings or scripts while operating machinery.

Epilogue

Some scientific-minded readers might need further proof that there is a highly effective, all-natural cancer cure that won't make you more sick, kill you, or give you more cancers, even beyond my medical reports and all the research I've provided in this book. I invite them to examine two reports: *History of Hoxsey Treatment*, by Patricia Spain Ward, PhD, and *Assessment of Outcomes at Alternative Medicine Cancer Clinics: A Feasibility Study*, by Mary Ann Richardson, Dr. Ph. Both of these reports provide convincing information about the efficacy of Hoxsey therapy.

In May of 1988, medical historian Patricia Spain Ward, PhD, who at that time was historian of the University of Illinois at Chicago, submitted a report titled *History of Hoxsey Treatment*. It had been commissioned by the Office of Technology Assessment (OTA) of the United States Congress. Although her work and her opinion was held in high esteem, her report was deemed to be biased toward Hoxsey therapy, so very little of the report was published in the OTA's 1990 publication, *Unconventional Cancer Treatments*. In the report, she states, "In actuality, except for work with mice done in the 50s by an outside contractor for the NCI, but never published in the scientific literature, it appears that Hoxsey's treatment has never been tested, either in animals or in humans." Her complete report may be found through the information provided in the Resources section of this book. At that web site, it is easy to print the report.

The other report, funded by an NIH grant under the NCCAM, is *Assessment of Outcomes at Alternative Medicine Cancer Clinics: A Feasibility Study*, by Mary Ann Richardson, Dr. Ph., Nancy C. Russell, MPH, Tina Sanders, MS, Robert Barrett, PhD and Catherine Salveson, RN PhD. It too is a powerful resource that documents the success of alternative cancer therapies. In it, both the Biomedical Center in Tijuana, Mexico and the Livingston Foundation Medical Center in San Diego were said to maintain high success rates for cancer recovery. This report was published in *The Journal of Alternative and Complementary Medicine*, vol. 7, no. 1, 2001, pp. 19–32.

This report is also available through the web site listed in the Resources section. The full report can be downloaded in pdf format.

Afterword

Conclusion

The determination to live longer and healthier lives is what drives the public to research alternative medicine therapies and natural cures that have few or no side effects. Often, traditional medicine doesn't provide all the answers or insurance companies won't pay for the better alternatives, because corporate America can't line their pockets with patented remedial fixes. This is why Americans have needed to become their own medical historians, or home pharmacists. Almost every household in the United States is now self-treating, using some form of home remedies that they've researched on their own. These extra measures and out-of-pocket expenses are those that we Americans are willing endure to keep ourselves healthy.

I feel sorry for America and its citizens, because medical politics have kept the Hoxsey clinics out of the country. The United States is supposed to be the most medically advanced country in the world, but because of medical politics, it lags way behind the health systems of many other countries. We're behind the times with a lopsided system that legally favors traditional medicine and ostracizes those who desire natural cures.

"Technology has surpassed our humanity." Albert Einstein

At least my government gives me the freedom to express my views without going to jail; for this reason, among many, I remain patriotic. Americans relish their freedoms, but we are jailed when it comes to natural cancer cures, because you cannot patent an herb or a diet to make money from it. Therefore, the best cancer cures, the natural ones, are not publicized or extensively utilized in this country. Because of this, millions of cancer patients needlessly die each year.

My purpose in writing this book is not only to save lives, but also to get the word out about natural cancer cures. I hate watching America damage her reputation as a world leader in medicine due to its impotent health care system bankrupting or killing its citizens who get sick. It's a sad commentary when we have to leave the country to get treated with alternative medicines that generally have a higher cure rate.

A system that makes our citizens poor and corporations rich, while the environment continues to deteriorate in the name of industrial progress and money-first values, MUST CHANGE. We must ask ourselves how long we will let the rich rule with money-and-greed-first policies. Our insurance companies are growing richer from our misfortunes. Due to politics and the environment, our ability to sustain life on this planet gets chipped away little by little, while the minority speaks out and the majority turns their backs!

Perhaps we can start voting conscientious people into office, who will run our government better. Maybe, if we have a vision, we can start sharing it more openly with other people, and with our children and grandchildren, and perhaps it will be passed on and accepted by the majority. We can make a difference if *each person who finds value in this book writes their congressional representatives and assists in calling for a congressional hearing.* We should not be afraid to be vocal about this, because our lives may depend on it as the incidence of cancer continues to dramatically rise.

In order to become a cancer survivor, however, we cannot continuously burden ourselves with these truths. Instead, we must speak our truths clearly and quietly until mankind is willing to hear them and do something about it.

We are each on a journey, orchestrated on a spiritual level; everything will turn out all right in the end. Most world religions, and modern-day prophets and mystics, predict that the world will have a complete spiritual awakening, and mankind will live 1000 years of peace. It's important to live with this faith, and keep the "kingdom of God within (us)," as Jesus of Nazareth recommended. Peace comes from within, where faith and hope lie waiting for us to tap into at any time.

My Travels and People's Stories

Chatting with Liz, the Clinic Director

On one of my most recent visits to the BMC, I chatted for an afternoon with the clinic director, Liz, Mildred's sister. We discussed many things. One of them a very interesting and popular story circulating among the staff at the BMC.

A woman was seeing a traditional oncologist in the United States for cancer therapy. She left his care to come to the Biomedical Center. After a while she was getting good results with Hoxsey therapy and then became cancer-free. Years later, at one of her annual check-ups at BMC, she was sitting in the waiting room when she noticed somebody she recognized. It was her oncologist from the states. She asked what he was doing there, and he told her that he had noticed that she got better, and now he had cancer and wanted the same benefit. However, he explained, if his colleagues or his state medical board found out about him coming to the BMC, he could be ostracized and would have difficulty practicing medicine. So he asked her to promise to never tell anyone that she saw him at the clinic. She agreed.

People Sharing in Belize

One of the time share exchanges we made involved a resort in Ambergris Caye, a remote island in Belize. After we arrived in Belize City, we took a ferry to San Pedro Island. From there, we had to transfer to another dock and wait for the resort to send a boat for us and take us to the northern part of the island. The resort was located a couple of hundred yards away from the world's largest living reef, a snorkeler's paradise.

While we were waiting for the resort boat, a woman with long blond hair was there with her husband, and they were talking to my wife. Occasionally she would puff on an inhaler; she seemed to have breathing problems. The conversation turned to this book. The woman told us that they were from Texas and they and another couple were staying at a nearby resort. Then the woman asked me if I had cancer.

I said I was a cancer survivor. She told me that she had stage four breast cancer. I asked her if she had tried the Hoxsey method, and described it to her, but she just kept smiling disinterestedly. After a short time, I realized that she had chosen traditional medicine and was at peace and ready to leave this world. This was her last trip to paradise on earth before she entered the next, more paradisiacal, world. Strangely, she radiated an unusual contentment most people lack in this world, as if she knew where she was going next.

Hearing our conversation, a man walked up and introduced himself as the couple's friend. Following him was a woman, who appeared to be his wife. He began discussing his extensive research into the same cancer-curing herbs that I had researched. I stopped him and asked, "How do you know all these things." He told us that his daughter had battled a form of sarcoma, one of the most difficult cancers to cure. She was given only months to live, but lived five years. He said that he grew blood root and not only used it as an external salve for killing the tumors under the skin, but also wadded up the resin into a ball, which she took throughout the day. At one point she was completely clean of her cancer. But when she went to college she went off the low animal-high plant diet that her father had put her on, ate dorm food, and passed away.

Her mother, his wife, was standing right behind him, with anguish on her face as if she wanted to say something, but didn't. Something like, "It was her time for God to take her," I suppose. Her mother and I stared at each other for a silent moment, knowing this truth, but not saying anything. Her father was trying to make sense of it all, as the researcher he was. It seems to be the way some fathers respond to illness in their families. This is their way of doing something about it.

Her father said that after their daughter's cancer came back they went to Sloan Kettering and the traditional medicines took her out rather quickly. As I boarded our boat I was thinking that nobody wants their child to outlive them.

Later that night, I remembered the benefit of getting a terminal illness. To act as if there was no tomorrow, to truly live a life of peace, integrity, and freedom of maintaining more distance from worldly cares...it's one of the gifts of the disease.

As I talked to the Belizean people about cancer, many of them laughed and claimed that cancer was not a big problem there because they didn't have the pollution problems of the United States and other industrialized countries, and all their sugar is natural, not processed. On hearing of my book project, they asked me if I planned to take the "medicine walk" outside Belize City. I found out that this is a rain forest path with significant curative plants growing along side of it that draws visitors and researchers from across the globe. I made a promise to myself to walk the medicine path in the near future.

A visit from Lou, the Local Handyman

Around the time I contracted cancer, there was a man named Jerry, a born-again Christian who took it upon himself to regularly minister to his neighbors. Jerry was a dependable and honest contractor, who could always be counted on to do good economical work. He built most of our wraparound deck. He would often check up on our family to see if we needed anything. Sometimes I'd have him haul away trash and wood, or things we no longer needed.

Jerry told me that his assistant, Lou, had prostate cancer that had spread to stage four, and his doctor gave him a maximum of two months to live. Lou was not a Christian, which bothered Jerry, but I told Jerry to send him up to my house to watch the Hoxsey videos, something I've done for other cancer patients, many of whom visited the clinic and recovered. But Lou never came to see me.

Several months later, Jerry showed up at my door. With him was Lou, grinning from ear to ear. Jerry said, "Look at 'im. He's cured! The doctor said he ain't got cancer no more." I asked Lou how he did it, and he said he knew an old man "up a holler" (a mountainous valley) who had prostate cancer and cured himself with herbs. He said the old man told him to send cash in an envelope to this PO box, and a bottle of herbal tonic would be returned. It is illegal in this country to claim that something cures cancer and sell it, so this is how it had to be done.

Lou sent the money as specified, then received his herbal medicine in a little dropper bottle. He took a few drops a few times a day, and was cured. I asked if he knew what herbs were in it, and he said that he thought there was blood root in it. I told him that I knew an herbalist who was aware of some underground research being conducted showing great success in curing cancer with blood root. I told him that the BMC used it for external cancers and that my sister was giving it to her daughter, after traditional medicine failed to help her daily debilitating migraine headaches. Her headaches were now manageable and often non-existent. Her daughter was just six years old. The name of the herbal remedy was *The Headache Remedy*. I began to realize that blood root has more curative powers than I'd imagined.

A Seminar Attendee's Confession

Near the end of 2005, I presented this recovery system to a group of holistic health professionals in Virginia Beach. Afterwards, a woman pointed to her lip and said, "You see this mark right here?" I said I did and she said, "I just came down with melanoma and I decided to use a form of what you refer to as escharotics. It's a salve I found on the internet called cancema. They manufacture it in either Canada or Australia, I think. It has blood root in it." She pointed to it again, "Look, this is where it was, now all you see is a small mark. It came out through the skin. Isn't that amazing?"

I agreed, then thought back to the photographs I saw in Ausubel's book demonstrating escharotics on an army general. I also recalled one of the older Hoxsey videos, which showed white blood cells forming a barrier around a breast tumor the size and shape of an egg and necrotizing it. Then the BMC doctors extracted it through the skin. I remembered Hoxsey's autobiography, which showed a photograph of a brain cancer that was lifted through the skull. It was covered on the radio and caused quite a controversy (see appendix B). I also thought of the many melanoma patients I met in Tijuana who returned to the BMC for escharotics every few years. I thought, "It's only a matter of time, before the secret cures for cancer are no longer a secret."

A Cancer Patient Looking for Answers but Finding Shysters

If I could, I would answer phone calls all day long from people who have cancer who are looking for alternative cancer therapies, to help them distinguish between the shysters and the credible sources for alternative natural cures, such as Hoxsey therapy. Although I generally don't have the time, I found it important to speak with a woman with squamous cell carcinoma who contacted my office.

She'd seen my article in the March 2006 issue of *Venture Inward* magazine. She explained that she'd been diagnosed with cancer two months ago and her conventional medical doctors and her family were urging her to start radiation on her tonsils immediately. She was afraid of the slight risk of ending up on a trachea tube and a feeding tube, because of the location of the cancer and the side effects of traditional therapy. So she refused treatment and began what I call "experimenting." In her search she found one popular natural cure book recommending colloidal silver. I told her that I was a naturopathic researcher and had found no benefit in such a cure.

She then told me that a doctor in Florida had a patient who got cured with a liver cleansing kit. I told her a liver cleanse may be helpful but was not considered a comprehensive cancer therapy. Then I asked her if this patient was using any other therapy, and she said she wasn't sure. This woman said she was supposed to send $600 in unmarked bills to this so-called doctor and that she would receive the kit in the mail. I asked her how long she was going to experiment with her life—until the point where she begins to lose it? When she complained about the money to fly to clinics such as the BMC, I told her that many churches have been known to chip in on airline tickets and a night's lodging for those who have cancer and request it.

From there, I told her what I would tell anybody who has cancer and is looking for a natural cure. Cancer is a multi-billion dollar industry. Because of this, she will find many people claiming to have cures who want a piece of the pie. A liver cleanse can be helpful in conjunction with a comprehensive cancer therapy; but it is not a cure by itself. When a person's life is at stake, he or she should investigate a therapy and look for independent research that verifies it. If independent research is scarce, then the clinic offering the therapy should offer a list of testimonials to contact. Preferably this list should be made up of people who had her same type of cancer and were cured.

Out of all the alternative cancer clinics that offer comprehensive therapies, the NIH has only discovered two with significant results: the Livingston Foundation Center in San Diego and the Biomedical Center in Tijuana, Mexico. I told her to tell her family about the report on the Hoxsey web site.

I told her that experimenting is not advisable. I reminded her that I was a naturopathic researcher and that was why I experimented with my own cancer, knowing I had a year and a half to whip this thing.

I told her that the BMC would educate her on a comprehensive cancer system, with a team of oncologists who were primarily from medical colleges in Mexico City—the same universities that many baby boomer medical students attended in the sixties when it was difficult to get into medical school in the states. Most of them returned to the states to practice after graduation.

I told her that the BMC has a track record of eighty years and eighty percent success, and the Livingston Foundation Clinic has a similar success rate, yet the BMC is the least expensive of all such clinics. Patients are generally seen for a full day, unless their cancer is well advanced, and then they stay longer. I explained what would probably happen during a full day visit at the BMC.

Then I asked her what she had to lose. If it didn't work, it would be evident in the tests done two months later at her next visit. The worst case scenario was that she could then do traditional medicine or try something else. She responded that her doctors said she had two years to live, so why not. She thanked me, and told me she would book a flight for San Diego, destination Tijuana, as soon as she hung up the phone.

Those Who Thank Me

Many people correspond with me. Some make appointments to see me for a naturopathic consultation or for a hypnotherapy session, wanting additional assistance with mind-body therapy. Some simply cross my path and thank me. For example, recently, Dr. Jans came to teach at the annual holistic health conference that my organization sponsors, and he was teaching a workshop titled "Cancer: The best thing that ever happened to me." (If you will recall, he was the person who was just weeks away from death when I recommended he travel to the BMC.)

I sat in the back of the room. Twice, when he came to the part of the story describing how I encouraged him to go to the BMC when he was on his last legs and his oncologist in the states had given up on him, he got choked up and couldn't go on. This thanks from him, and from other people, is what makes all this work so worthwhile. It's not easy to talk about the subject of cancer all the time, promoting this book and this therapy, so I want to thank *you* for thanking *me*.

Updates—Before Going to Press

Hoxsey in America

Just before going to press, I did a final web site search for herbal cancer cures that may be available in the United States and logged on to www.altcancer.com. The host for the site is Alpha Omega Labs, located in Lake Charles, Louisiana. This company manufactures Hoxsey, essiac, cancema (a topical blood root paste), and other natural cancer cures. When I got to the site, I was saddened to find out they had shut down their on-line store and appeared to be out of business. I phoned the number on the site and discovered they'd been shut down by the FDA September 17, 2003. It appears that anything with the Hoxsey name on it still creates attention, controversy, and a battle that may never end. Those Americans who don't want to go to Mexico, or another country, for obtaining natural cancer cures may have to make their own herbal medicine tinctures. Perhaps, as a safeguard, we should consider ordering the book *The Herbal Medicine Maker's Handbook*, by James Green.

US Heat on the BMC

Two days before gong to press, I discovered that US government officials were putting pressure on the government of Mexico to create difficulties for their most popular alternative medicine clinics, including, of course, the BMC. When I heard the news, I was afraid that the herbal tonics may not be available anymore. After phoning them, I discovered that they simply had to reorganize areas within the clinic to fit newly imposed guidelines. The Mexican government's primary concern was the Hoxsey tonic. Again, the word "Hoxsey" continues to raise controversy, because it cures cancer at a very low cost to the consumer.

A Farewell to My Mother

Jane Chips felt so strongly about this book, that when she was dieing from a massive stroke a week before this book went to press, I flew out to show her the cover, reminding her who it was dedicated to (her). She was coherent enough to point to the cover with the one arm that she could still move, indicating that this was an important purpose for me. Tears were shed, and they continue to roll.

I have great joy in releasing this three year project to the public, but I also feel a great loss from losing the woman who loved me unconditionally and gave me a solid, unshakable psychology with which to approach life. I have faith that she will assist me with what I need to do to contribute to the Hoxsey therapy crusade. As in the movie Star Wars, when Obe Wan Kenobi surrendered his life for the sake of helping others in a greater capacity, I'm sure she will provide assistance from the other side. She was a saint.

The Purpose for Writing This Book

Personally, I feel that God and the BMC have given me my life back. This book is my way of repaying the favor.

The cover of this book represents the fact that each of us has a clock that's ticking from the day we're born, and that those who have a life-threatening illness become uniquely aware of this fact. Most cancer survivors would tell you that the result of surviving is *carpe diem*, which is Latin for "seize the day." If we watch for this opportunity, no matter how difficult life gets, we can make the best of each day. Even in the most difficult days, we can find the gem in the rough, the one blessing we can look back on at the end of each day that tells us that it was a day worth living.

The thing I don't doubt any more is that God's herbs and natural foods are curing this illness we call cancer, which humankind gives to itself through its negligence. I am 100 percent positive that the "war on cancer" that the National Cancer Institute waged decades ago had already been won by a man called Harry Hoxsey and his herbal therapies, which have already cured hundreds of thousands of people.

The truth is that if people were disciplined about taking their herbs and supplements, and staying on the diet, the Hoxsey approach's average success rate would be higher than 80 percent. It also seems that when Hoxsey patients make the five year mark cancer-free, they never have to worry about cancer again. It seems that this approach rebuilds the immune system in the process of eliminating the malignancy, almost as if the Hoxsey patients have undergone some sort of inoculation. Although no cure for cancer can be effective for everyone, an approach with an 80-plus percent success rate, or 90 percent if followed to the letter, in my book qualifies as a cure.

I couldn't take more than one chemotherapy treatment, because of losing my memory, my personality changing, and potentially losing my writing and teaching ability. If the natural method had not worked for me, I wouldn't be here, and this book wouldn't have made it into existence. So for me, the all-natural approach was the only choice.

Now, having written this book, I feel I've accomplished my purpose, the whole purpose for my contracting the illness. Thank you for having considered this approach and may God bless you on your journey, the one journey that has no end.

Appendix A

Select Pages from...

The Visitors Registry
at the Biomedical Center

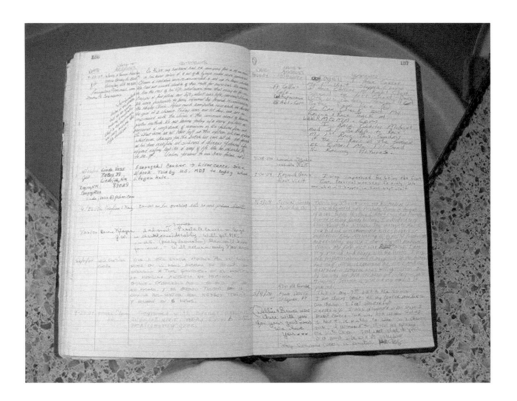

The following pages from of the visitors registry were selected by
Aida and the author for the following reasons:
1) Their ability to allow the visitors to remain anonymous
2) Their ability to show a wide range of cancers and results
3) The stories demonstrating clarity and legibility
4) Showing return visitors who report the status of their condition

Date	Name & Address	
		(malignant ameloblastoma & lupus)
March 3/03		This is my 5th visit for a rare form of bone cancer. My
J.W.	B.C. Canada	last visit showed that the tumors have reduced their size by 83%! I was in stage 4 when I began coming here. I am nervous and excited to get my newest results. Jehovah has sustained me through this journey, and I sincerely pray for all who embark on their own journey of recovery. Blessings to you all!!
March 4/03	Fairfield, CA	1st Visit! Excited & looking forward to God's healing with this Center. The people here have been wonderful & my husband, kids & I know that the lord led us here for a complete healing from Stage 4 Breast Cancer, metast. to liver, bones, etc... God Bless you all & Good Luck!
3-5-03 J.W.	ESCONDIDO CA.	1ST Visit To See iF This will woRK insteAd oF SuRgeRy FoR Colon cancer. we aRe oPtomistic & our hope is in Jah, as Jesus said "with God all Things are Possible".
3-5-03	MOAB. UTAH	8TH time BACK. GREAT REPORT NO CANCER.
3-5-03	Nucla, Colorado	Great Results!
3-5-03	Montrose Colo	First Visit Breast Cancer
3-5-03	Montrose CO.	2nd Visit - doing great - Good luck to all who visit, you won't be sorry!
3. March 03	Ranchos de Taos N.M.	It is my first time here and I am soo delighted about the atmosphere and approach of the professionals. It is simple but logical and yet professional. I have a lot of hope that the condition I am fighting for 14 yrs. will come to a wonderful end. Thank you spirits!

NAME + ADDRESS

21-03   Montgomery, Al.

1st Visit Soft tissue Sarcoma in my ethmoidal Sinus.

21-03   Stage 1 oral cancer. Past history breast cancer, had a lumpectomy, stem cell transplant, chemo & radiation. Didn't want to go through that again, have a friend who has come to the Hoxsey Clinic & has been successful.

1/03   This is our second trip and Carl is feeling much better. We have met a number of nice people. The only thing we found difficult is the diet, but we are getting better at finding new ways to prepare dishes. We wish everyone the best of luck.

26/03   1st Visit with Ovarian Cancer diagnosed '95. I have been thru chemo, radiation and surgery and by the Grace of God I am still here. Smarter now and willing to try this wonderful clinic that I've heard so much about so I can get my life back.
   Prayers and love to all who come thru these gates...

22/03   Curepe, TRINIDAD   1st Visit just for a check-up. Impressed by the quality of medical examinations.

/10/03   Riverside Ca.   Well, here we are again on our second visit, 4 months later. my mom is still alive & well, she had a small relapse but nothing super tonic can't take care of. Jehova has blessed us so much & alot of it has to do with this place. im sure everyone will find alot of hope here.
   never fear Jehova is always near. stay strong brothers & sisters. Rev 21:4 !!!   p. se go next time.

/10/03   Coming to the clinic for 7 years prostate cancer. Doing well. Thank Jehovah Psal 33:24

/10/03   3rd Visit Colon Cancer diagnosed 11-02. Coming to the clinic since this time. I feel good, healthy and positive. My energy level is high! Stay on the Tonic Never Give up!   Jehovahs Love,

Date	Name + Address	(JW)
4/3/03		My first visit with a sister From Long Beach my DX 3/10/03 multi myeloma, I too am so encouraged
	L.A. CA.	So many witnesses have been here and are healed and now are cancer free, I met so many sisters of Bro that have given me information to fight this disease. I'm with Jehovah's Org and am up for this fight will keep in touch
4/3/03	San Diego, CA	(JW) My visit here is for chelation therapy (for angina) and I fully expect to be pain free because I have met so many encouraging people that have gone thru varied treatments and are doing well and are so willing to share tips and experiences that are upbuilding. WAZ Z UP
		I have come for treatment of Colon cancer + liver problem. Many brothers + sisters of Jehovah's Witnesses have given me much confidence of the good work of this clinic.
4/7/03	Nucla Colorado	2nd visit doing good - 2 cancers cured (Skin cancer) by Hoxey pomade salve
4-9-03	+ re 9	Breast Cancer since Feb. 1999 - still hanging in there
4-9-03	Birmingham, AL	This is my fourth visit to the clinic. I feel so good from the diet + the treatment I can't believe it
4-9-03	Corning CS	2nd visit & now cancer free! (Breast Cancer)
4-11-03 JW	Philip, SD.	My first visit! Drs gave me 2 wks - 3 mo to live last Oct. Refused their chemotherapy + radiation but was doing some natural therapies. My chiropractor loaned me a video of Bio Medical Clinic, my daughter knew some in her com coming out so they let me come along. I am encouraged by the warm reception here!
	Danail	I went to the moon in ninty sixty AIA and I died
4-11-03 JW	FT. Bridger Wy.	Third visit. Doing Fine. Hope to be here some time with
4-14-03 (7th on 8th visit)	Stockton, CA LCS	Started here in about 1985 for skin cancer on face. After two treatments cancer healed up in 3 weeks with nearly invisible scar. Another on shoulder healed in 2000. Have read You Don't Have to Die by Dr. Hoxey. Thank God for this clinic and The Nelson sisters.
4-14-03	Pond Rd. VA	first visit: When we heard of this clinic I knew it would work for my mom breast cancer! Thankyou for (Jam

Date	Name & Address	
		We will be back for second visit in July. Diagnosed with DCIS + Stage 2 Invasive Carcinoma with 2-3 cm lump in my right breast. I pray for what God promises us to claim in our perfect health + healing! Receive + Believe! I Thes. 5:16-18 Always be Joyful!
4/15/03	Sylmar, CA.	1st time visit. - 34 yrs old Hodgkins Lymphoma. We were recommended by a brother (JW) that was treated here. We hope to have the same results as others in this book. It's very encouraging to read through. We continue to pray to Jehovah for strength and comfort during these hard times. Started with non-Hodgkins Lymphoma Stage 2 12/01 then 4/03 cancer re-appeared, had a big lump in my neck, and alot of lower back pain. I have been diagnosed with Hodgkins Lymphoma now (Stage 3) I am currently being treated with chemotherapy in U.S. but hope to have great results here!
4/15/03	Seattle, WA	Am doing so well that I will now be able to slowly wean off the tonic. Thank you to all the Staff at Bio Medical - next visit will be in 1 year!
4/16/03	Centralia, WA	Doing well - been here 2 yrs, come down every 6 mos. These Dr's know what they are doing - Diet is critical.
4/16/03	Round Lake Illinois	When I was here for a check up, it was discovered that I have melanoma in my system. Melan in the urine. Went on Tonic, diet & suggested vitamins. Today, 3 months later - the urine test is clean. I will stay on the program completely and return in a year. This program really works!! If I can do it so can you!! Good Luck.
4/21/03 Bladder Cancer (J.W.)		First visit. Bladder Cancer doctor in Albuquerque NM wants to remove bladder. Referred Sister Karen Payne (Reg. Cong.)
4/21/03 -Tracy CA		*Six visit* All is well. Still cancer free, thank Jehovah. Continuing therapy + diet. Good luck to all those beginning the journey.
J.W. Colo Springs.		My Mom came here in the 80's with cervical cancer. She is alive and well. During the treatment she was pregnant with me and I am well, too. My mother, father, grandmother, grandfather, me, brother and aunt are all here for check ups. All is well. No cancer!

Date	Name & Address	
Apr. 23/03	J.W.	It is now my 5th visit to the clinic, I was diagnosed with prostate cancer in Apr. 17th 1995, My 1st visit was in Oct. of 1995, My P.S.A. was 89.7 when first found. Before finding out about Hoxsey, I had radition and experanced 2nd degree burds throughout all my internal organs.
		Dr.s at hoxsey put me on the tonic and gave me shots of B12 for radition burns, within 6 mo. my P.S.A. was down to about 10-12 within a yr. my P.S.A. was down to 0.1
		In Oct. of 1999 I had been out of my tonic for 6 mo. was then told, I had spots on my lungs, liver, & Kindey & P.S.A. had again elivated. 6 mo. later after tonic no spots
		I am back now with the same condition as in 99, I've been out of tonic for 6 mo. And spots are back, but I Know in 6 mo. I will be cancel free once again in my lungs, liver, Kidney & P.S.A. will be down again.
		Take care my bro. & sisters with Agape love, your bro, Chuck Havelton
		P.S. Call if your ever in Cow Town U.S.A. and remember, everything in this system is only temporry even up to the point of death. Rev. 21: 3H4
April 25, 2003		CHECK UP TODAY WITH BLOOD WORK XRAYS, VISIT WITH NEXT MEDICAL
J.W.	LOVELAND, CO	DOCTOR ELIAS GUTIERREZ, M.D. BLOOD TESTS & CHEST X-RAYS ALL LOOK A-OK. AA WILL COME ANY 2 OR 3 DAYS ON 4-3-03 PSA < 2.2. PROSTATE CANCER IS IN REMISSION NOW FOR PAST 7 YEARS. 1ST EXAM FEBRUARY 1993 PSA < 7.4 WITH 4 BIDAYS ALL PATATKING NOW, I FEEL MUCH BETTER TODAY IS MY 4th VISIT.
April 30/2003		
May 5/03		this is our 1st visit here, we heard about this place through brothers in our cong- & through an article in the awake magazine, my mom Maria has gone through chemo therapy for one year now and doctors said to continue chemo. i dont think my mom could withstand another therapy. on may 4th i learned about this wonderful place through alot of prayer to Jehovah and faith, he has blessed us & answered my prayers brothers, sisters & friends remember psalms
	Riverside ca Jehova's Witness Arlington Cong.	

Date	Name & Address	
5-7-03	Seligman, AZ	I was diagnosd with stage 3 Breast Cancer a little over a year ago I have had 3 sugeys and to day the Dr has taken me off of some of my meds and I'm doing so much better - thanks Doxey treatment and the good Lord. I recomend this treatment for any one. You go girl - I love you!
	Seligman Az.	
5-7-03		Wonderful Clinic Drs so kind. first time here. Wonderfully everyone feels as good as I do.
5-8-03	(J. W.)	1st Visit had colon Cancer Tumor Removed U.S one cancer cell in 1 of 18 Lymphnode Removed. so nice Dennis pick up - Relief Tension
5-8-03		1st visit tumor left breast (J. W.)
		ALSO CFS & FIBRO - PLEASE WRITE catalina wild rose @ netscape.net
5-5-03		Diagnosed with uterine cancer & because of serious bleeding was operated on Oct 29 2002. Dr. said I had to have very strong chemo for many months & then chemo. Instead I came here Dec 10th (or near that date) Today, my second visit here, all my tests were perfect. The Lord has been so good to me. May God bless you too. If anyone would like to talk to me my phone no. is
5-12-03	T.W.	Have Had Cancer in the Past. About 10 yrs. ago Came here & became Cancer free. Breast cancer this year again. Back on tonic & Diet.
	Raymond, Wa	feeling real good again. Thanks Don my wonderful Hubby & Best Human Friend
5-16-03		I was diagnosed with Kidney Cancer but 4. I am back for my three month check up and I feel wonderful. I had a tumor on the side of my head the size of an orange and after taking hoxsey for 2 weeks the tumor was gone. I have followed the diet and have never felt healthier.
5-19-03		Little Rock, Arkansas.
5-19-03		Bklyn, N.Y.
	Newton Parkside Camp	
5-19-03		doing fine, looking forward to a long and happy life serving my Creator Jhoval
5-22-03	BC. Canada	This is my 7th visit to Bio Medical Clinic. I came here in a wheel chair diagnosed with lung cancer not treatable - not operatable. given 3 months to live - today I feel wonderful. Thankyou Bio Medical Centre. Every day is a bonus.

Date	Name & Address

stensland. We just found out that the cancerous mass that has decided to grow in place of her removed uterus/ovaries has now spread into her fatty tissue. She has done everything right and still the cancer is as tenacious as she is. I just hope that she doesn't give up. Hoxsey has worked great for my other grandma Rochell Davies, so I still have hope for Marlene. I love her so much.

Good Luck!

7/7/03

Today was my first time at the Center. I'm very happy to be here and know this therapy will work. I was told on 6-4-03 that I have breast cancer. With the help of my mother, relatives and friends the traditional method of medicine was outruled and the experiences of others (   ) helped me decide this was the best, safest and most productive means to get well. So here we are — my mom and I sitting here at this clinic waiting for my Hoxsey! I know I'll return, and I'm looking forward to it and certainly getting well. You can be sure I will help many others to do the same. Thank you Connie for telling about those you knew who came here also.

Thanks to all,

7/8/03

2nd visit. First visit 2/18/03. Came after receiving diagnosis of breast cancer. Doctor wanted to remove large portion of breast — possibly all — and follow with radiation/chemo. I had a friend's mother who came to Hoxsey 45 years ago with breast cancer and is alive and healthy today at age 92. I take my time and stick to my diet precisely. I pray always. I thank my Heavenly Father for guiding me here and for the wonderful people at the clinic. May they be blessed.

DATE	NAME ADDRESS	
7-15-03 JW	(_____)	Prostate Cancer - diagnosed 6/03. Gleason score 8. Oncologist says this is a very aggressive cancer & gave me 6 months to live. PSA went from 3.5 to 5.8 in 6 months. This is my first visit here
7-23-03	Bret + Krystin Kelly P.O. Box 15056 Farmington NM 87401	1st Visit for both) Krystin checkup for asthma + an old kidney problem. Bret for heart + thyroid.
7-23-03 Bladder Cancer JW		2nd Visit 3 month check-up I have stuck strictly to the diet 7 days after I started the diet my energy went up so much I could hardly believe it. I would sleep 3/4 of the time now I work like I did when I was 30 yrs old. Dr. says, Dr Says no Cancer spots! Ha HoBo! 6 months come back.
8-5-03	Tracy Ca.	1st visit. Diagnosed w/ Prostate cancer. PSA of 5. Biopsy positive Rejected complete prostate removal. My sister was here 6yrs ago w/ lymphoma. 6 months later she was cured. My wifes mother lived 11yrs after treatment here for bone marrow cancer. I have confidence in clinic and faith in Jesus to help me thru this.
8-6-03	Matt Russell	3d visit - Dx- Stomach cancer. After chemo - Surgery - cancer still evident - After starting Tonic + Herbs No Signs of cancer after 2 CTs + 1 Endoscopy w/ biopsy. Chaxean is feeling + looking great. Her spirits are good - Praise God for blessing us + sending us here. There is Hope here. God Bless - Matt + Chaxean
8-6-03	Tehachapi, CA	1st visit - Metastatic breast cancer to Liver Lung - very (Will return 11/03 for Vac) Herceptin X
8-7-03	Madera, CA	1st Visit my mother was diagnosed with brain tumor doctors suggest she needs and operation to take out most of the tumor and start radiation and chemo, but she wants to try this out to see if it helps she has faith in god and the virgin Mary, Guadalupe that she will get cured and live many years more.
8-21-03	Smith Doniphan Mo.	Our 1st visit to BMC - We were So comforted to learn of this place - the Staff + Doctors were most kind - thorough + Professional we'd recommend it to anyone & if any patients want to use Natural Organic garden + lawn products we produce them + will sell @ mfgrs direct pricing if the patient mentions BMC when they call or
mfgr's of		

DATE	NAME ADDRESS	
9-12-03		3rd visit - diagnosed GIST (stomach cancer) spread to Liver
	Cottage Grove, OR	2-03. Started Hoxsey 3-03. Just got CT scan report - cancer
		is going away! I haven't had 1 sick day. I feel great!
		I know I am healing in my whole body. I am thankful
		every day for the gift of life + look forward to that
		report that says - "All clear" - soon.
9-15-03		
		Here for the first time. Colon cancer 1½ yrs
	Fordville N.D.	ago. now returned in the Liver and Lymph nod
		around Kidney. Am looking forward to treatment
		from Hoxsey. Hope it helps.
9-18-03		from Plumas, Manitoba, Canada
		This is my fourth trip. Had breast
		cancer diagnosed in Jan 2002. Am
		doing fine on the tonic and pills.
9-23-03		Well here for visit #6. and guess
		what?! The doctors believe that
	( )	where the ugly and destructive
	J.W.	cancer festered in my jaw, a
malignant ameloblastoma	scar is all that remains! A scar!
(rare form of bone	new bone is forming AND I made
cancer in jaw).	enough of a recovery to fall madly
		in love and get married in June!
		I am able to care for my babies
		(9 + 3) as well as my husband. I
		still get a little tired but I
		figure its ok, in exchange from
		being bedridden and dying to
		being a full time wife + mother
		and most importantly LIVING!
		Jehovah, my congregation and my
		amazing support system here at
		the clinic sustained me and now I
		am able to start giving back.
		Blessings to you all! See you
		in 6 months for my check-up!
9-23-03		1st Time here - diagnosed w/ Prostate Cancer.
	Cathedral City, CA	received the Special Tonic along w/ 3 other
		medications - due back in three months
		will update then! Everyone here
		is a great tribute to what Mildred
		started. Thank you Jesus Christ for
		referring us here!

DATE	NAME ADDRESS	
11-3-03		2nd visit, mets breast cancer, to bones + liver, feeling good & still positive about beating this. God is giving me patience to let this tonic work. We are sure it will with His help. Have more energy than ever and we just love the staff here. God Bless + Good luck to you all.
11-6-03	Burbank, CA	Dx Breast Ca 7/2000. Declined Surgery, Chemo & rad. This is my 9th visit. No sign of cancer. All tests normal. We are each in charge of our own health. Thank you, God.
11·7·03	Pomona, CA J/w	I've been on the tonic for about 3 years. Was diagnosed w/ ovarian cancer. my CA125 has been going up so I started getting chemotherapy again An oncologist told me that the tumor is back & im scheduled for surgery in 3wks. I hope that even a modification in my treatment will stabilize my cancer again thanks to Jenw's help im feeling great!..
11·07·03	San Bernardino, CA J/w	I'm Elena's sister, I also have have ovarian cancer. I've been cancer free! I'm just here for a check-up. about 2 yrs.
11·07·03	→	Prostate - Bone - Lymph Gland I came here after surgery for prostate cancer 6 weeks later PSA kept going up. Doctor said come back in 6 months. 1½ weeks Later came to mexico and they knew exactly where cancer was! It will be 9 years Jan 2004. I'm doing great. Enjoying Life To God be the Glory!! Refer back to 11-09-01 — 1-21-99. 7-3-02!! I asked God for 5 years HE has given me nine already. P.t.L.
11-0703		I was diagnosed with Non-Hodgkins Lymphoma in August of 1998. Ron told me about the Hoxey Clinic and I came here for the first time 2 years ago. The tumors have stopped growing and are shrinking. I feel great and thank God for the doctors here who minister to so many people and are seeing good results. God is so-so good!

DATE	NAME + ADDRESS	1st. treatment
12/03/03	St. Louis, Mo	TRANSITIONAL CELL CARCINOMA — Bladder, left hip, small of the back
12/4/03 (JW)	New Ulm, MN.	— 3RD VISIT CHECKUP & TREATMENT FOR PROSTATE CANCER GOING VERY WELL. SEE YOU NEXT YEAR
12/5/03 (JW)	Phoenix, AZ	1st Treatment for breast lump and facial carcinoma, skin lesions. Was referred here by a friend who was cured of breast cancer and other testimonials. Will be back.
12/8/03 (SW)		1st Treatment — Colon Cancer
12/10/03	Granada Hills, CA	7th visit. Started Dec. 2000 w/breast cancer (Two tumors). In 5 mos, no sign of cancer. No mastectomy, no chemo, no radiation. After 3 yrs. still on program. No more headaches. Good diet I am very strict w/diet.
12-10-03		1st TREATMENT ovarian cancer Diagnosed with ovarian cancer with great chance of metastases and fluid in the lung — I never thought I would be a patient in days of the Bio Medical Clinic. I have known of the clinic or more than 20 years and have recommended treatment to anyone who speaks of cancer. The experience I am about to undertake will be hard but its reward will be great!
12-10-03		YO ESTOY DIAGNOSTICADO CON CANCER EN LA LARINGE CUERDA VOCAL IZQUIERDA ES UN CANCER BIEN DIFERENCIADO. DESPUES DEL DIAGNOSTICO DE MI MEDICO EN HILLW SON DE OPERAR Y CORTAR CUERDAS VOCALES DECIDI POR RECOMENDACION DE UN AMERICANO DE APELLIDO CALVIN ME ENTERE DE ESTA CLINICA Y AQUI ESTOY CONFIANDO QUE SU DIAGNOSTICO SEA BUENO PARA MI. GRACIAS.
12-11-03 JW	Gilford, NH.	1st visit, we are encouraged and have had our hope restored. Life is a gift from Jehovah. We are thankful for this opportunity to restore a measure of health, hopefully more.
12-13-03		Eleven years with prostate Cancer came here with PSA 55.5 down as low as neg 3
12-15-03		My nombre es Angelica Maldonado es

Appendix B

Excerpts from Harry Hoxsey's Autobiography

You Don't Have To Die
Originally Published in 1956

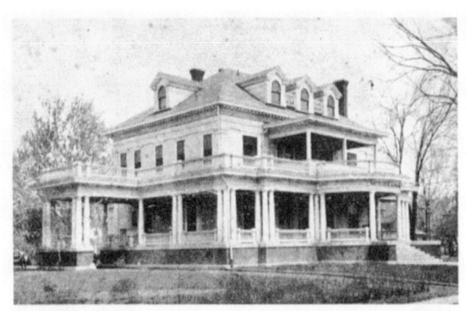

The Hoxide Cancer Sanitarium, one of the landmarks of Taylorville, Ill. in 1924.

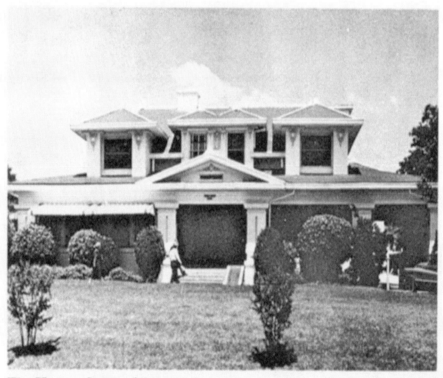

The Hoxsey Cancer Clinic—a 60 room converted residence about a mile from the heart of downtown Dallas.

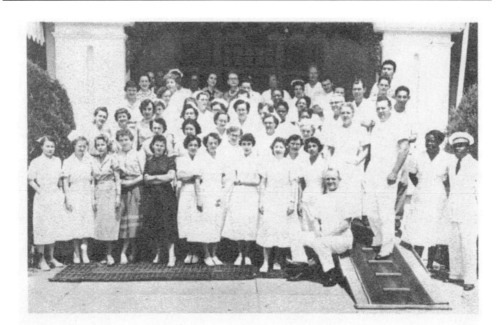

The staff of the Hoxsey Cancer Clinic at Dallas, Texas. Among the 60 employes are 7 doctors, 26 nurses, 8 x-ray technicians and 5 laboratory technicians.

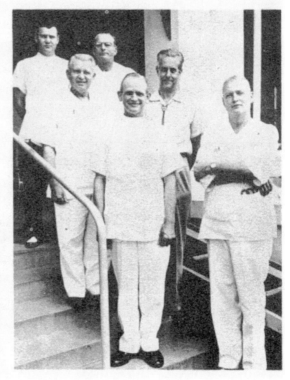

Doctors at the Clinic are (first row) Dr. Benjamin A. Harry and Dr. Douglas C. Logan; (second row) Dr. Alfred H. Staffa and Dr. Donald Watt; (back row) Dr. Charles P. Barberee and Dr. William E. Stokes. Not shown is Dr. Walter F. Pickett, M.D., who recently joined the staff.

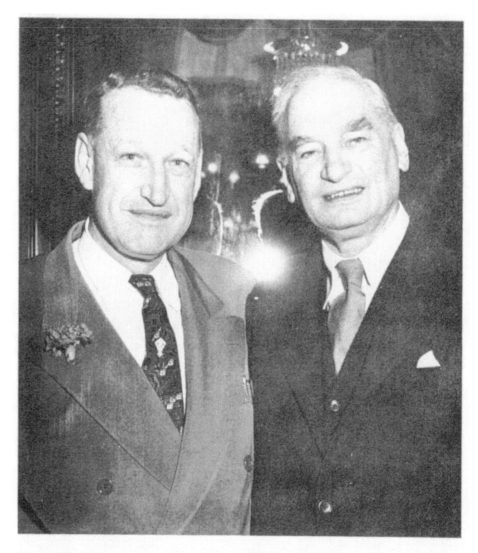

Harry M. Hoxsey with U.S. Senator William Langer, after latter introduced bill for Congressional investigation of treatment.

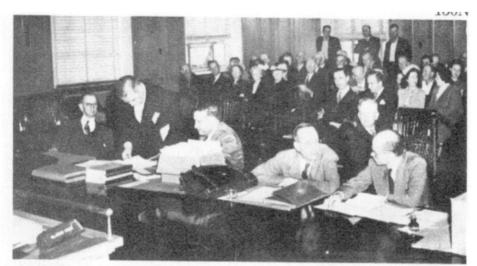

Counsel table at trial of libel and slander suit vs. Hearst (Chapter 15). Bending over table beside Hoxsey is his principal counsel, Herbert Hyde.

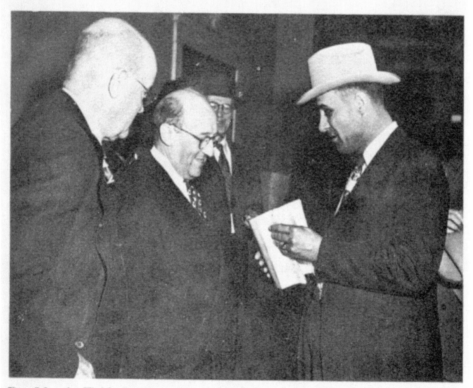

Dr. Morris Fishbein, "surprise" witness in the Hearst case, is handed summons to defend himself against libel and slander charges.

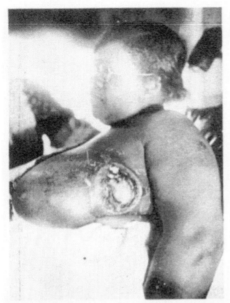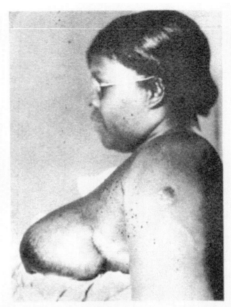

Mrs. Ethel Dennis of Philadelphia, treated for cancer of the breast in 1934 (Chapter 12). Before and after treatment. Biopsy report below, from well-known laboratory, attests that this patient had cancer when our treatment began.

LELAND BROWN LABORATORIES
422 CENTER BUILDING
6916 MARKET STREET
UPPER DARBY, PA.

PHONE, BOULEVARD 4222

June 27, 1934.

Dr. E. M. Hewish,
2131 Columbia Ave.,
Philadelphia, Pa.

Dear Mr. Hewish,

      Examination of piece of tissue, taken from breast of Mrs. Dennis, 2040 Turner Street, Philadelphia shows the presence of cords of cancer cells arranged in rows with infiltration of the cells into the surrounding tissue. The stratified squamous epithelium is intact.

      DIAGNOSIS: Tubular carcinoma.

                  Very truly yours,

                  LELAND BROWN LABORATORIES,

                  By:

                              Pathologist.

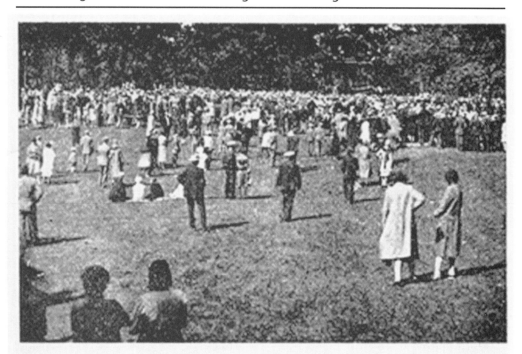

32,000 people turned out in a demonstration at Muscatine, Iowa on May 30, 1930, to witness the "resurrection" of Mandus Johnson (Chapter 11). Cancer covered entire top of his skull (left). Fully healed (right) he lived on for 30 years.

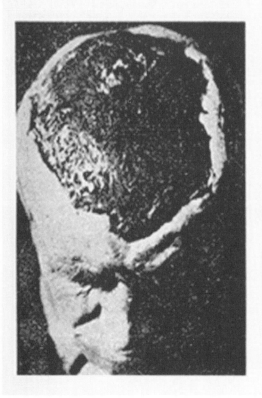

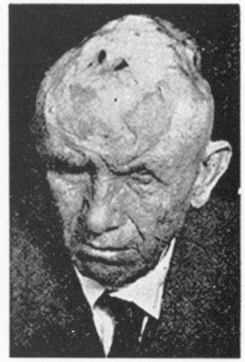

Resources

Books

Cancer Diagnosis: What to Do Next/Alternative Medicine Guide, by W. John Diamond, MD, W. Lee Cowden, MD, and Burton Goldberg

Cancer Medicine From Nature, by Roger Bloom

Clinical Hypnotherapy: A Transpersonal Approach, 2ed, by Allen Chips, DCH

Edgar Cayce on Diet and Health, by Anne Read, Carol Ilstrup, and Margaret Gammon, edited by Hugh Lynn Cayce

The Edgar Cayce Handbook for Health Through Drugless Therapy, by Harold J. Reilly and Ruth Hagy Brod

Encyclopedia of Natural Medicine, by Michael Murray, ND and Joseph Pizzorno, ND

The Lord's Answer To Your Every Need, compiled by Dr. A. L. Gill

The Natural Pharmacist: Your Complete Guide to Reducing Cancer Risk, by Richard Harkness

PDR for Herbal Medicines: The Information Standard for Complementary Medicine Third Edition, by Jeorg Gruenwald

Politics In Healing: The Suppression and Manipulation of American Medicine, by Daniel Haley

The Ph Miracle, by Robert Young, PhD, and Shelley Redford Young

Prescriptions for Nutritional Healing, by James F. Balch, MD and Phyllis A. Balch, CNC

Reducing Cancer Risk, by Richard Harkness, Pharm., FASCP

Script Magic: A Hypnotherapist's Desk Reference, 2ed, by Allen Chips, DCH

Ten Essentials of Highly Healthy People, by Walt Larimore, M.D.

When Healing Becomes a Crime, by Kenny Ausubel

You Don't Have To Die, by Harry Hoxsey

Audio Recordings

Self-Hypnosis and Meditation CDs
Cancer Recovery, by Dr. Allen Chips
Available at: www.holistictree.com

Videotapes

Quacks Who Cure, by Kenny Ausubel
Available at: www.Hoxsey.com (video), or www.Altcancer.com (download)

The Patient Experience, by Bernie and Carol Main
Available at: www.Hoxsey.com

Note: These may also be available soon on www.holistictree.com

Related Organizations and Clinics

Alpha Omega Labs
www.altcancer.com

Alliance for Natural Health
www.alliance-natural-health.org.

American Cancer Society
www.cancer.org
(800) 227-2345

American Holistic University
www.AHUonline.us
(800) 296-MIND

Association for Research and Enlightenment (ARE)
Health and Rejuvenation Center
(757) 437-7202
www.EdgarCayce.org

Baar Products
(800) 269-2502
www.baar.com

Biomedical Center (BMC) The Hoxsey Clinic
Ph: (01152664) 684-9011
Fax: (01152664) 684-9744
www.Hoxsey.com
BMC@telnor.net

Heritage Products
(800) 862-2923
www.caycecures.com

In Pursuit of Tea
www.InPursuitOfTea.com

Lombardi Cancer Center
(202) 784-4000

M.D. Anderson Cancer Center
(800) 392-1611
(713) 792-3245

Mannatech Inc.
www.GlycoScience.com

National Center for Alternative and Complementary Medicine (NAACM)
under the National Institutes of Health
(888) 644-6226; (301) 519-3153
www.NCCAM.org

National Association of Transpersonal Hypnotherapists
540-997-0325
800-296-MIND
www.holistictree.com

National Cancer Institute
(800) 4-Cancer
www.cancer.gov

NutriCology
(800) 545-9960
www.allergyresearchgroup.com

Second Option Newsletter
by Dr. Rowen
(800) 728-2288; (770) 399-5617

Spring Wind Herbs (pharmacy)
(800) 588-4883

World Health Organization
www.WHO.org.

Articles of Scientific Proof

"History of Hoxsey Treatment," by Patricia Spain Ward, PhD. A report commissioned by the Office of Technology Assessment (OTA) of the United States Congress, May, 1988.
Available at: www.cancersalves.com/botanical_approaches/ historic_practioners/Hoxsey_treatment.html

"Assessment of Outcomes at Alternative Medicine Cancer Clinics: A Feasibility Study," by Mary Ann Richardson, Dr. Ph., Nancy C. Russell, MPH, Tina Sanders, MS, Robert Barrett, PhD and Catherine Salveson, RN, PhD. *The Journal of Alternative and Complementary Medicine,* Vol. 7, #1, 2001, pp. 19-32, Mary Ann Leibert, Inc.
Available at: www.Hoxsey.com

Educational Opportunities

American Holistic University offers a variety of online educational workshops, designed for both the general public and natural health practitioners. Topics revolve around a variety of natural health arts and sciences. In addition, topics in transpersonal psychology, hypnotherapy, and other mind-body interventions are discussed. Log on to AHU's web site (listed is this segment) for more information.

Order Form

Order this book, and others at
TranspersonalPublishing.com
or send the following order form in with
__check
__money order
__credit card_____
exp._____   Zip Code for CCd_____

Killing Your Cancer Without Killing Yourself: Using Natural Cures that Work

____books at $24.95=
discount for 2 or more copies   Less 10%   _____
NC Residents add 8% sales tax   _____
plus $2/1 copy or $3/2 copies   Ship&Hdl   _____

                                       Total Due   _____

*All shipping is U.S. and must be media mail
Phone for priority or international shipping: 800-296-MIND.
Free shipping for 3 or more copies
Discount cannot be combined with other offers
Prices and availability subject to change without notice

Make Checks and money orders payable to
Transpersonal Publishing
PO Box 7220
Kill Devil Hills, NC 27948

Note to Wholesalers and bookstores:
Contact the publisher directly at 800-296-MIND
or TranspersonalPublishing.com

Related Books

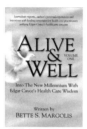
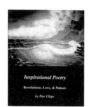
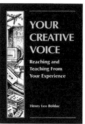
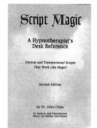
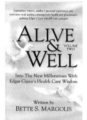
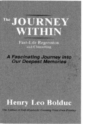
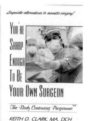
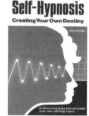
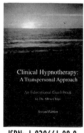
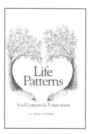
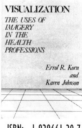
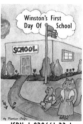
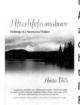
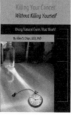

INDEX

"What lies behind us and what lies ahead of us
are tiny matters compared to what lies within us."
-Anonymous, variously attributed to
Thoreau, Emerson, and Holmes